Immersive Virtual and Augmented Reality in Healthcare

The book acts as a guide, taking the reader into the smart system domain and providing theoretical and practical knowledge along with case studies in smart healthcare. The book uses a blend of interdisciplinary approaches such as IoT, blockchain, augmented reality, and virtual reality for the implementation of cost-effective, real-time, and user-friendly solutions for healthcare problems.

Immersive Virtual and Augmented Reality in Healthcare: An IoT and Blockchain Perspective presents the trends, best practices, techniques, developments, sensors, materials, and case studies that are using augmented and virtual reality environments with the state-of-the-art latest technologies like IoT, blockchain, and machine learning in the implementation of healthcare systems. The book focuses on the design and implementation of smart healthcare systems with major challenges to further explore more robust and efficient healthcare solutions in terms of low cost, faster algorithms, more sensitive IoT sensors, faster data communication, and real-time solutions for treatment. It discusses the use of virtual and augmented reality and how it can provide user-friendly and interactive communication within healthcare systems. Illustrated through case studies, the book conveys how different hospitals and healthcare equipment providers can adopt good practices found in the book to improve the performance/productivity of their staff and system. The content is rounded out by providing how IoT, blockchain, and artificial intelligence can provide the framework for designing and/or upgrading traditional healthcare systems by increasing security and data privacy.

A valuable resource for engineers working with systems, the healthcare professionals involved in the design and development of healthcare devices and systems, researcher scholars, multidisciplinary scientists, students, and academics who are wishing to explore the use of virtual and augmented reality in new and existing healthcare systems.

ARTIFICIAL INTELLIGENCE IN SMART HEALTHCARE SYSTEMS

Series Editors: Vishal Jain and Jyotir Moy Chatterjee

The progress of the healthcare sector is incremental as it learns from associations between data over time through the application of suitable big data and IoT frameworks and patterns. Many healthcare service providers are employing IoT-enabled devices for monitoring patient health care, but their diagnosis and prescriptions are instance-specific only. However, these IoT-enabled healthcare devices are generating volumes of data (Big-IoT Data), that can be analyzed for more accurate diagnosis and prescriptions. A major challenge in the above realm is the effective and accurate learning of unstructured clinical data through the application of precise algorithms. Incorrect input data leading to erroneous outputs with false positives shall be intolerable in healthcare as patient's lives are at stake. This book series addresses various aspects of how smart healthcare can be used to detect and analyze diseases, the underlying methodologies, and related security concerns. Healthcare is a multidisciplinary field that involves a range of factors like the financial system, social factors, health technologies, and organizational structures that affect the healthcare provided to individuals, families, institutions, organizations, and populations. The goals of healthcare services include patient safety, timeliness, effectiveness, efficiency, and equity. Smart healthcare consists of mHealth, eHealth, electronic resource management, smart and intelligent home services, and medical devices. The Internet of Things (IoT) is a system comprising real-world things that interact and communicate with each other via networking technologies. The wide range of potential applications of IoT includes healthcare services. IoT-enabled healthcare technologies are suitable for remote health monitoring, including rehabilitation, assisted ambient living, etc. In turn, healthcare analytics can be applied to the data gathered from different areas to improve healthcare at a minimum expense.

This book series is designed to be a first choice reference at university libraries, academic institutions, research and development centres, information technology centres, and any institutions interested in using, design, modelling, and analysing intelligent healthcare services. Successful application of deep learning frameworks to enable meaningful, cost-effective personalized healthcare services is the primary aim of the healthcare industry in the present scenario. However, realizing this goal requires effective understanding, application, and amalgamation of IoT, Big Data and several other computing technologies to deploy such systems in an effective manner. This series shall help clarify the understanding of certain key mechanisms and technologies helpful in realizing such systems.

Next Generation Healthcare Systems Using Soft Computing Techniques
D. Rekh Ram Janghel, Rohit Raja, and Korhan Cengiz

Immersive Virtual and Augmented Reality in Healthcare
An IoT and Blockchain Perspective
Edited by Rajendra Kumar, Vishal Jain, Garry Han, and Abderezak Touzene

Immersive Virtual and Augmented Reality in Healthcare

An IoT and Blockchain Perspective

Edited by
Rajendra Kumar,
Vishal Jain, Garry Tan Wei Han, and
Abderezak Touzene

CRC Press
Taylor & Francis Group
Boca Raton London New York

CRC Press is an imprint of the
Taylor & Francis Group, an **informa** business

Designed cover image: © TBC

First edition published 2024
by CRC Press
2385 Executive Center Drive, Suite 320, Boca Raton, FL 33431

and by CRC Press
4 Park Square, Milton Park, Abingdon, Oxon, OX14 4RN

CRC Press is an imprint of Taylor & Francis Group, LLC

© 2024 selection and editorial matter, Rajendra Kumar, Vishal Jain, Garry Tan Wei Han, Abderezak Touzene; individual chapters, the contributors

ISBN: 978-1-032-37261-7 (hbk)
ISBN: 978-1-032-37406-2 (pbk)
ISBN: 978-1-003-34013-3 (ebk)

DOI: 10.1201/9781003340133

Typeset in Times
by Apex CoVantage, LLC

Contents

Chapter 6   AR/VR Revolutions in Future Healthcare 96

Dr. Pawan Whig, Shama Kouser, Ankit Sharma,
Ashima Bhatnagar Bhatia, and Rahul Reddy Nadikattu

*Sandhya Avasthi, Ayushi Prakash, Tanushree Sanwal,
Shweta Roy, and Shelly Gupta*

Preface

This book focuses on design and implementation of smart healthcare system with major challenges to further explore more robust and efficient healthcare solutions in terms of low cost, faster algorithms, more sensitive IoT sensors, faster data communication, real-time solution for treatment. With use of wearable devices and their connectivity with smartphones, the users are very much conscious regarding their health status. The AR/VR technology provides a pleasing interaction with the healthcare devices, while technologies like IoT and blockchain provide faster and secure communication. Such kind of systems is very much required for disabled and senior citizens living independently. This book is targeted to a variety of readers, like scholars and academic persons, industry peoples involved in manufacturing healthcare devices and providing infrastructural support connecting the devices and sensors over wide area networks, application developers and data analyst of healthcare devices like different scanners and wearable healthcare devices. The book also aims to network with electronic data processing administrators managing healthcare data and users' credentials and keeping the system free from intruders. The use of virtual and augmented reality provide user-friendly and interactive communication with healthcare systems. The major technologies involved are healthcare 5.0, convergence of IoT, blockchain and AR/VR, cloud computing, 3D printing in healthcare, robotics in healthcare, wearable and transplantable healthcare devices, and case studies.

Smart healthcare system is a need of today's life. It is equally beneficial for healthcare workers and patients both. Smart sensors can analyze the health status of peoples so they can adopt a healthy lifestyle, as recommend by healthcare wearable devices at a low cost. The medical insurance companies can have the status of their customers online. The treatment of patients can be done by specialist doctors from remote locations using such systems. IoT sensors may reduce the cost involved in visiting doctors and hospitals. The development of expert systems will help people to get cured at minimum expenditure. Using smart healthcare, people can be educated about their health status and keep themselves health-aware using healthcare applications in their smartphones. The technologies like augmented and virtual reality, IoT, blockchain, Vehicle-to-Everything, etc. may have great contribution towards technological and infrastructural support in implementation of smart healthcare.

The augmented reality works on real-world movements of human parts. Therefore, augmented reality may help medical practitioners get a better way of drawing blood, using a handheld near infrared scanner to project over the skin for showing the positioning of veins in the patient's body. Many times, it becomes very difficult to trace the right vein to inject the medicine. Several other medical cases can be visualized using augmented reality.

Virtual reality in healthcare has a very wide scope, like simulation of surgical applications for providing training and demonstration to medical students. This may help a lot to visualize the parts in 3D representation to make training easy and cost-effective. Once this kind of simulation is prepared, it can be used any number of times anywhere. This may also help the patient and his/her family to know how exactly the doctors are going to operate the patient and post-operation precautions. The animation or simulation has more impact than verbal briefing.

The major applications of augmented and virtual reality in healthcare include the increasing demand of robotic surgeries and cardiovascular surgeries. This visualizes the depth where there may be chances of making mistakes in the surgery.

Adopting the increased use of cognitive and artificial intelligence platforms several potential applications can be developed for healthcare. The use of data mining, pattern recognition, natural language processing may replicate the way the human brain works and thinks.

The cognitive computing systems may lead to processing massive amounts of data instantly for answering specific inquiries and making customized AI advice. Cognitive computing in healthcare may also link the different functions of the human where machines and the human brain may indeed overlap for improving the human decision-making.

The last few years have witnessed the development of virtual and augmented reality devices that are increasingly capable of offering an immersive experience much closer to reality. With the technological advancements almost all devices are decreasing their sizes with increased productivity and are easier to handle. Such devices are giving contributions in almost all areas, like robotics; the interest and application possibilities for them increase. In the healthcare sector, there is an infrastructure, games, training using huge potential, and use of virtual reality. This is because of multidisciplinary approaches that technology is allowing to present the things using virtual reality devices giving a realistic presentation and internal functionality supported by the latest technologies like IoT, blockchain, machine learning, etc.

The immersion of IoT, blockchain, machine learning, etc. in virtual environments is still required to do a lot in many daily life activities, including people's health powered by smart healthcare offered by hospitals and wearable self-care devices.

The book *Immersive Virtual and Augmented Reality in Healthcare: An IoT and Blockchain Perspective* is aimed to present the trends, best practices, techniques, developments, sensors, materials, and case studies that are using augmented and virtual reality environments with state-of-the-art latest technologies like IoT, blockchain, machine learning in the implementation of healthcare systems and to present challenges observed.

Positive user experiences with the use of wearable healthcare devices equipped with IoT sensors, secured by encryption algorithms and blockchain, data privacy, and safety from intruders, and healthcare case studies are presented by the contributors of the book.

The target readers of this book are the healthcare professionals involved in the design and development of healthcare devices and systems, researcher scholars, multidisciplinary scientists, students, and academia who are wishing to explore the use of virtual and augmented reality in new and existing healthcare systems.

Our book is aimed to use artificial intelligence, blockchain, and Internet of Things (IoT) in virtual and augmented reality averment for design and development of healthcare systems, analyzing the healthcare data. The use of IoT, blockchain, and artificial intelligence provides the framework for designing and/or upgrading the traditional healthcare systems by increasing the security and data privacy. Better ideas from contributors of the book will help to design and manufacture more user-friendly and sustainable, wearable, and transplantable healthcare devices. The edge cognitive computing provides a framework for designing and developing healthcare systems for visualization of brain, blood vessels, and other parts' activities using augmented reality. This book presents new horizons for future research in healthcare and multidisciplinary areas.

Chapter 1 discusses uses of AR/VR-based technology and its related 3D animation tools in preventive health education. A systematic review of past records is conducted, covering topics such as the concepts of IR4.0, technological shifts in healthcare settings, IoT sensors for smart healthcare, AR in sports science as a digital tool for health science education, and Minecraft worlds that illustrate virtual healthcare systems. Exemplary cases are also presented to elaborate on current trends in the field, such as the use of 3D printing, wearable devices to promote health education, and robotics for smart healthcare implementation.

Chapter 2 is about applications of healthcare informatics, particularly applications of IT and computing in the healthcare sector and medical sciences emphasizing virtual reality. Various latest technologies from these subfields are also emerging and rising globally, and among the latest technologies, important are cloud computing, big data, IoT, artificial intelligence, ML (machine learning) and DL, virtual reality (VR), blockchain technologies, etc.

Chapter 3 reviews the general applications of VR. It includes the review of healthcare applications of VR and new age technology, namely: IoT, AI, digital twin, big data, blockchain, and more. The chapter proposes a model for healthcare systems based on IoT and blockchain, which is really helpful in simplifying and amalgamating the diverse applications of VR, IoT, Digital Twin, blockchain, and machine learning.

Chapter 4 discusses recent ML techniques used to model cancer progression. A variety of supervised ML approaches, predictor features, and datasets are used to create the predictive models described here. ML methods are increasingly being used in cancer research.

Chapter 5 discusses the platform architecture based on the Internet of Things and blockchain, making it easier for patients to properly manage their diabetes on their own and helps doctors monitor it more effectively. The architecture combines IoT and blockchain technology to gather patient data and safely and quickly share it with the medical team while maintaining patient privacy.

Chapter 6 discusses about popularity of AR in healthcare, revolutionizing the way medical professionals and patients interact with medical information and technology. It also discusses how AR is improving patient outcomes by providing education and accurate information, and the technology has significant potential in the field of medicine.

Chapter 7 discusses the implications of AR technologies in V2X, as well as the challenges and future directions in the implementation of these emerging technologies. Vehicle-to-Everything (V2X) has emerged as a new hybrid type of communication between transport vehicles (V2V), pedestrians (V2P), infrastructure (V2I), and networks (V2N), which requires the features of the 5G network to provide application connectivity and for citizens' new mobile services. V2X uses cases/applications that enable vehicles to connect and exchange data with other vehicles, traffic lights, parking spaces, nearby people, and services to coordinate traffic flow and environmental safety.

Chapter 8 elaborates on the authors' initiatives to develop a road map for PHC (with a special focus on health education and health promotion) integrating augmented reality (AR) and virtual reality (VR)-based technology in achieving sustainable development goal (SDG) no. 3 (Good health and well-being) and no. 4 (Quality education).

Chapter 9 discusses the application of various algorithms to study the characteristics of the effect of press physiotherapy on the bio-signals of the lieges. The analysis' main goal is to look for a possible attenuation of alpha rhythm in each patient. Common spatial structure are calculated to enhance alpha-power before or after stimulation or post- over pre-simulation for each trial involving cross-validation.

Chapter 10 discusses overview of blockchain technology, recent trends in mHealth, smart healthcare applications, and augmented reality. Blockchain has a lot of uses in healthcare because electronic medical records and other ICT-based tools create so much medical data. It gives flexibility, connectivity, accountability, and a secure way to access data. As privacy is important for health records, the use of blockchain became one of the obvious solutions. Blockchain can protect health data and prevent common risks due to its decentralized nature.

Chapter 11 explores implementing a blockchain in the healthcare system by discussing a use case. Specifically, it focuses on current (technical and nontechnical) limitations of implementing blockchain technology in current systems, with exhaustive possible use cases and one use case for the prevention of counterfeit drugs using supply chain management concepts in particular with the possible implementation of it.

Editor Bios

Rajendra Kumar is presently Associate Professor in CSE Department at Sharda University, India. He holds a PhD, MTech, and BE (all in computer science). He has 24 years of teaching and research experience at various accredited institutes and universities like Chandigarh University (NAAC A+). His fields of interest include IoT, deep learning, HCI, pattern recognition, and theoretical computer science. He has authored five textbooks, edited seven conference proceedings, chaired three sessions in international conferences, published more than 30 papers, three patents, and two monographs. He is the reviewer of *Medical & Biological Engineering & Computing*, *Expert Systems with Applications*, etc.

Vishal Jain is presently Associate Professor at the Department of Computer Science and Engineering, Sharda School of Engineering and Technology, Sharda University, Greater Noida, U. P. India. Before that, he has worked for several years as an associate professor at Bharati Vidyapeeth's Institute of Computer Applications and Management (BVICAM), New Delhi. He has more than 16 years of experience in the academics. He obtained a PhD (CSE), MTech (CSE), MBA (HR), MCA, MCP, and CCNA. He has more than 850 research citation indices with Google Scholar (h-index score 14 and i-10 index 25). He has authored more than 95 research papers in reputed conferences and journals, including *Web of Science* and *Scopus*. He has authored and edited more than 35 books with various reputed publishers, including Elsevier, Springer, DeGruyter, Apple Academic Press, CRC, Taylor and Francis Group, Scrivener, Wiley, Emerald, and IGI-Global. His research areas include information retrieval, semantic web, ontology engineering, data mining, ad hoc networks, and sensor networks. He received a Young Active Member Award for the year 2012–2013 from the Computer Society of India, Best Faculty Award for the year 2017, and Best Researcher Award for the year 2019 from BVICAM, New Delhi.

Garry Tan Wei Han is Associate Professor at the UCSI Graduate Business School, UCSI University. He has been acknowledged as the world's "10 Most Productive and Influential Authors in Mobile Commerce and Applications" in 2016, "Top 3 Authors in the World" in Mobile Commerce in 2017, "World's Top 10 Core Authors" in Social Commerce in 2018, and "Top 5 Most Productive Authors in the World" in the area of Mobile Commerce in 2019 and 2021. He was also the recipient of the National Outstanding Reviewer (2019) by Private Education Co-operative (Malaysia), Outstanding Reviewer Award (2019) by Internet Research, Emerald (UK), Top Downloaded Technological Forecasting and Social Change Article (2019) by Elsevier (US), Emerald Outstanding Contribution Award (2020) by Emerald (UK), Top Reviewer Award (2020) by Sustainable Production and Consumption (Elsevier) (US), Most Cited Telematics and Informatics Article (2021) by Elsevier (US), Most Cited Expert Systems with Application Article (2021) by Elsevier (US), Highly Cited Paper (2022) by Clarivate Analytics (US), Most Cited Journal of Computer Information System Article (2022) by Taylor and Francis (UK), and Most Cited Technology in Society

Article (2022) by Elsevier (US). His work is cited over 5,100 times with a current h-index of 35.

Abderezak Touzene is Full-Time Professor of Computer Science at the College of Science, Sultan Qaboos University, Muscat, Sultanate of Oman. He has more than 30 years of teaching and research experience. Prior to joining Sultan Qaboos University, he worked at King Saud University, Saudi Arabia, and Grenoble Institute of Technology, France. He obtained his PhD from Institut Polytechnique de Grenoble, France (1992), MSc from Paris-11 (Orsay) University, France (1989), and BSc from University of Technology Houari Boumedien, Algeria (1987) [all in Computer Science]. His areas of interest include smart systems, cloud computing, cybersecurity, machine learning, big data analytics, IoT, etc. In the last five years he has written 23 journals and 11 conference publications, and he has received eight research grants. He also serves as an editorial board member of MDPI, CNCIJ, etc., a referee of several journals and conferences, and an advisor on the WARSE board.

Contributors

Abderezak Touzene
Sultan Qaboos University, Oman

Anant Bhardwaj
Delhi Technological University, India

Ankit Sharma
VIPS-TC, India

Ashima Bhatnagar Bhatia
VIPS-TC, India

Ayushi Prakash
ABES Engineering College, Ghaziabad, India

Babita Panda
KIIT Deemed to be University, India

Corrienna Abdul Talib
Universiti Teknologi Malaysia, Johor, Malaysia

Deepak Kumar
Faculty of Engineering and Technology, Manav Rachna International Institute of Research and Studies, Faridabad, India

Devendra Kumar
University of Technology and Applied Sciences-Shinas, India

Eng Tek Ong
UCSI University, Kuala Lumpur, Malaysia

Faiza Al Salti
Sultan Qaboos Comprehensive Cancer Care and Research Centre, Oman

Faiza Rashid Ammar Al Harthi
Sultan Qaboos University, Oman

Fei Ping Por
Wawasan Open University, Penang, Malaysia

Girish Kumar Sharma
Delhi Skill Entrepreneurship University, India

Himani Mittal
Goswami Ganesh Dutta Sanatan Dharma College, India

Jing Hang Ng
MAHSA University, Selangor, Malaysia

K. S. Tiwary
Raiganj University, West Bengal, India

Kamalambal Durairaj
SEAMEO RECSAM, Malaysia

Khar Thoe Ng
SEAMEO RECSAM, Malaysia

Kumar Avinash Chandra
Birla Institute of Technology, Mesra, Ranchi, India

Manoj Singhal
G. L. Bajaj Institute of Technology, Greater Noida, India

Naeem Hannoon
Madya, Consultant, Malaysia

Nasser Alzeidi
Sultan Qaboos University, Oman

Nelson Cyril
PondokUpeh Secondary School,
   Penang, Malaysia

P. K. Paul
Raiganj University, West Bengal, India

P. S. Aithal
Srinivas University, Mangalore, India

Pawan Whig
VIPS-TC, India

Prabhat Kumar Upadhyay
Birla Institute of Technology, Mesra,
   Ranchi, India

Rahul Reddy Nadikattu
University of the Cumberland, USA

Rakesh Kumar Dhaka
ITM University, India

Reza Setiawan
SEAMEO QITEP in Science, Bandung,
   Indonesia

Ritam Chatterjee
Raiganj University, West Bengal,
   India

Sampurna Panda
ITM University, India

Sandhya Avasthi
ABES Engineering College,
   Ghaziabad, India

Shah Jahan Assanarkutty
SEAMEO RECSAM, Malaysia

Shama Kouser
Jazan University, Kingdom of Saudi
   Arabia

Shelly Gupta
CST Department, Manav Rachna
   University, Faridabad, India

Shobha Tyagi
Faculty of Engineering and Technology,
   Manav Rachna International Institute
   of Research and Studies, India

Shweta Roy
ABES Engineering College, Ghaziabad,
   India

Shwetank Arya
Gurukul Kangri Vishwavidyalaya
   (Deemed), Haridwar, India

Sivaranjini Sinniah
SEAMEO RECSAM, Malaysia

Sucheta Chakraborty
Raiganj University, West Bengal, India

Sushil Sharma
Texas A&M University Texarkana, USA

Tanushree Sanwal
KIET Group of Institution, Delhi-NCR,
   Ghaziabad, India

Yee Jiea Pang
UniversitiTeknikal Malaysia, Melaka,
   Malaysia

Ying Li Thong
SEAMEO RECSAM, Malaysia

1 Industrial Revolution (IR) and Exemplary AR/VR-based Technological Tools in Preventive Health Education
The Past, Present, and Future

Eng Tek Ong, Yee Jiea Pang, Corrienna Abdul Talib, Reza Setiawan, Jing Hang Ng, and Fei Ping Por

1.1 INTRODUCTION

1.1.1 THE CHANGING LANDSCAPE OF GLOBAL LIVING CONDITIONS

The advent of the fourth Industrial Revolution (IR4.0) has significantly impacted the global landscape of using digital tools for communication in education, industry, and especially the healthcare settings. This section first elaborates on how the landscape of education was affected by IR4.0 and the rationale for writing this chapter.

1.1.1.1 What Is Industrial Revolution (IR) 4.0?

The world is ruled and impacted by digitalization, particularly the Industry Revolution 4.0 (IR4.0) technologies. Emerging IR4.0 technologies in healthcare, such as artificial intelligence, cloud computing, big data, virtual reality/augmented reality, 3D printing, robotics, nanotechnology, and the Internet of Things (IoTs), are dramatically reshaping healthcare systems. The adoption of IR4.0 technologies in healthcare over the years has led to more precise diagnosis and treatment of patients. Healthcare is the most important area of all the benefited sectors from adopting IR4.0 technologies. It improves the quality of life, and it has saved many lives.

IR4.0 technologies improve understanding of complex medical and physiological issues and decrease the barriers to delivering care directly to patients. For instance, telehealth allows clinicians to interact with patients in different locations, decreasing the cost of medical and diagnostic imaging and improving access to high-quality medical care. Besides, the mundane tasks that previously had to be done by humans are automated and extended with the adoption of IR4.0 technologies. As a result,

DOI: 10.1201/9781003340133-1

healthcare professionals can focus their time and efforts on research and development to upgrade the quality of medical treatment.

In an operating room, IR4.0 technologies also play a prominent role, ranging from preoperative planning to performing surgeries to monitoring outcomes. For example, virtual 3D reconstructions are performed in trauma patients, which help guide the medical team on where to make the most accurate incisions or bony reconstructions with plates. The images can be reviewed beforehand without making a single incision to plan the surgeries. Another example is using infrared technology to monitor blood flow in the flaps used in breast or head and neck cancer reconstruction. Implantable devices are also available to send real-time blood flow data directly to the phones of medical professionals. In the wake of the advancements brought on by telemedicine, the capabilities of surgical techniques have made a considerable contribution. Robotics can treat patients virtually controlled by surgeons who are not directly in the operating room [1].

Rather than replacing humans with technologies, IR4.0 provides a new way to enhance how humans collaborate efficiently and effectively with technologies. For instance, IoTs and big data make tracking patients' medical records more accurate and faster. As a result, the personalization of healthcare needed can be exact. It can be accomplished by analyzing individuals' data and presenting care, coaching, and health recommendations that precisely address their conditions, goals, and lifestyles instead of offering a set of treatments that fits a broad solution.

With a proper digital agenda and strategies that harness the power of technology and people, the healthcare sector will confidently leap to the forefront of global competitiveness. The healthcare sector is intrigued by the potential of IR4.0 in medical technologies, which poses huge contributions to the general well-being of people's lives.

1.1.1.2   How Did the Past (e.g., IR1.0 to IR3.0) Influence the Present Healthcare Settings?

Before the information age in the digital era, the first Industrial Revolution (IR1.0) used natural resources such as water and steam power to mechanize production. [2] reported that Healthcare 1.0 used mechanical engineering and automation. Later when there was a growth in population, electric power was used in order to achieve mass production during the second Industrial Revolution (IR2.0). Hence, Healthcare 2.0 was electrically energy-oriented, as reported in [2]. Then, the third Industrial Revolution (IR3.0) used electronics and information technology to automate production. Therefore, it is not surprising that telecommunication and information communication technology (ICT) was seen in Healthcare 3.0. Finally, with the advent of IR4.0, as reported in section 1.1.2, there is the intelligent device deployment in Healthcare 4.0 [2].

1.1.2   RATIONALE AND FOCUS OF THIS CHAPTER

This chapter outlines some examples of such tools, focusing on AR/VR-based technology and its related 3D animation tools or applications in preventive health education. Since primary healthcare involves all walks of life, such knowledge must be disseminated. Health education should also be one of the major focuses in the educational system; hence this chapter is written by co-authors who are mostly educators/learners at secondary and tertiary levels.

1.2 REVIEW OF RELATED LITERATURE

1.2.1 Systematic Review

This section outlines the systematic review of the past records on topics including the concepts of IR4.0 and technological shifts in healthcare settings. Among the topics being outlined (Table 1.1) are AR in biological science and sport science education as an exemplary digital tool for preventive health education, IoT sensors for smart healthcare, Minecraft worlds that illustrate virtual healthcare systems, 3D printing for health science education (HSE) models, wearable devices, and robotics for smart healthcare, to name a few.

1.2.2 Exemplary AR/VR-based Technological Tools in Health Science Education and Healthcare Settings

Elaboration with exemplary cases will also be made on the current trends, including 3D printing, wearable devices to promote health education, and robotics for smart healthcare implementation.

TABLE 1.1

Exemplary Digital Tools/E-Platforms for Virtual Learning (VL) in Health Science Education (HSE) in the Past and Present

Tools/Platforms *(Features/Functions)*	Researchers	
	2000 to 2015	**2016 to Present**
Digital (Learning) Tools		
AR in Biological Science Education (*Animation on various health related functions/systems*)	[3–6] [Refer 2.2.1]	[7], Augmented Reality (AR) VL tool [Refer 2.2.1] [8]
AR in Sport Science Education (*Illustrations of animated paths of the travelling of balls*)	[9]	[10–12] for AR Sport Science Education [Refer 2.2.2]
IoT Sensors and Robotics for Smart Healthcare (*Communication*)	[13–15]	[16–19]
Minecraft Worlds in Health Settings (*Illustration/Demonstration in virtual word*)	N/A	[Refer Appendix A]
3D Printing for HSE models (*Modelling/ Visualizing complicated models*)	N/A	[Refer Appendix B]
Apps (*Promoting healthy lifestyle/monitoring health status*)	N/A	[Refer Appendix C]
E-platforms		
Learning Activities Management System (LAMS) (*Monitoring and evaluating health education*)	[20] [Refer 2.2.3]	[21] [Refer 2.2.3]
Video/Web-based Learning (*Visualizing/Analyzing 3D learning*)	[22, 23] [Refer 2.2.4]	[24–28] [Refer 2.2.4]

1.2.2.1 Augmented Reality (AR) in Biological Science Education

In the past, augmented reality (AR) has been gaining so much interest in various fields, especially in health science education, due to its potential to provide contextual learning experiences by connecting the nature of information in the real world. Based on the results of studies that have been collected, there are a few examples of AR application usage in health science education. The topics discussed are related to anatomy, forensic medicine, and clinical skills.

Anatomy learning with the help of augmented reality application has been proposed by Galvao and Zorzal named MuscleView Projector and MuscleView Portable. These projects use the mirror idea that gives users the impression that they are viewing inside their bodies and provide direct feedback to the students. For MuscleView Projector, by installing software, an image representing the human body is displayed with the aid of a projector (see Figure 1.1). There are several areas that can be selected by the users allowing the selected area to be changing its scale, shape, or angle where a new screen will be displayed. MuscleView Portable has the same concept as MuscleView Projector but with the aid of a mobile device (see Figure 1.2). The mobile device's background will be images in real time captured by the mobile device. The muscle image displayed can be controlled and positioned over body part. By using the AR application, the students can learn about human anatomy.

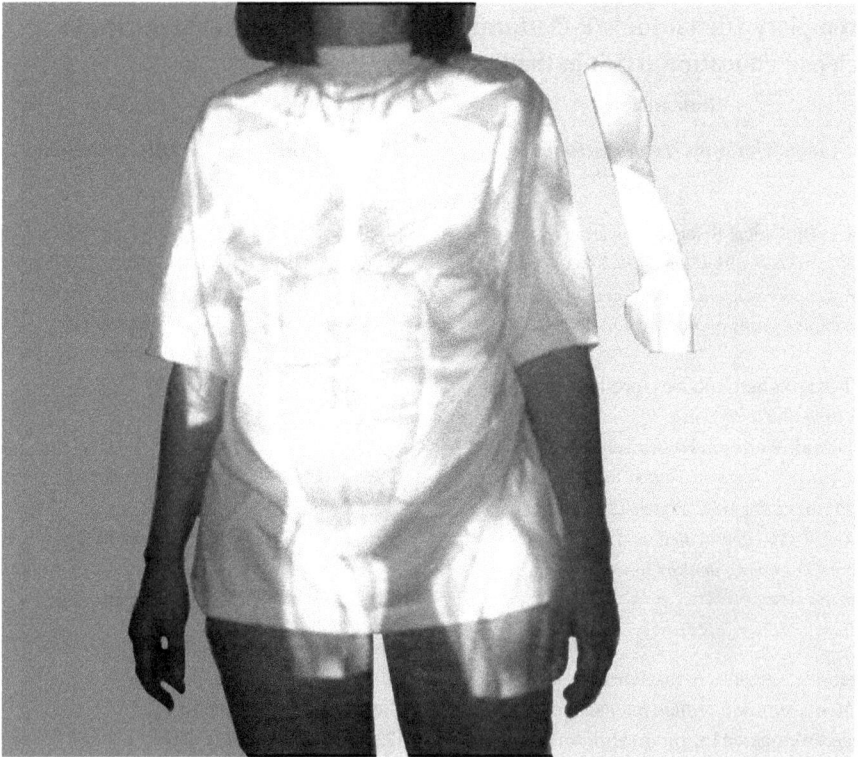

FIGURE 1.1   MuscleView Projector

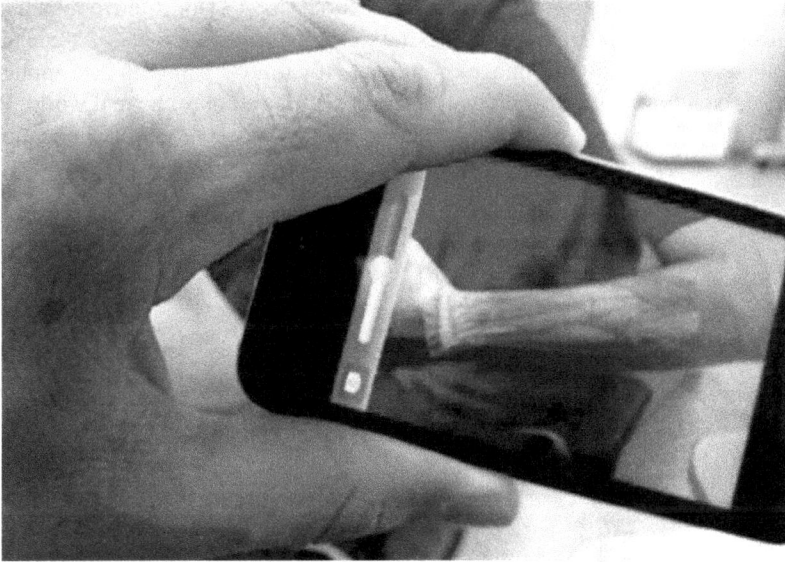

FIGURE 1.2   Image of forearm muscle superimposed onto a person using a mobile device

1.2.3   EXEMPLARY AR/VR-BASED TECHNOLOGICAL TOOLS IN HEALTH SCIENCE EDUCATION AND HEALTHCARE SETTINGS

Elaboration with exemplary cases will also be made on the current trends including 3D printing, wearable devices to promote health education, and robotics for smart healthcare implementation.

Some projects integrate mobile augmented reality (mAR) for educational purposes. This is possible because the mobile device has a camera and sensors. Through this application, information related to health can be delivered in real-time with a more interesting approach by integrating 3D virtual objects into the real world.

Albrecht et al. provided an example of mobile augmented reality with the aim to compare the effect of mAR blended learning environment (mARble) and textbook material on students' knowledge gain and changes in an emotional state. It was found that third-year medical students that use mARble gain more knowledge compared to students that use textbook material to learn forensic medicine related to gunshot wounds. This is due to mAR concepts that boost students' interest in learning the topic. In this module, predefined markers representing wound patterns found in forensic medicine can be detected. An image of the corresponding wound pattern will be overlaid when the mobile device's camera acquires the image of the marker placed on the student's body. There is also multimedia content such as audio, video, and images that can be accessed through a virtual flashcard system included in mARble. As a result, students are motivated to learn the topic due to new learning experiences, as realistic wound patterns can be viewed as entirely different from conventional learning.

Another example of AR application in health science education has been developed by VisualMed Systems Group, according to [29]. Various visualization and interactive features are provided in this application. Compared to conventional learning material, 3D visualization provides more realistic features. Thus, students can learn anatomy by taking an image of an anatomical atlas using an AR application (Figure 1.3). Additional information is also superimposed onto the real world. Based on the evaluation survey, students and teachers highly accept the AR application.

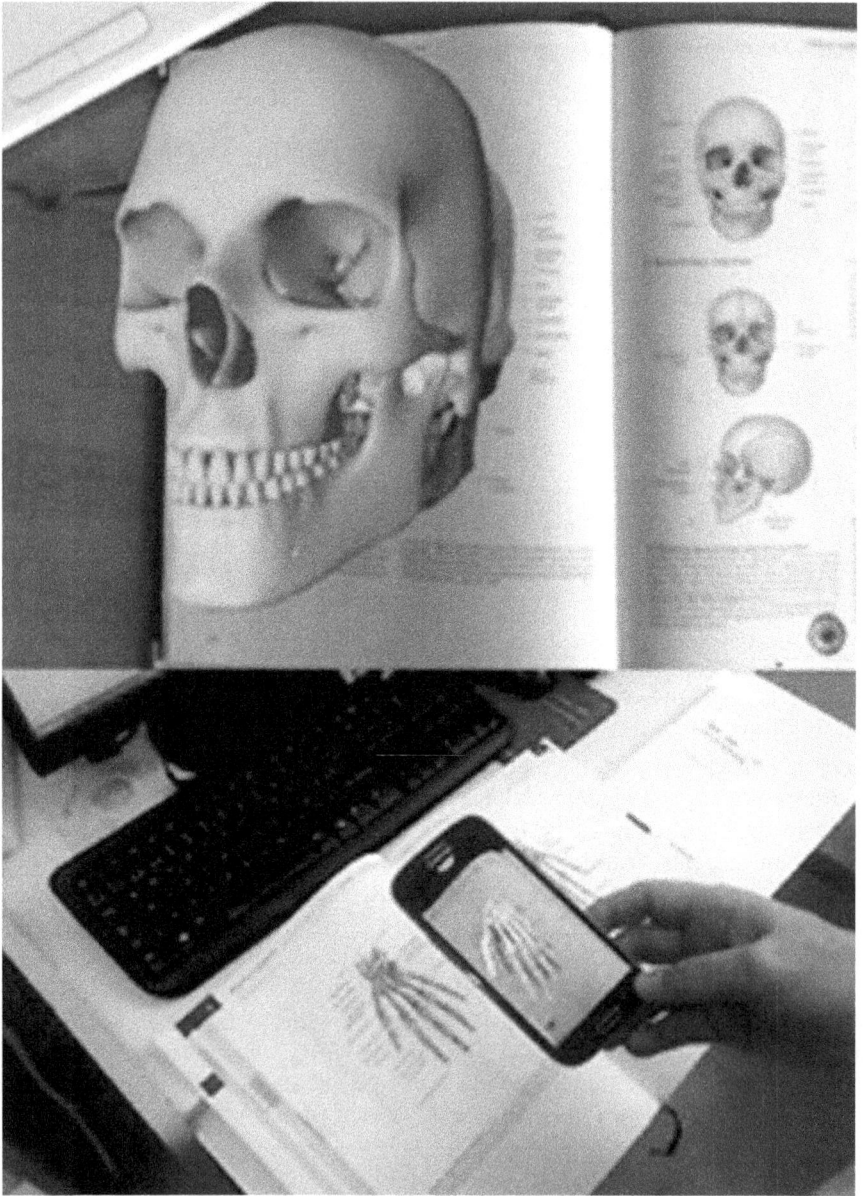

FIGURE 1.3   Anatomy study by using augmented reality application

A study by [30] has been conducted on 72 undergraduate nursing students with the aim of investigating the potential of mAR technologies in enhancing clinical skills learning in the lab. The study found that students are satisfied with the application as self-directed learning is supported, and clinical skills are reviewed. This AR application supports constructivist learning. Students must explore various resources and link the concepts learned using hyperlink materials. It also requires social interaction and practice reflection. To use the application, students need to scan the AR-tagged equipment and resources using a mobile device (see Figure 1.4 and 1.5). Then, students can explore various multimedia resources related to nursing equipment and skills by clicking on the call-to-action button.

In more recent years, based on the results of studies from several references that have been collected, there are several examples of the use of AR media applications in science learning related to health science education. Some topics discussed related to health education include the concept of influenza, the introduction of types of teeth and their treatment, and learning related to stroke. In addition, these media are prepared for users with various target age ranges, ranging from early-childhood students and elementary school students to adults.

As has been developed by [7] named "The Bad Effect of Influenza" (Figure 1.6), this project was designed to encourage students to pay attention to learning science concepts through games and animated 3D web-based activities. This science learning media was developed using Kellers' attention, relevance, confidence, satisfaction (ARCS) model to motivate students' learning.

This media uses AR technology to increase students' learning motivation regarding the concept of the influenza virus and the symptoms that will be experienced by a

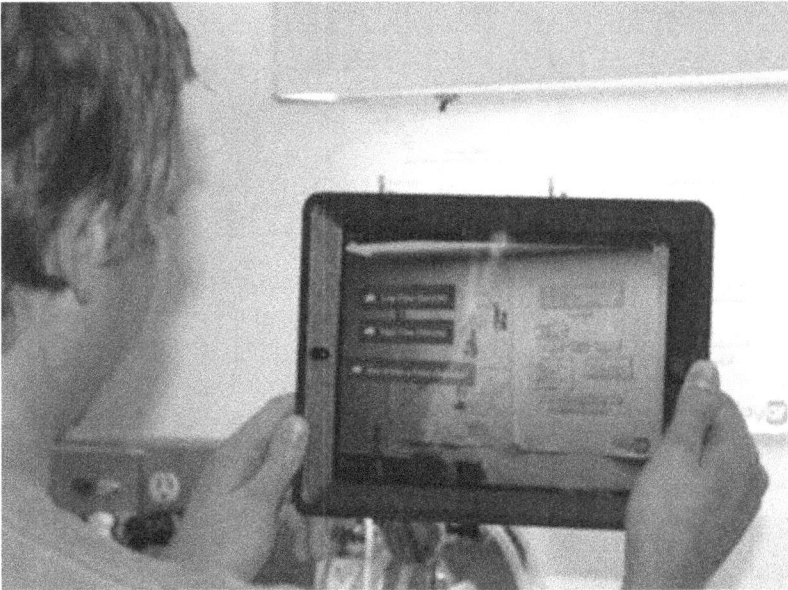

FIGURE 1.4 View of AR call-to-action buttons augmenting a poster on a tablet screen

FIGURE 1.5   View of AR call-to-action buttons using a QR mark on a mobile device

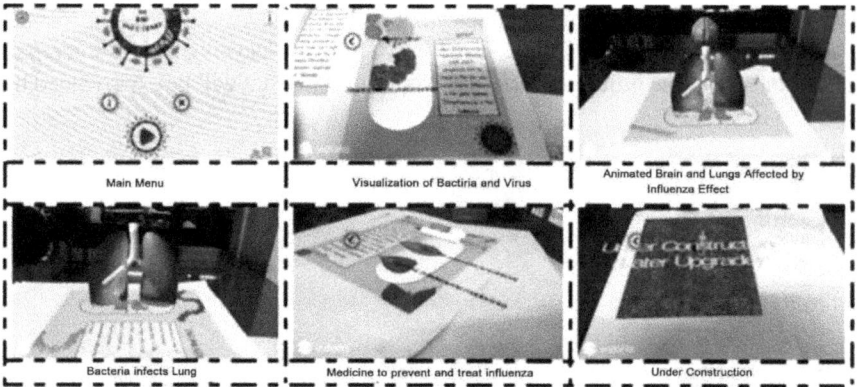

FIGURE 1.6   Screenshots of Augmented Reality 3-D models

person if infected with the virus. The picture in the next section shows the AR media students use to learn the concept of influenza. In addition, AR media provides various animations such as the shape of the influenza bacteria, the symptoms caused in several body organs, such as the lungs and brain, and medical procedures to prevent and treat the disease.

In [31] "Application of Augmented Reality Technology as a Model of Dental Health Education Media for Children," another sample was provided regarding AR application in health literacy education related to the introduction of dental health. This AR media is integrated into a book (Figure 1.7) targeted at users with an age range of children aged 4–7 years or early childhood to grade 2 elementary level school. This AR media complements the information provided in the book by introducing various types of teeth, such as canines, molars, and incisors, as well as the proper procedure for brushing teeth.

It would be best to install a smartphone with the APKtoolKit application to use this AR media, which is also provided as a package in the book. Once installed, the application can be used immediately by pointing the marker (Figure 1.8) on the

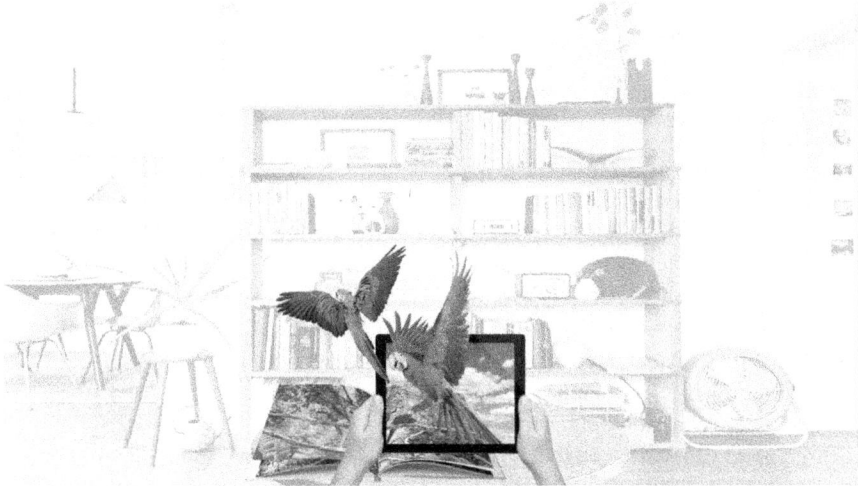

FIGURE 1.7 Cover page of the book containing an AR feature

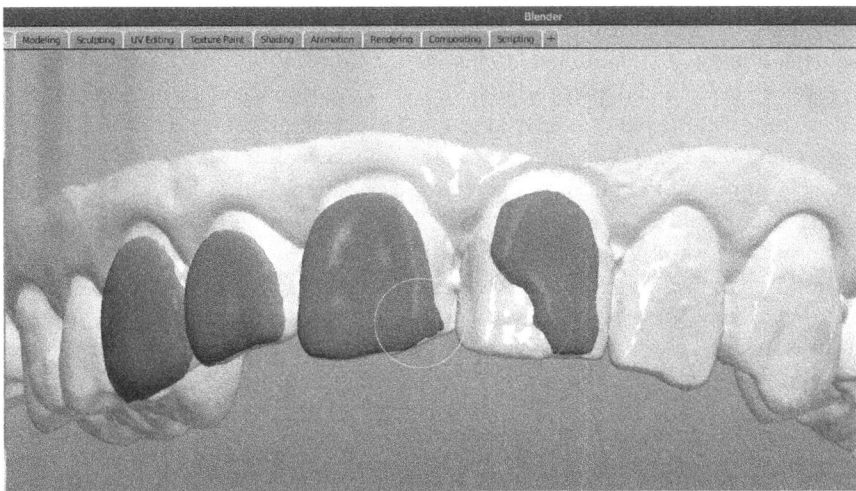

FIGURE 1.8 Marker for showing incisor tooth 3D model

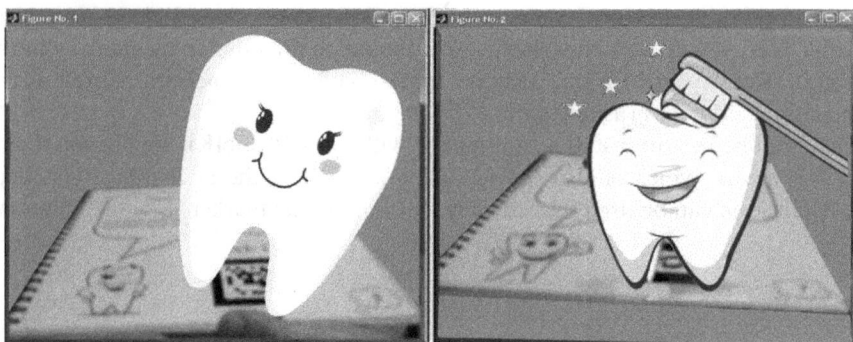

FIGURE 1.9   Screenshot of 3D teeth model using the AR app

smartphone camera, the marker will automatically be read, and 3D objects will appear on the screen (Figure 1.9).

From the results of learning trials using AR media, compared to conventional learning through lectures, even though both modes can provide a good understanding of dental health, children are more interested and enthusiastic in seeing a visual packaged with animation. [8] provided other samples of AR in health science education. This study investigated the effectiveness of augmented reality (AR) compared to a written pamphlet for enhancing the understanding of stroke and underlying stroke mechanisms, anatomy, and physiology.

Targeted at users aged 18 to 25, this tablet-based AR learning media uses interactive 3D brain images and is equipped with audio streaming narration that provides information related to stroke pathophysiology, the anatomical structure of the human brain, and stroke management. To use the media, the user must hold a cube-shaped device to complement the AR media. This cube has dimensions of 6 cm by 6 cm with different color patterns on each side. The device recognizes this pattern, and when the cube is placed in front of the camera, the screen replaces the cube with augmented reality as a brain model (Figure 1.10).

A voice narration will play through the user's smartphone when the media is used. Along with that, the relevant areas discussed appear in different colors to attract the user's attention. The 3D brain model will rotate in real-time when the user rotates the cube. Layers of the brain can be removed by tapping the screen (Figure 1.10) so that the user can learn how the anatomy of the human brain is structured according to the various layers.

Based on the results of this research study, it was found that although both AR media and conventional pamphlets can help users understand concepts related to stroke, using AR media can provide a better and richer experience. This makes AR technology effective for improving health literacy and understanding certain diseases such as stroke.

1.2.3.1   Augmented Reality (AR) in Sports Science Education

An observation made was that there are various ways that football can travel in the air before reaching goal post on land. This observation was captured in the form of

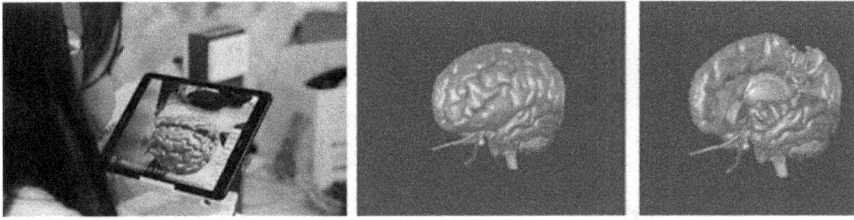

FIGURE 1.10 Leftmost image: A participant takes part in the AR application. Middle and Right images: Screenshots of the brain model during development, showing the ability to remove layers.

a sketched drawing. Therefore, the fifth author was also involved in blended-mode training on using digital tools and e-platforms during school co-curriculum activities. The activities were completed before drawing the path of the 3D model on the Blender tool for Augmented Reality (AR) and reported by the team members as part of the project team's output submitted end of the blended-mode training. The AR tool allows the sketching of paths of the moving ball to be reflected as an animated object, such as football, before reaching the football post. Exemplary AR learning output is accessible from http://bit.ly/footballAR, names of application files Football. apk and Footballpost.apk, to name a few [32]. Hence the amateur footballer learned to predict the paths of football travelling in the air by using AR tools to sketch how the ball travels in the air, starting from either one of the four ways to kick the ball, that is, "Robona shot" (Figure 1.11).

During the LearnT-SMArET e-course series (2017–2018), a project titled "Movement in the air (e.g., football travelling in the air), water and land" [32] was prepared by Malaysian students to promote learning of physics/mathematics concepts (e.g., Newton's law of motion, speed, force, angle, trajectory, or the path followed by a projectile flying or an object moving under the action of given forces, etc.) contextually supported by digital tool and e-platforms, as reported by [12].

1.2.3.2   Learning Activities Management System (LAMS)

The Learning Activity Management System (LAMS) has been applied in healthcare and medical education, providing educators with the ability to experiment with different learning design approaches [33]. LAMS facilitates the visualization of sequences of learning activities or educational processes, with configurable instructions and resources [34]. In addition, students' progress can be monitored, allowing for necessary interventions. A study by [35] designed LAMS templates for scientific stream modules, which included coursework on the Scientific Basis of Medicine, for undergraduate medical students at the University of Western Sydney. The study utilized LAMS's online activities, with one of the topics being cardiovascular disease and risk factors. The templates include learning activities, questions and answers, feedback, resources on the disease, patient data, and assignments, all using LAMS's tools and features. LAMS allows educators to plan and discuss scientific stream modules without restrictions due to its user-friendly interface.

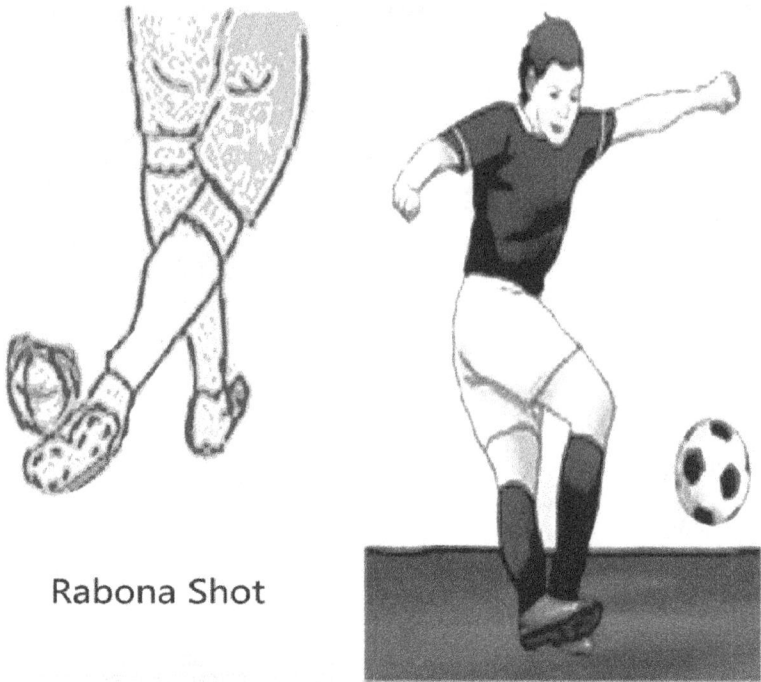

Rabona Shot

FIGURE 1.11   Diagram on sample football path (Robona shot)

In recent years, LAMS has also been used to facilitate team-based learning (TBL) sessions in health and social care programs, as reported by a study conducted by [36]. In this approach, students receive TBL materials, such as clinical scenarios, through LAMS. The effectiveness of the program was evaluated, and the results showed a significant improvement in the students' readiness to participate in interprofessional learning after the TBL sessions.

1.2.3.3   Video/Web-based Learning Platforms

Video and web-based learning are popular platforms in education due to their ability to help students visualize and understand complex concepts. According to literature, these platforms have been commonly used in discussing topics related to diseases and clinical skills. In a study by [37], a web-based learning platform called Picmonic Learning System (PLS) was developed and used by medical students to support their learning of medical sciences. The study compared students' memory retention of disease topics between PLS and traditional text-based materials. Eighty-eight first-year medical students participated in the study, and the results showed that students who used PLS had better memory retention than those who used traditional text-based materials.

PLS utilizes audiovisual mnemonics designed to provide significant and relevant information related to medical science concepts. A keyword mnemonic strategy

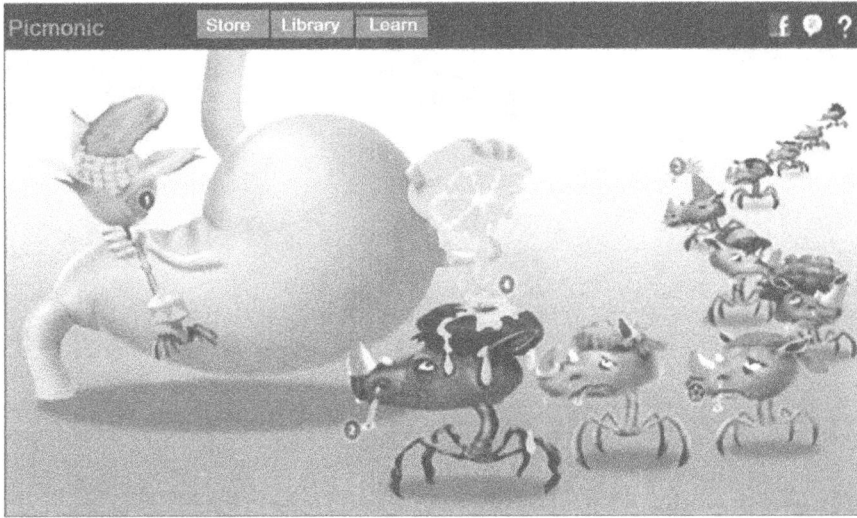

FIGURE 1.12 Screenshot of the Picmonic Learning System (PLS)

is used to encode important attributes of the disease topic into memorable characters. These characters are connected and illustrated as pictures, and audio files are recorded. Students can access these files in PLS along with a summary of the topic and each attribute's text-based definition (Figure 1.12). The audiovisual mnemonics contain interactive components that allow students to enlarge specific attributes in the picture, and students can also self-assess their understanding of the disease topic.

Video-based learning has been widely used in medical education, particularly for teaching clinical skills. In a study by [38], 411 (Year 3 and Year 4) medical students were surveyed to investigate their use and perception of clinical videos in learning clinical skills. The study found that the videos were effective and had a positive impact on learning clinical skills, particularly for basic clinical skills such as physical examination skills and clinical procedures. These videos were available on e-MedEdu, an online platform for medical education.

Video and web-based learning have become increasingly popular in recent years due to the rapid development of digital technology. There are several examples of using videos or web-based learning platforms in health science education, as evidenced by the results of several works of literature. These topics include the anatomy of the pharynx and larynx, surgical procedures, and chronic diseases such as type 2 diabetes (T2D) and obesity.

One study by [39] investigated the use of videos related to the pharynx and larynx in first-year anatomy curriculums. The study aimed to evaluate medical students' motivation levels for self-directed learning of pharynx and larynx anatomy using videos compared to those who only attended lectures, practical classes, and tutorials. The results showed that students who used videos enjoyed learning the anatomy and demonstrated a high level of motivation for self-directed learning compared to their counterparts. The

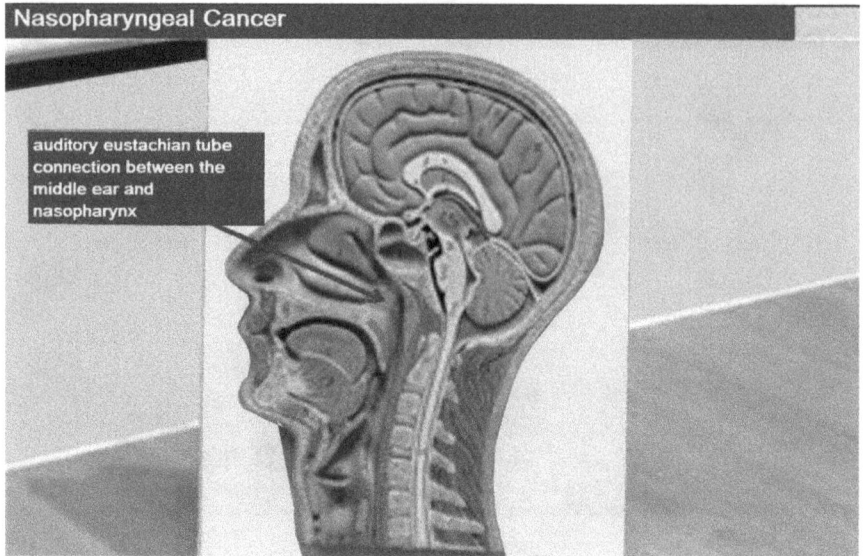

FIGURE 1.13   Screenshot of video embedded in learning anatomy of larynx

videos in the anatomy curriculum included an introduction, demonstration, self-test using plastic anatomical models, and clinical anatomy, as shown in Figure 1.13.

Another example of a video-based online platform has been implemented in surgical education in a study by [40]. This platform was designed for medical students to learn surgical topics. Surgical procedures are video recorded, including clinical case information and medical background information. The students that use the video-based online platform achieve better scores in written exams than those that use conventional textbooks to learn surgical topics.

For web-based learning, web-based educational activities on type 2 diabetes (T2D) and obesity have been developed and can be accessed on the medical education website, according to [26]. The activities consist of videos that address the learning objectives. For example, the first activity, touchIN CONVERSATION, focuses on managing specific patient cases. In contrast, the second activity, named touchMDT, focuses on T2D and obesity. It was found that the participants that use these web-based educational activities show significant enhancement in knowledge, competence, and performance.

1.3   DISCUSSIONS AND CONCLUDING REMARKS

1.3.1   Issues Encountered

Even though video, web-based learning platforms, and AR usage in health education bring many positive effects, a few challenges can be identified. First, a digital device such as a smartphone or computer is required. Students from low-income families might need help affording digital devices and are left behind in their studies. School facilities might be available for them. However, they cannot use the AR application outside the school session.

Next, pedagogical issues need to be considered in using these technologies. When AR is adopted in the learning process, it might result in constraints among teachers. In the current curriculum, many topics must be completed within a certain period. As a result, AR usage only allows certain concepts to be covered, and other important concepts may be omitted. In addition, the content in the AR system is fixed. This inflexibility does not allow the teacher to make changes to accommodate students' needs.

Teachers and students must have the digital skills to use these technological tools in the teaching and learning process. The inability to use these tools will prevent achieving the learning objectives, and students will feel the content learned is more complex. Using videos and web-based learning platforms might affect students' social interaction as they focus on technological tools. The students will rely more on technology to interact with others, affecting their confidence and communication skills.

While there are numerous, varied, and keep-expanding applications of augmented reality and virtual reality in health education that we could harness in making teaching and learning much more meaningful and pedagogically effective, there are also, nevertheless, certain issues which need to be highlighted and be aware of. The following are some issues, especially in AR/VR-based technological tools in preventive health education.

1.3.1.1 Technical Glitches

When health education is conducted using AR and VR technology, technical glitches often occur, which undoubtedly affect the functionality of the virtual learning activity. For example, when there is a problem with the hardware, it could be due to a malfunctioning of the device or even due to the problem of connectivity to a local server, which inhibits students' accessibility and completion of the learning activities. Additionally, if it is due to the content glitches, then the 3D objects in the augmented reality would not anchor appropriately in front of the learners and function in the way they are expected to function during a learning activity.

1.3.1.2 Security Threat and Privacy Breach

Privacy constitutes one of the biggest security threats of AR and VR-based technological tools. Given that augmented reality "augments" or enhances the real world by overlaying or adding digital elements—visual, auditory, or sensory—to the real-world view, a user's privacy may be compromised because AR technologies can track the user's activities. For example, AR tracks and collects lots of information about who the users are and what activities they have undertaken, so much so that the tracking is much more compared to the social media networks such as Facebook, Instagram, or other forms of technology. This, in turn, raises a number of concerns, particularly the following:

1. Where the companies would store the augmented reality data—on the device itself or in the cloud, and if it is the latter, would it be encrypted.

2. How the companies would use and secure the gathered information of the users.
3. Whether or not the collected data would be shared with third parties, and if affirmative, how these third parties would use the data.
4. The extent of potential loss of privacy if hackers were to gain access to the technological device.

Meanwhile, the security threats from VR are slightly different from that of AR's simply because VR is limited to its own cyber environment, which involves only an interface such as a headset or goggles and not the real physical world. Therefore, the danger arises if a hacker takes over the device. Just manipulating the content by the hacker may cause health hazards like dizziness or nausea to the users. Additionally, a major VR privacy issue is the highly confidential and personal nature of the data collected. Biometric data such as retina or iris scans, handprints and fingerprints, voiceprints, and face geometry are examples of "personally identifiable information" (PII). These biometric data are nearly impossible to anonymize, so a real security problem would arise should the VR systems be hacked.

1.3.1.3 High Cost

There is no doubt that virtual reality (VR) has been used in health and medical education, given the numerous benefits deriving from its use [41, 42]. For example, the training in health education has relied on virtual reality technology to simulate the human body. Additionally, virtual reality (VR) and augmented reality (AR) have been effectively employed in the training of enhancing cardio-pulmonary resuscitation (CPR) skills [43, 44]. However, substantial costing or budgeting is needed in procuring and setting up the hardware in addition to the costly software platform, which makes the use of AR and VR unattractive.

1.3.1.4 Reduced Human Interaction

When virtual applications such as AR and VR are employed in health education, it entails much mechanization of education and training. We often hear the phrase "robots cannot replace teachers." In the same vein, AR and VR also cannot replace teachers. The reasons for that are many; for example, teachers are considered mentors, supporters, and inspirers. Hence, the significance of direct interaction and the often-emphasized positive relationship between the students and the teacher underlines the great importance placed on direct conversations and direct face-to-face promotive interaction. In short, the more connected the students are to technology, the more disconnected they are—physically—from their peers and the teacher.

1.3.1.5 Lack of Real-Life Experience

Particularly in medical education, a real-life experience where the training uses human beings and real medical tools or apparatus is critically important. The training using AR and VR rests upon the assumption that all the learning activities that took place in the virtual environment transfer to their corresponding real-world activities or environments. The extent to which the training from the virtual world is successfully transferred to real-world environments has yet to reach a clear empirically supported conclusion, even though there are anecdotal pieces of evidence. [45] concluded in their study that the transfer of learning from a virtual and simulated environment to a real clinical setting does not occur automatically and unswervingly. Instead, numerous factors affect the transfer of learning, and these factors are categorized into 3 categories: learner-related, educational-design related, and clinical environment-related factors.

1.3.2 IMPLICATIONS AND SUGGESTIONS FOR THE WAY FORWARD

1.3.2.1 Implications

The preceding issues related to the use of AR and VR have implications that one needs to be mindful of while managing, planning, and implementing health education. First, it is undeniable that technical glitches arise and should be expected with any virtual learning program using advanced learning technologies. However, technical glitches could be alleviated if we were to run a virtual pilot program with a selected group of learners. By running the pilot, the facilitator, teacher, or lecturer can identify the problems and difficulties that the learners face and subsequently come up with some solutions before the program-wide rollout or implementation.

Pertaining to the security threat and privacy breach, ensuring cybersecurity is in place is very important. Virtual reality systems, like any other connected system, are the targets of cyber threats. Therefore, two types of cybersecurity need to be given full attention: protocol and product security. In the former (i.e., protocol security), the data sent while in transmission are protected. For example, the data sent to and from a VR headset are encrypted and authenticated so as to protect confidentiality and ensure the authenticity of the data. Meanwhile, the system is protected from hacking in the latter (i.e., product security). For example, the secure boot would verify that only authorized firmware can run on a VR headset; failing which, a compromised headset or vice versa would infect the laptop.

While it is not an end-all solution, the issues of reduced human interaction and lack of real-life experience could be addressed using a blended training approach, where different modalities are used. In order to ensure which training modality fits or suits the needs of the students in which topic or learning outcome, a training needs analysis should be conducted. Undeniably, the students are less immersive when accessing the AR training using their smartphones or tablets compared to the training via virtual reality (VR) experience. AR and VR-based training provides much less human interaction than face-to-face, real-life physical training. Therefore, if blended learning uses different modalities, students will get the best out of the blended approach.

1.3.2.2 Suggestions for the Way Forward

No matter how much technological advancement was seen to have happened, the digital divide and cybersecurity are still important factors that contribute to the issues mentioned previously that deter the implementation of AR/VR in health education. Hence, apart from examining all the issues mentioned previously before implementation, the authors suggest that policy makers consider all factors before implementing, especially in countries that still lack Internet access. Moreover, since human interaction and real-life experience are two important aspects to be considered in education especially starting from the early years, it is advisable that curriculum developers should consider the use of multi-mode approaches to devise a curriculum that could integrate the use of digital tools with contextual learning or outdoor studies to ensure a balanced education for all considering physical, psychological, and social aspects.

1.4   CONCLUSION

In conclusion, the fourth Industrial Revolution has brought about significant changes in various fields, including education, industry, and healthcare. The use of AR/VR-based technology and 3D animation tools has been highlighted as a powerful tool for preventive health education. The systematic review of past records has covered the concepts of IR4.0, technological shifts in healthcare settings, IoT sensors for smart healthcare, AR in sports science, Minecraft worlds, 3D printing, wearable devices, and robotics for smart healthcare implementation. Exemplary cases were presented to elaborate on current trends in the field. However, there are possible issues and implications of these digital tools, and further discussion and research are needed to address these concerns. Overall, the use of AR/VR-based technology and 3D animation tools in preventive health education has great potential to revolutionize healthcare and promote better health outcomes for individuals and communities.

ACKNOWLEDGMENTS

The authors would like to express their heartfelt gratitude to all who contributed to the successful completion of this study. We give special thanks to our co-researchers, proofreaders, and coordinators, including Prof. Dr. Yoon Fah Lay from Universiti Malaysia Sabah; Ms. Nurul Nazatul Shahizah bt Mahamad Shobri from Universiti Teknologi Malaysia; Adjunct Asst. Prof. Dr. Khar Thoe Ng from UCSI University; Dr. Subuh Anggoro from Universitas Muhammadiyah Purwokerto, Indonesia; and Dr. Rajendra Kumar from Sharda University, India. We also extend our appreciation to all students, administrators, teachers, and stakeholders involved in various training, research, and development activities that contributed to the success of the studies related to the topics covered in this chapter.

REFERENCES

[1] Scherman, J. (2019, May 20). *5 Ways Technology in Healthcare Is Transforming the Way We Approach Medical Treatment.* Rasmussen University. Retrieved from www.rasmussen.edu/degrees/health-sciences/blog/technology-in-healthcare-transformation/.
[2] Nayyar, A. (2022). *Healthcare 1.0, 2.0, 3.0 and 4.0.* Retrieved October 31, 2022, from www.researchgate.net/figure/Growth-of-the-healthcare-industry-from-version-10-to-version-40_fig2_343400503.

[3] Galvao, M., & Zorzal, E. (2013). Augmented reality applied to health education. In *Proceedings of the 2013 15th Symposium on Virtual and Augmented Reality, SVR 2013* (pp. 268–271). https://doi.org/10.1109/SVR.2013.54.

[4] Albrecht, U., Folta-Schoofs, K., Behrends, M., & von Jan, U. (2013). Effects of mobile augmented reality learning compared to textbook learning on medical students: Randomized controlled pilot study. *Journal of Medical Internet Research*, *15*(8), e182. doi:10.2196/jmir.2630.

[5] Juanes, J. A., Ruisoto, P., Prats, A., Cabrero, F. J., Framiñán, A., Paniagua, J. C., & Gómez, J. J. (2013). Visualization and interactive systems applied to health science education. In *Proceedings of the First International Conference on Technological Ecosystem for Enhancing Multiculturality—TEEM '13* (pp. 49–53). https://doi.org/10.1145/2536536.2536545.

[6] Garrett, B., Jackson, C., & Wilson, B. (2015). Augmented reality m-learning to enhance nursing skills acquisition in the clinical skills laboratory. *Interactive Technology and Smart Education*, *12*(4), 298–314. https://doi.org/10.1108/ITSE-05-2015-0013.

[7] Narulita, S., Perdana, A. T. W., Annisa, N. F., Darmakusuma, M. D., Indarjani, & Ng, K. T. (2018). Motivating secondary science learning through 3D interactive technology: From theory to practice using Augmented Reality. *Learning Science and Mathematics Online Journal*, *13*, 38–45. Retrieved from http://myjurnal.my/filebank/published_article/83604/2018_3_SN_3845.pdf.

[8] Moro, C., Smith, J., & Finch, E. (2021). Improving stroke education with augmented reality: A randomized control trial. *Computers and Education Open*, *2*, 100032. https://doi.org/10.1016/j.caeo.2021.100032.

[9] Bozyer, Z. (2015). Augmented reality in sports: Today and tomorrow. *International Journal of Science Culture and Sport (IntJSCS)*, *3*(4), 376–390. Retrieved from www.researchgate.net/publication/282840597_Augmented_Reality_in_Sports_Today_and_Tomorrow.

[10] The Barça Innovation Hub Team. (2019, September 2). *The Use of VR/AR/MR to Improve Performance in Sports*. Retrieved from https://barcainnovationhub.com/the-use-of-vr-ar-mr-to-improved-performance-in-sports/.

[11] Ohio University. (2020). *Virtual Training for Football Is Becoming a Reality*. Retrieved from https://onlinemasters.ohio.edu/blog/virtual-training-for-football-is-becoming-a-reality/.

[12] Ng, J. H., Kumar, R., Ng, K. T., et al. (2020). Visual learning tools for sports and physical health education: A reflective study and challenges for the ways forward. In *The Proceedings of the 5th International Conference on Management, Engineering, Science, Social Science and Humanities (iCon-MESSSH'20) (Virtual)* (pp. 81–91). Retrieved from www.socrd.org/wp-content/uploads/2020/12/Proceedings_iCon_MESSSH20.pdf.

[13] Kolici, V., Spaho, E., Matsuo, K., Caballe, S., Barolli, L., & Xhafa, F. (2014). Implementation of a medical support system considering P2P and IoT technologies. In *2014 Eighth International Conference on Complex, Intelligent and Software Intensive Systems* (pp. 101–106). IEEE.

[14] Kolici, V., Spaho, E., Matsuo, K., Caballe, S., Barolli, L., & Xhafa, F. (2014, July). Implementation of a medical support system considering P2P and IoT technologies. In *2014 Eighth International Conference on Complex, Intelligent and Software Intensive Systems* (pp. 101–106). IEEE.

[15] Catarinucci, L., De Donno, D., Mainetti, L., Palano, L., Patrono, L., Stefanizzi, M. L., & Tarricone, L. (2015). An IoT-aware architecture for smart healthcare systems. *IEEE Internet of Things Journal*, *2*(6), 515–526. doi:10.1109/JIOT.2015.2419411.

[16] Vippalapalli, V., & Ananthula, S. (2016, October). Internet of things (IoT) based smart health care system. In *2016 International Conference on Signal Processing, Communication, Power and Embedded System (SCOPES)* (pp. 1229–1233). IEEE. doi:10.1109/SCOPES.2016.7955904.

[17] Ahad, A., Tahir, M., Aman Sheikh, M., Ahmed, K. I., Mughees, A., & Numani, A. (2020). Technologies trend towards 5G network for smart health-care using IoT: A review. *Sensors, 20*(14), 4047. doi:10.3390/s20144047.

[18] Ghazal, T. M., Hasan, M. K., Alshurideh, M. T., Alzoubi, H. M., Ahmad, M., Akbar, S. S., . . . Akour, I. A. (2021). IoT for smart cities: Machine learning approaches in smart healthcare—a review. *Future Internet, 13*(8), 218. doi:10.3390/fi13080218.

[19] Gyrard, A., Tabeau, K., Fiorini, L., Kung, A., Senges, E., De Mul, M., . . . Tsukamoto, M. (2021). Knowledge engineering framework for IoT robotics applied to smart healthcare and emotional well-being. *International Journal of Social Robotics, 13*(1), 1–28.

[20] Dalziel, J. (2003). Implementing learning design: The learning activity management system (LAMS). In G. Crisp, D. Thiele, I. Scholten, S. Barker & J. Baron (Eds.), *Interact, Integrate, Impact: Proceedings of the 20th Annual Conference of the Australasian Society for Computers in Learning in Tertiary Education (ASCILITE), Adelaide, Australia 7–10 December 2003* (pp. 593–596). Australasian Society for Computers in Learning in Tertiary Education.

[21] Chan, L. K., Ganotice, F., Wong, F. K. Y., Lau, C. S., Bridges, S. M., Chan, C. H. Y., Chan, N., Chan, P. W. L., Chen, H. Y., Chen, J. Y., Chu, J. K. P., Ho, C. C., Ho, J. M. C., Lam, T. P., Lam, V. S. F., Li, Q., Shen, J. G., Tanner, J. A., Tso, W. W. Y., Wong, A. K. C., Wong, G. T. C., Wong, J. Y. H., Wong, N. S., Worsley, A., Yu, L. K., & Yum, T. P. (2017). Implementation of an interprofessional team-based learning program involving seven undergraduate health and social care programs from two universities, and students' evaluation of their readiness for interprofessional learning. *BMC Medical Education, 17*(1), 221. doi:10.1186/s12909-017-1046-5.

[22] Goel, H., Yang, A., Bryan, M., Robertson, R., Lim, J., Speicher, M., & Islam, S. (2014). The Picmonic® learning system: Enhancing memory retention of medical sciences, using an audiovisual mnemonic Web-based learning platform. *Advances in Medical Education and Practice, 5*, 125–132. doi:10.2147/AMEP.S61875.

[23] Jang, H. W., & Kim, K. (2014). Use of online clinical videos for clinical skills training for medical students: Benefits and challenges. *BMC Medical Education, 14*, 56–56.

[24] Ang, E., Talib, S. N., Thong, M. K., & Charn, T. C. (2017). Using video in medical education: What it takes to succeed. *Medical Education, 51*(1), 94–96. https://doi.org/10.1111/medu.13124.

[25] Schmitz, S. M., Schipper, S., Lemos, M. et al. (2021). Development of a tailor-made surgical online learning platform, ensuring surgical education in times of the COVID19 pandemic. *BMC Surg, 21*, 196. https://doi.org/10.1186/s12893-021-01203-5.

[26] Ho, C., Yeh, C., Wang, J., Hu, R., & Lee, C. (2021). Curiosity in online video concept learning and short-term outcomes in blended medical education. *Frontiers in Medicine, 8*. doi:10.3389/fmed.2021.772956.

[27] Talib, C. A., Nazratul, S. B., Marlina, A., Ng, K. T., & Zawadzki, R. (2017, November). Video-based learning in chemistry education: Issues and challenges. In K. T. Ng (Ed.), *Learning Science and Mathematics On-line Journal* (Volume 12, pp. 34–50). Retrieved from http://myjurnal.my/public/article-view.php?id=135421 OR www.recsam.edu.my/sub_LSMJournal/images/docs/2017/(4)CAT%20p35–51_final.pdf.

[28] Parimalah, L., Talib, C. A., Ng, K. T., Faruku, A., & Zawadzki, R. (2019, December). Implementing technology infused gamification in science classroom: Systematic review and suggestions for future research. In K. T. Ng & M. Rajoo (Eds.), *Learning Science and Mathematics On-line journal* (Volume 14, pp. 60–73). Retrieved from http://myjurnal.my/public/article-view.php?id=138896 OR www.recsam.edu.my/sub_LSM-Journal/images/docs/2019/2019_5_PL_6073_Final.pdf.

[29] Kirriemuir, J. (2002, April). The relevance of video games and gaming consoles to the Higher and Further Education learning experience. *ResearchGate*. Retrieved from www.researchgate.net/publication/316856694_The_relevance_of_video_games_and_gaming_consoles_to_the_Higher_and_Further_Education_learning_experience.

[30] Garrett, B., Jackson, C., & Wilson, B. (2015). Augmented reality m-learning to enhance nursing skills acquisition in the clinical skills laboratory. *Interactive Technology and Smart Education, 12*, 298–314. doi:10.1108/ITSE-05-2015-0013.

[31] Martini, E., Purwanto, B., & Subagyo, A. (2019). Application of augmented reality technology as a model of dental health education media for children. *International Journal of Engineering & Technology, 8*(1.9), 36–38. doi:10.14419/ijet.v8i1.9.14847.

[32] Soh, J., Khoo, H., & Ng, J. H. (2018, October to December). *Movement on the Earth, Water, in the Air and Space. Storybook Submitted for Augmented Reality Online Training*. RECSAM.

[33] Ellaway, R., Dalziel, J., & Dalziel, B. (2008). Learning design in healthcare education. *Medical Teacher, 30*(2), 180–184. doi:10.1080/01421590701874066.

[34] Baniasadi, T., Ayyoubzadeh, S. M., & Mohammadzadeh, N. (2020). Challenges and practical considerations in applying virtual reality in medical education and treatment. *Oman Medical Journal, 35*(3), e125. https://doi.org/10.5001/omj.2020.43.

[35] Dalziel, B. (2007). *Designing LAMS Templates for Medical Education*. Proceedings of the 2nd International LAMS Conference 2007: Practical Benefits of Learning Design, pages 43–49.

[36] Chan, L. K., Ganotice, F., Wong, F. K. Y., Lau, C. S., Bridges, S. M., Chan, C. H. Y., Chan, N., Chan, P. W. L., Chen, H. Y., Chen, J. Y., Chu, J. K. P., Ho, C. C., Ho, J. M. C., Lam, T. P., Lam, V. S. F., Li, Q., Shen, J. G., Tanner, J. A., Tso, W. W. Y., Wong, A. K. C., Wong, G. T. C., Wong, J. Y. H., Wong, N. S., Worsley, A., Yu, L. K., & Yum, T. P. (2017). Implementation of an interprofessional team-based learning program involving seven undergraduate health and social care programs from two universities, and students' evaluation of their readiness for interprofessional learning. *BMC Medical Education, 17*(1), 221. doi:10.1186/s12909-017-1046-5.

[37] Goel, H., Yang, A., Bryan, M., Robertson, R., Lim, J., Speicher, M., & Islam, S. (2014). The picmonic® learning system: Enhancing memory retention of medical sciences, using an audiovisual mnemonic Web-based learning platform. *Advances in Medical Education and Practice, 5*, 125–132. doi:10.2147/AMEP.S61875.

[38] Jang, H. W., & Kim, K. (2014). Use of online clinical videos for clinical skills training for medical students: Benefits and challenges. *BMC Medical Education, 14*, 56–56.

[39] Ang, E., Talib, S. N., Thong, M. Y., & Charn, T. C. (2017). Using video in medical education: What it takes to succeed. *Medical Teacher, 39*(6), 632–639. doi:10.1080/01421 59X.2017.1309377.

[40] Schmitz, S. M., Schipper, S., Lemos, M., Lammers, W., Prins, H., & van den Dobbelsteen, J. J. (2021). Development of a tailor-made surgical online learning platform, ensuring surgical education in times of the COVID19 pandemic. *BMC Surgery, 21*, 196. https://doi.org/10.1186/s12893-021-01203-5.

[41] Halbig, A., Babu, S. K., Gatter, S., Latoschik, M. E., Brukamp, K., & von Mammen, S. (2022). Opportunities and challenges of virtual reality in healthcare—a domain experts inquiry. *Frontier in Virtual Reality, 3*, 837616. https://doi.org/10.3389/frvir.2022.837616.

[42] Kuyt, K., Park, S. H., Chang, T. P., Jung, T., & MacKinnon, R. (2021). The use of virtual reality and augmented reality to enhance cardio-pulmonary resuscitation: A scoping review. *Advances in Simulation, 6*(11), 1–8.

[43] Madison, D. (2018). The future of augmented reality in healthcare. *The Journal of Health Management, 18*(1), 42–45. doi:10.1177/0972063417749988.

[44] Nas, J., Thannhauser, J., Vart, P., van Geuns, R. J., Muijsers, H. E. C., Mol, J. Q., Aarts, G. W. A., Konijnenberg, L. S. F., Gommans, D. H. F., Ahoud-Schoenmakers, S. G. A. M., Vos, J. L., van Royen, N., Bonnes, J. L., & Brouwer, M. A. (2020). Effect of face-to-face vs virtual reality training on cardiopulmonary resuscitation quality: A randomized clinical trial. *JAMA Cardiology*, *5*(3), 328–335. https://doi.org/10.1001/jamacardio.2019.4992.

[45] Masoomi, R., Shariati, M., Labaf, A., & Mirzazadeh, A. (2021). Transfer of learning from simulated setting to the clinical setting: Identifying instructional design features. *Medical Journal of the Islamic Republic of Iran*, *35*, 90. https://doi.org/10.47176/mjiri.35.90.

Appendix A: Minecraft Worlds in Health Education Settings

(Using Minecraft tool to illustrate sustainable future city including organic farming, sustainable energy through solar panels, etc.)

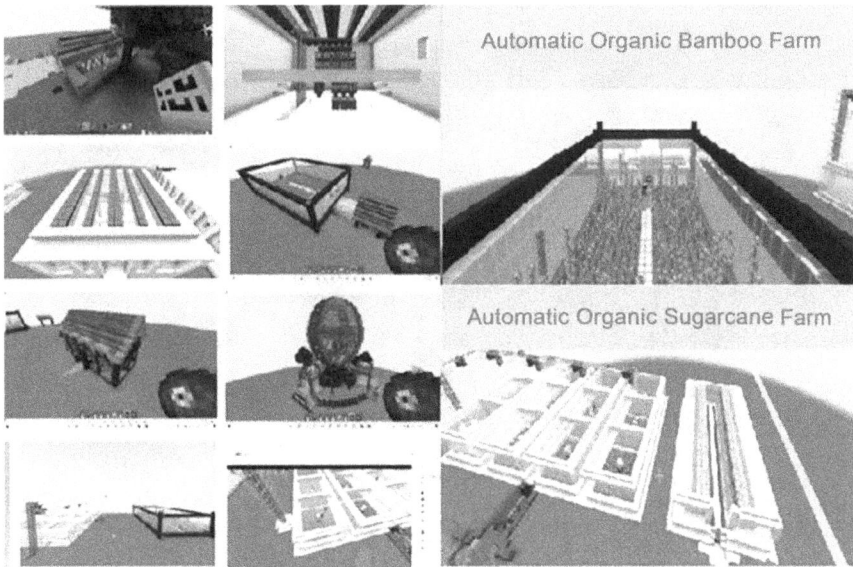

APPENDIX A   Minecraft worlds in health education settings

Prepared by: Foo, L. Z. H., Ho, J. S., Teh, Y. Q., Tan, Y. X., Ngoh, X. W., Tan, Z. B., Pang, Y. J. and Ng, K. T. *Sustainable Future City in Minecraft.* Project prepared for dry run during Heritage Immortalized Minecraft Championship (e-sport 18 September) 2022 and "LearnT-SMArET incorporating Technology in Values-based Sustainable Education (VaBSE) and Local Wisdom through Basic Education" e-course series (October–November 2022) organized by SEAMEO RECSAM.

Appendix B: 3D Printing for HSE Models to Promote Healthy Living

(Using 3D printing to illustrate ideal smart home with features that promote healthy living)

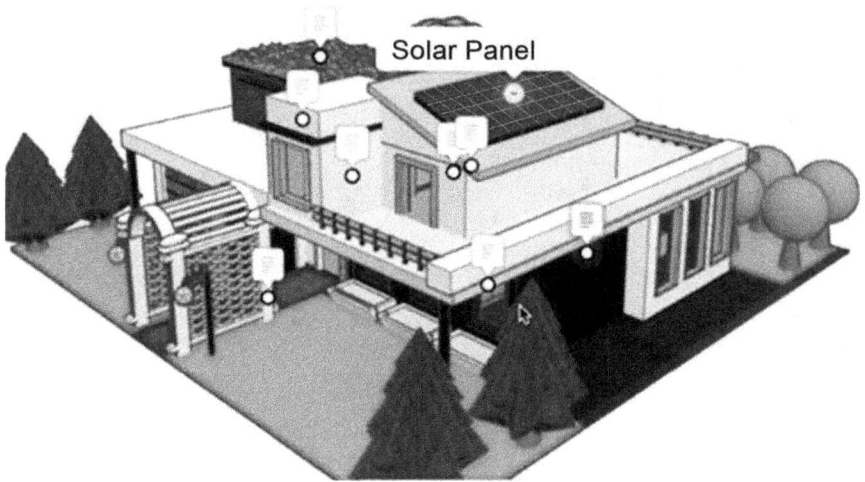
Solar Panel

APPENDIX B   3D printing for HSE models to promote healthy living

Produced by: C. Hoh, J. Ong, and D. Woon. *Smart House in 3D Design.* Project submitted for National STEM Carnival (*Karnival STEM Kebangsaan*) 2022 organized by Ministry of Education, Malaysia (October–November 2022).

Appendix C: Apps in Promoting Healthy Lifestyle

(Using Smartphone "Pacer" Apps to trace the running distance and path)

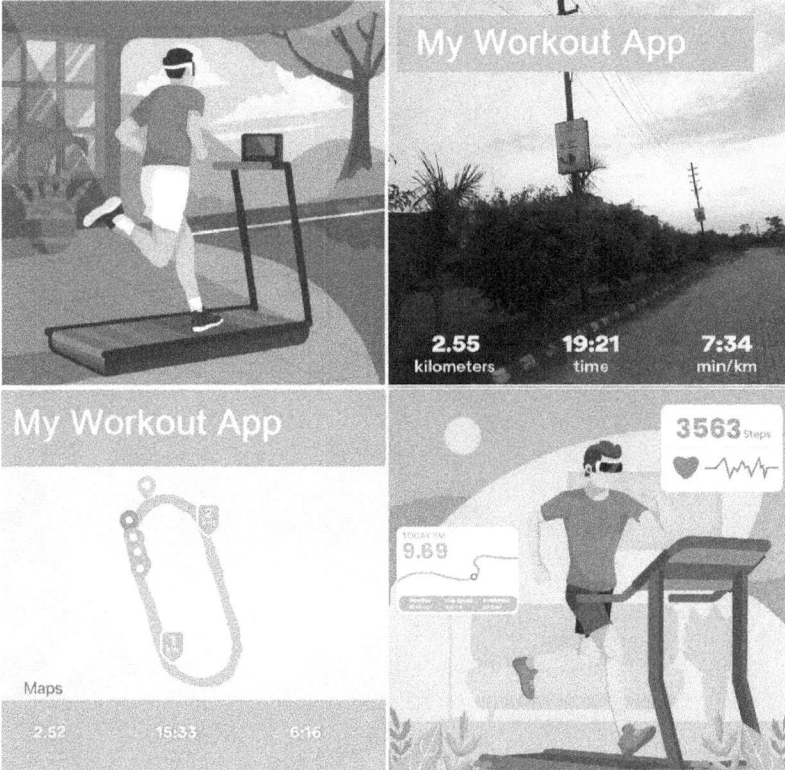

APPENDIX C1   Apps in promoting healthy lifestyle

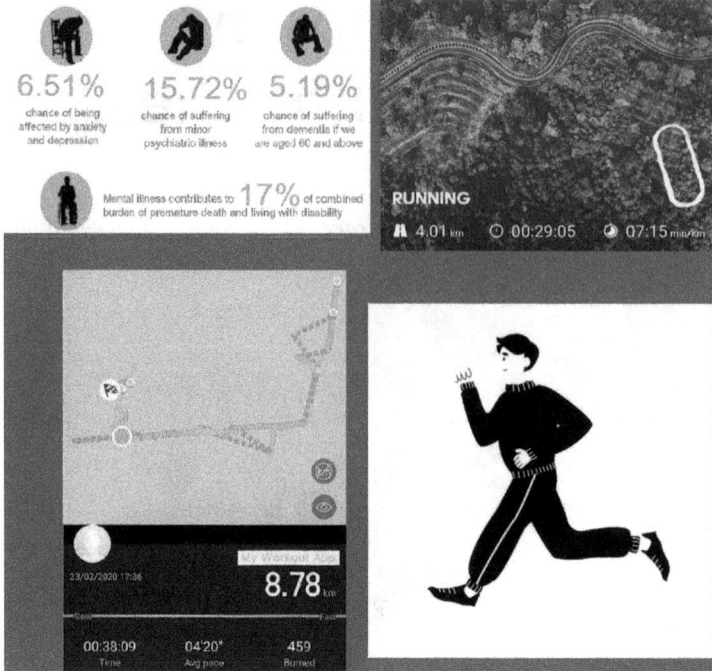

APPENDIX C2

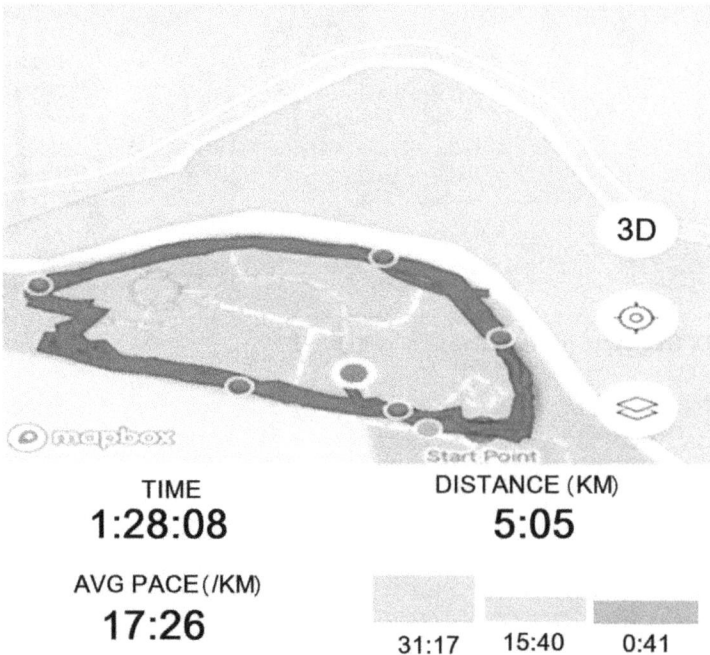

APPENDIX C3

NURIN Fatini
Today at 7:08 AM · North Seberang Perai District, Penang

Morning Run

Distance	Pace	Time
5.05 km	8:45 /km	44m 16s

Congratulations, this activity is your longest run on Strava!

Start and end hidden

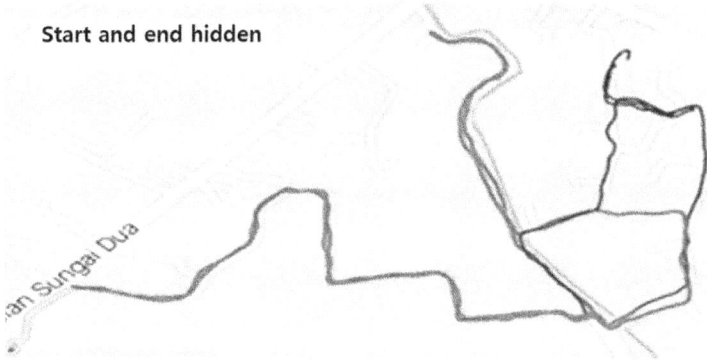

APPENDIX C4

Average	Total
6180	**488205**

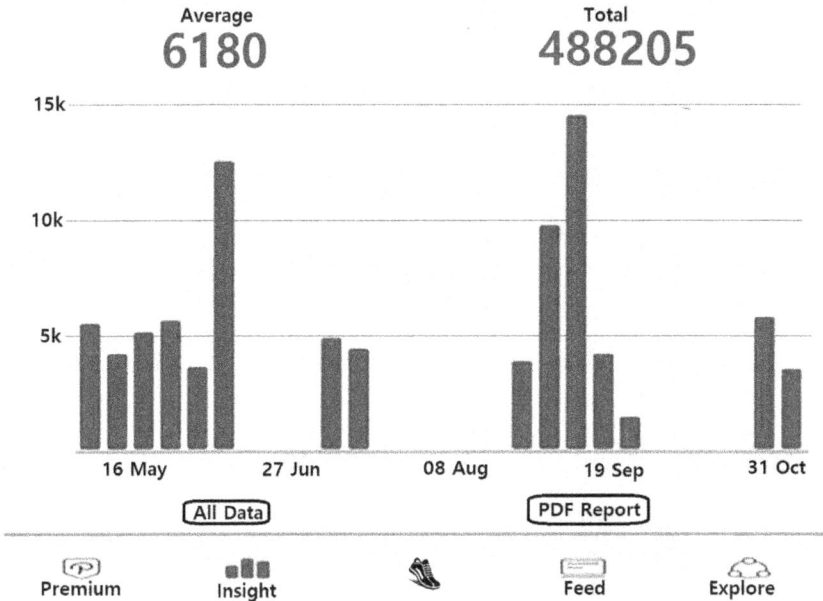

16 May　　27 Jun　　08 Aug　　19 Sep　　31 Oct

All Data　　　PDF Report

Premium　Insight　　　　Feed　Explore

APPENDIX C5

2 Advanced Healthcare Informatics Practice Vis-à-Vis Virtual Reality Implications—*A Scientific Overview*

P. K. Paul, Ritam Chatterjee, Sucheta Chakraborty, K. S. Tiwary, P. S. Aithal, and S. Sharma

2.1 INTRODUCTION

Information Technology (IT) has ever changed the way of handling today's digital period. This has become the most important source for development in this digital world. There are lots of factors under the marquee of IT, which are like a game changer in this digital society. Some of the arising technologies in the sphere of information technology are as follows (also refer to Figure 2.2):

- Software Technology
- Network Technology
- Database Technology
- Multimedia Technology
- Security Technology

Some of the advantages of using these rearmost technologies are the capability to cipher data, to store and manipulate large complex datasets in a structures format, to bear authentication to pierce it, to give the chance of penetrating these data in any time from any place and to lock it down under layers of security so bad actors cannot fluently get to it [1, 2]. Because of these wider benefits, nearly every sector or association is using IT, and healthcare sector is one of them. Here in Figure 2.1 some of the benefits are widely depicted. Technology and drugs have gone hand and hand for numerous times. Virtual reality is an alarming emerging technology in the area of computing and IT, and abbreviated popularly as VR, it allows users, including medical professionals and patients, to simulate a particular situation related to healthcare or experience. It offers an interactive but computer-generated environment. In the VR, simulation is immersive, and here the use of special 3D goggles can be seen

DOI: 10.1201/9781003340133-2

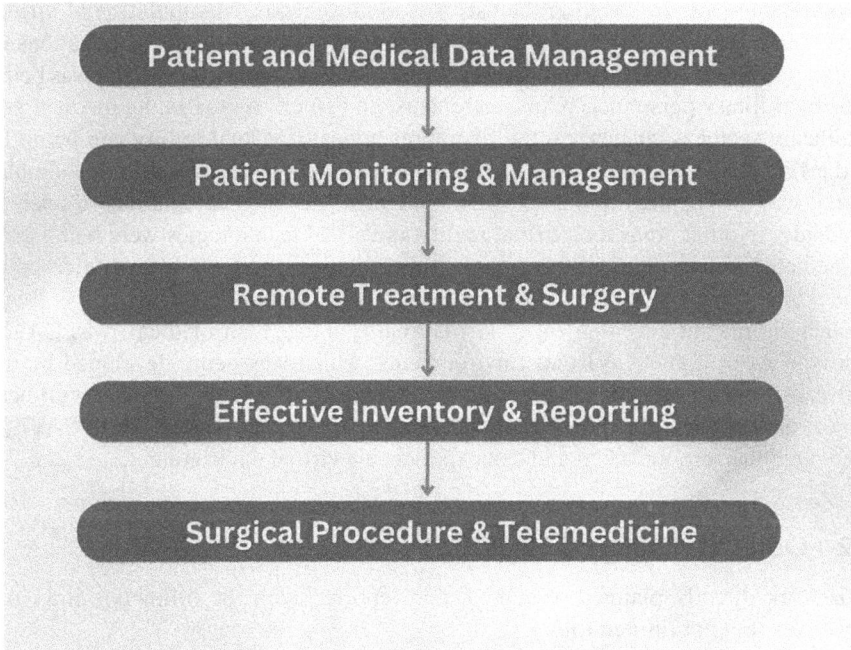

```
┌──────────────────────────────────────────────┐
│      Patient and Medical Data Management      │
└──────────────────────────────────────────────┘
                        ↓
┌──────────────────────────────────────────────┐
│       Patient Monitoring & Management         │
└──────────────────────────────────────────────┘
                        ↓
┌──────────────────────────────────────────────┐
│         Remote Treatment & Surgery            │
└──────────────────────────────────────────────┘
                        ↓
┌──────────────────────────────────────────────┐
│        Effective Inventory & Reporting        │
└──────────────────────────────────────────────┘
                        ↓
┌──────────────────────────────────────────────┐
│      Surgical Procedure & Telemedicine        │
└──────────────────────────────────────────────┘
```

FIGURE 2.1   The ultimate benefit of the digital healthcare systems

with a big LED screen, or sometimes gloves, which offer a sensory feedback and also offer a virtual world. In the healthcare and medical domain, lots of areas can be noted having interaction with information technology and computing. But virtual reality has many significant uses, such as in medical education and training, patient treatment, marketing of healthcare organizations, educating people to inform about a topic or medical situation or condition [3]. The market share in virtual reality will increase in the coming years in different sectors and areas. In the year 1987 the term VR was first coined by Jaron Lanier, though the aspects and philosophy of virtual reality (VR) can be stated as landmark by Morton Heilig, who was a cinematographer that time, for his ideas on virtual reality in the stories. In the year 1960 he included stereoscopic color display called "Sensorama." It came with the features of wind, odor emitters, stereo for audio, simulating moving chair—though the entire system was not that much interactive and advanced. Gradually other products have been developed in the area of virtual reality. In the year 1961 Philco Corporation developed the head-mounted display (HMD), which is integrated with the features of video screening, tracking systems, and also connected with the closed circuit camera system. In the military training and operations, HMD was being used. It was initially a surprising tool integrated with real and remote based viewing. To see fields and pictorial views, HMD was used by the helicopter pilots.

Sword of Damocles was developed in the year 1966 by Ivan, and this too was being used with an HMD connector to visualize the virtual world. In real time, such system works by tracking the user's head movements. Manipulation of virtual objects in a realistic way was also possible with that system. Early applications of virtual reality also were noted in the designing of vehicle simulators, and it was being used by military personnel, pilots, astronauts, and so on. As far as the medical and healthcare sector is concerned, the first applications of virtual reality can be noted in the 1990s, and this was being used in colonoscopy as well as endoscopy simulation. It was also applied in the teaching and learning of medical and health science. Gradually in other areas too, virtual reality and allied technologies were being used in medicine viz. in physical therapy and rehabilitation, recovery from addiction, in fitness and marketing, virtual surgery, telemedicine, and so on. During the 1990s another significant development in virtual reality (other than medical) was CAVE, that is, Cave Automatic Virtual Environments, which was being developed by the University of Illinois, USA. This was a useful tool in displaying images with near projection technique for showing walls, floors, ceilings, small rooms. With CAVE, a user can move into the room and can experience a virtual environment.

2.2   OBJECTIVE OF THE WORK

This work directly planned, executed, and reported with the following aims and objectives (but not limited to):

- To learn regarding healthcare informatics with features and characteristics with reference to IT and its components in healthcare practice.
- To know about the fundamentals of virtual reality, including its historical foundations, basic applications of virtual reality in healthcare systems.
- To learn about the emerging applications and trends on virtual reality in health informatics practice particularly in medical and clinical aspects, including administrative activities.
- To know about the sector-specific applications of healthcare informatics in different places and context.
- To find out the basic healthcare informatics applications in India with reference to the issues and challenges of virtual reality applications in Indian context.

2.3   METHODS

This chapter titled "Advanced Healthcare Informatics Practice Vis-à-Vis Virtual Reality Implications—*A Scientific Overview*" is a conceptual work and theoretical in nature. This chapter was basically prepared from secondary sources such as books, encyclopedias, and other documentary sources. In conducting this work journals were also collected and analyzed and, lastly, reported scientifically. Aims, objectives, and current scenario of different healthcare units, organizations, and associations have also been analyzed by their white papers, trend report, and website analysis regarding finding the latest practice and technologies. Since this is conceptual only and offers the overview of healthcare informatics, particularly virtual reality applications, therefore it does not lie on any primary data collection from the field.

2.4 REVIEW OF LITERATURE

Health informatics is an interdisciplinary subject practiced by many subject experts, ranging from biology, information technology, management science, healthcare administrators, and so on. Some of the notable works have been listed here with major findings.

Alotaibi, S. R., 2020 [4] in the research paper titled different aspects of AI in medical context, the experimenter described the necessity and operations of artificial intelligence as well as big data in the field of health informatics. This paper explains the topmost uses of mHealth to serve the humanity with the help of new and arising technologies in healthcare sectors. Experts study the operation of artificial intelligence and data analytics to give drug addicts awareness and planning ability, especially using checkout for specific challenges in mHealth, and AI and big data in mHealth. We propose a model based on analysis. Beam, A. L., and Kohane, I. S., 2018 [5] in their work discussed big data and machine learning trends, tools, and technologies in the field of health informatics. They showed that big data and machine knowledge go hand-in-hand with traditional statistical models that the best clinicians can perceive, thus generating algorithms like human cattle. Freeman, D. et al., 2017 [6] in their research paper related to the VR mentioned aspects of advanced healthcare informatics. Experts believe that with the help of virtual reality (VR) and computer-generated interactive environments, individuals are constantly witnessing problem situations and reason-based brain training on how to overcome the difficulties of internal problems. This paper aims to demonstrate that the technology's ability to generate new realities may ameliorate problems during treatment, as VR can also assess neuroimaging-worthy attention. Javaid, M., and Haleem, A., 2020 [7] in the research paper titled "Virtual reality applications toward medical field," the experimenters explained that the operation of this VR technology in the medical field is getting fashionable with better acceptability among millions. This exploration paper mentions that the scholars and croakers can inversely interact with the mortal body with the VR widgets and take all attention, and they can gain experience with the holographic images using VR headsets, which can surely increase the treatment systems. Moro, C. et al., 2017 [8] in their research paper described the aspects of anatomy where release of virtual (VR) and augmented reality (AR) biases allowed learning through practical and immersive gestures, making deconstruction research more appropriate using virtual reality tools. At the end of this study, they asked whether structural deconstruction of literacy through VR or AR exercises was as effective as tablet-based manipulation and whether these modes enabled improved student literacy, engagement, and outcomes. Samadbeik, M. et al., 2018 [9] in their work described how virtual reality is in fact one of the topmost generation that has been considerably used within the fitness subject these days, and it is implemented in a huge variety of conditions. Thus, it is important to become aware of the operations of digital fact generation for schooling in the clinical groups. Zhao, R. et al., 2019 [10] in their studies have defined how data pushed gadget fitness tracking to become fashionable in ultramodern production structures because of the huge deployment of low-priced detectors and their connection to the Internet and additional features given particular importance, especially deep literacy, which affords beneficial gear for processing and assaying those large ministry data. The foremost reason of this paper is to check and epitomize on the springing up of exploration paintings of deep literacy on gadget fitness tracking, to locate operations of deep literacy in gadget fitness tracking structures with the assistance of latest gear, like bus encoder (AE) constrained Boltzmann machines, deep Boltzmann machines (DBM), deep belief network (DBN), convolutional neural networks (CNN), intermittent neural networks (RNN), etc.

2.5   ADVANCED HEALTHCARE INFORMATICS PRACTICE

Healthcare technology refers to any IT tool or software designed to boost sanitarium and executive productivity, give new perceptivity into drugs and treatments, or ameliorate the overall quality of healthcare handed. Uses of smart and advanced technology in the medical and healthcare sector is changing and advancing telehealth, telemedicine, remote care, and health monitoring technology. Be it covering on the case, tracking once conditioning of the case is on, or storing the health updates and records of drugs, each and every situation is now handled by IT tools and technologies [2, 12, 18]. Many of the foremost technologies which are spreading their blessings in healthcare sectors and saving millions of lives are mentioned in Figure 2.2 (but not limited to):

FIGURE 2.2   Emerging technologies of IT in the healthcare sector

Apart from these technologies, healthcare sectors also use some other technologies as follows:

- Artificial intelligence
- Machine learning
- Robotics
- Augmented reality
- Human computer interaction (HCI) and so on

The applications of the major emerging technologies in the area of health informatics are as follows:

2.5.1 CLOUD COMPUTING AND HEALTHCARE

Cloud computing comes under the sphere of network technology, which literally saves stoner's time as well as cost by furnishing the access authority of information from anywhere and anytime [4, 13, 14]. Cloud computing technologies offer an innovative system of delivering IT services efficiently. It gives the chance to nearly store any kind of data and gives authorization to have the right of using tackle, software, platform, infrastructure without actually copping the whole thing. The main operations of cloud computing in the medical field are as follows:

2.5.1.1 Cost-Effective Treatment

Using advanced technologies, basic healthcare providers as well as hospitals will no longer need to purchase data storage devices and software [15, 16]. Also, there are no explicit fees associated with the healthcare cloud. You pay only for the resources you actually use. The use of all computing technologies in healthcare provides the perfect terrain for scaling [4, 13, 17].

2.5.1.2 In eHealth and Telemedicine

A key requirement for healthcare cloud services is real-time availability of computer cash registers, as well as data storage and computing power. It is now extensively used for eHealth, which refers to furnishing healthcare services electronically through the Internet [13, 15]. The cloud technologies allow different medical professionals to unite and give their input on complex medical cases, similar as tele-surgery, tele-radiology, etc.

2.5.1.3 In Drug Discovery

Cloud computing plays a significant part in medicine recovery because medicine recovery requires a large number of computing coffers for discovering different composites from billions of chemical structures [1, 18].

2.5.1.4 In Healthcare Information System

The healthcare assiduity uses cloud computing tools and technologies in health information systems to give better patient care, manage mortal coffers, better querying services, and billing and finance [2, 15, 16]. Cloud computing in healthcare assiduity is also used to develop, test, and emplace these systems.

2.5.1.5 Personal Health Records

Cloud technology operation in healthcare is managing access to particular health records (PHR) and electronic health records (EHR). With cloud computing techniques for PHR, druggies can fluently pierce and manage the PHR database and share data [6, 19, 20]. These programs have advanced participating features that give druggies high control over participated data.

2.5.1.6 Clinical Decision Support System (CDSS)

CDSS is an advanced system that uses the knowledge and jester of a medical professional to give advice on case record analysis. This system is used for diagnosing conditions and defining drugs. Cloud computing can be used to produce similar systems that give better patient care. Also, with the advancement of technology, smartphones and fitness trackers now cover heart rate, diabetes, and blood pressure [13, 20, 21].

These are few applications related to the cloud technologies in medical and healthcare sector, which not only saves time, gives security, but also provides better treatment environment and also provides the chance to interact with doctors without even going to the clinic or hospital.

2.5.2 BIG DATA, ANALYTICS IN THE CONTEXT OF HEALTH INFORMATICS

Big data or data analytics falls under database technology. It holds promise in many business areas, and healthcare is turning to big data to provide answers to many age-related problems, insanity, and the treatment of habitual ailments [4, 17]. Big data as far as healthcare is concerned is being used to manage the complex as well as vast amount of information created through the transfer of digital technology to collect case (patient) records and help manage nursing home performance. It differs from being too large and complex for conventional techniques [5, 14, 22]. There are many positive and life-saving aspects to performing big data analytics in medical and healthcare. Some of the key operations of big data analytics in healthcare include (but are not limited to):

2.5.2.1 In Health Data for Sound Strategic Planning

The application of big data in medicine enables strategic planning, and such credit must go for better perception of people's provocations. Nurse directs and can analyze test results for people in different demographic groups to determine factors that prevent people from receiving treatment [5, 17].

2.5.2.2 In Effective Individual and Remedial Ways

Medical reports and gossip meetings generate vast amounts of data every day. Using big data tools and technologies such as PowerBI and Tableau, croakers can analyze data to validate treatment processes and medication efficacy and even predict fetal perceptions of cases [17, 23]. Using the proper system, one can easily do a proper identification of the treatment possible in a particular condition. Ineffective treatments and processes can be eliminated to achieve desired results. Health analytics can use big data for the identification of patient enrollment trends as well as specific times of the day. Moreover it is worth it to use in scheduling the right number of staff during peak or off-peak hours.

2.5.2.3   In Electronic Health Records (EHRs)

It is the most comprehensive application of big data in medicine. Each person has their own digital file containing demographics, history of medical records, dislikes, test results, and more. Files are shared through secure information systems and are available to both public and private sector providers [24]. Each dataset consists of adaptive trains. This means croakers can apply changes over time without the pitfalls of paperwork and data duplication [4, 5, 18].

2.5.2.4   In Real-Time Waking

The real-time awakening in healthcare is one of the most important installations of big data analytics. As far as healthcare is concerned, CDS (Clinical Decision Support) related software basically analyzes medical data on the fly and advises physicians as they form conventional opinions [1, 4, 25]. This information is also fed into a public health database. This allows cloakers to compare this data in socially beneficial domains and change their deployment strategies accordingly.

2.5.2.5   In Reduces Fraud and Abusive work

A major area of healthcare fraud and abuse is false claims. Data analytics tools are being used in finding fake documents and understand implicit fraud patterns. Careful monitoring of discrepancies between product offerings and billing data can help identify erroneous billing.

2.5.3   INTERNET OF THINGS (IoT) AND HEALTH INFORMATICS

The Internet of Things is truly transforming the sodality of healthcare, redefining the space of bias and people commerce in the delivery of healthcare results. IoT helps in better and healthy healthcare monitoring, opening up opportunities to keep cases safe and sound, enabling roach to deliver superior care [4, 5, 26]. There are healthcare businesses that benefit patients, families, barks, hospitals, including various kinds of insurance companies, some of which are listed in the next section and shown in Figure 2.3.

2.5.3.1   In Virtual Patient Monitoring

Remote and virtual monitoring is the most common operation of healthcare IoT devices. Gadgets such as fitness bands, as well as other wirelessly connected biases like smart shoes and smart rings, draw individual attention to the case [12, 27–29]. These can automatically collect health criteria such as heart rate, blood pressure, and temperature from cases that are not in-person present at a medical facility, eliminating the need for cases to travel to providers or collect the cases themselves.

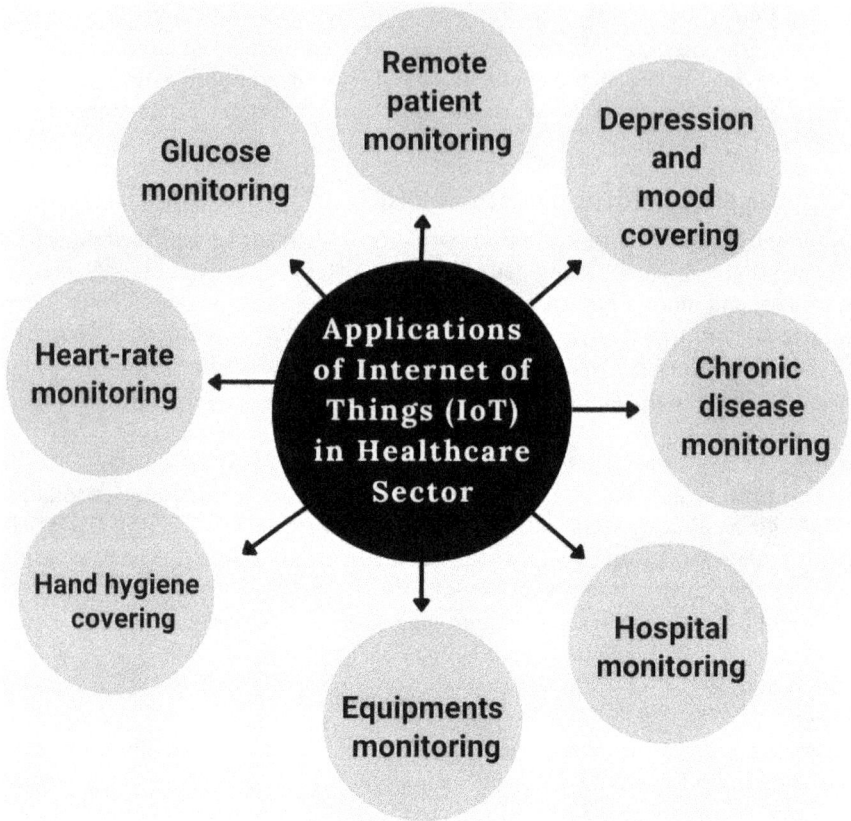

FIGURE 2.3   Some applications of IoT in healthcare sectors

2.5.3.2   Blood Glucose Monitoring

Internet of Things bias is helpful in finding challenges by enabling uninterrupted and also automatic and intelligent monitoring of glucose status in certain cases. Glucose monitors eliminate the need to manually keep records and can alert instances when glucose conditions are problematic [30, 31]. In fact, when you sleep at home with this device, you can send health updates directly to Quakers. Quakers can also review actions and act accordingly, if desired.

2.5.3.3   Heart Rate Monitoring

Heart rate monitoring can be tiring for patients actually staying in a medical facility. Regular heart rate checks do not protect against rapid heart rate fluctuations. Also, the traditional bias against continuous cardiac monitoring used in hospitals keeps cases connected to wired devices at all times, affecting patient mobility [2, 32, 33]. Different IoT devices are available for the heart rate monitoring, allowing patients to move as they please with continuous coverage of the heart.

2.5.3.4   In Hand Hygiene Covering

Historically, there has not been an effective way to guarantee that staff members and individuals inside a healthcare facility washed their hands properly to reduce the risk of spreading infection. The device can provide guidance on how to sanitize to reduce a specific danger in a specific situation [10, 14, 28].

2.5.3.5   Depression and Mood Covering

Another category of data that has historically been difficult to continuously gather is information about depression symptoms and the general mood of the case. Healthcare professionals might occasionally inquire about patients' moods, but they were ill-equipped to predict unexpected mood swings [34, 35]. Tense in disposition, by gathering and analyzing data comparable to heart rate and blood pressure, IoT devices can address these issues [27, 36]. These items can suggest details about the internal state of a case.

2.5.3.6   In Parkinson's Complaint Monitoring

Healthcare professionals must be capable of evaluating how the rigidity of their patients' symptoms change throughout the day in order to handle Parkinson's cases most effectively [12, 37, 38]. The constant collection of information about Parkinson's symptoms by IoT devices is expected to make this job much simpler.

2.5.3.7   Hospital and Equipment Monitoring

Beyond covering patient health, there are many other areas where IoT devices can really help in hospitals. Tagged with detectors, these things are used to track the real-time location of medical equipment such as wheelchairs, defibrillators, nebulizers, oxygen pumps, and other monitoring equipment. Distributed medical staff can also be analyzed in real time [12, 33, 39]. IoT gadgets are also useful for asset management, such as managing drugstores, and environmental monitoring, such as checking the temperature of refrigerators and controlling humidity and temperature.

2.6   VIRTUAL REALITY IN PROMOTING HEALTHCARE AND HEALTH 5.0

Virtual reality is revolutionizing the healthcare system. It gives a new dimension to the existing healthcare system. Using different technologies it creates various sensory simulations which provides interactive and realistic environment to the healthcare professionals. It provides many opportunities to the healthcare system.

Virtual reality technologies are used to cure various *problems of the children*. Virtual reality technologies are mainly used in three types of treatment for the children—such as motor impairment, pain management, and pediatric anxiety management [1, 40, 41]. Virtual reality technologies are very much useful to the children who have motor impairment. Various types of activity-based game helps in the movement of the muscle and the joints. It also helps to detect the actual location of the pain and help in pain management [1, 18, 42]. It is a common problem of the children that they may feel anxiety and depression. Many interactive games are used to reduce the anxiety label of the children and make them happy. Virtual reality techniques have performed well in *pain management*. Various types of pain can be managed by VR techniques. It creates a virtual environment which may have a beautiful landscape, may have hill environment, may have sea, may have waterfall, may have animals, may have bird sound, and so on [6, 7, 26]. Different types of virtual reality games give you real-life gaming experience, which directly gives you the benefit of physical exercise so various types of pain can be controlled by this method. Various VR technologies have been used in pain management. It is used in chronic pain management, acute pain management, regarding aspects and pain control, managing mental pressure including relief from the anxiety and comprehensive pediatric pain management.

Among different valuable uses of the virtual reality, an important one is *medical training purpose*. Virtual reality creates a virtual environment where the medical professionals can experience real-life situations in a simulation format. The trainee doctor can see a human body from various angles. They may be able to practice their professional skills with no limitations. The doctor may be able to practice the operations or may replace organs of a human body virtually [11, 14, 43]. The nurses may also virtually practice the profession of skills like pushing an injection or giving saline to a patient and many more tasks. Virtual reality technologies is also helpful in medical education [44]. The medical students get a very clear concept about the subject [12, 18, 45]. Using a 3D model, the medical students can visualize the human organs in any skeleton, which makes anatomy learning easy. It also helps in the development of medical social skills. Various types of surgery can perform the medical student virtually, which increases their professional skills. Another important use of virtual reality technologies is that it will help to learn operating techniques of various medical equipment. The students are able to operate different types of medical equipment, such as an ECG machine, CT-Scan machine, USG machine, and so on.

Virtual reality technologies are helpful in improving the *mental health problem* of children, adolescents, adults, and elderly people. It first detects the symptoms and tries to find the problem and the reason behind that. Virtual reality technologies counsel the people, and it provides the cognitive behavioral therapy for the improvement of mental health [18, 27, 46]. It improves the attention span and the mental stability of the user. It also helps to reduce specific phobias likes fear of heights, different animal and insect phobia, panic disorder, fear of driving, fear of crossing the road, and so on. It also helps to improve some learning disorders like dyslexia, dysgraphia, problems in number counting, and so on.

Haptic gloves are one of the important elements of virtual reality. Haptic gloves are a special type of gloves which have many of micro fluidic actuators. If you touch any object virtually, it will give you a physical touch feeling with your own skin. Different complex sensations like pressure, texture, and vibration can also be simulated by these gloves. This glove is very useful for robotic surgery, for remote surgery, or for orthopedic impaired patients. Multisensory experience is another feature of virtual reality technologies [4, 13, 47]. Various sensors and actuators work together to provide the real-time sensory experience for the virtual environment. Virtually the doctors may touch the patient's body, or the patient may feel the touch of the doctor and react accordingly.

Smart glasses are another important element of virtual reality technology. It is very useful for medical professionals. At the time of patient meeting, the doctor can see the previous health record of the patient. Big data analytics and the data mining technologies will help the doctor to get the patient-related information that are stored in the database so the diagnosis of the problem becomes easier [4, 5, 16].

Global teleportation can be achieved by virtual reality technologies. It can hypothetically transfer anything without traversing the physical space. Any medical instrument can be used globally for the benefit of the patient [12, 33]. Thus the knowledge, skills, and technologies can be teleported globally at any time and from anywhere.

Virtual reality technologies create a huge opportunity in *dentistry science*. Virtual reality technologies help to distract the patient's focus and actually help to reduce the anxiety level of the patient and also with the pain. Virtual reality technologies help the dentist to visually explain the teeth condition of the patient before operation so that it could be easily understood by the patient. The virtual reality technologies also help the doctor to find the problem. Before performing any action, the doctor could design the model virtually and show the prototype to the patient [1, 7, 25]. If there is concern from the patient, the doctor can actually perform the action virtually, such as replacing the cavities with basic fillings or simply design and fit dental prosthetics which include the bridges, crowns, and dentures. The patients also get a visualization for the choice of false teeth. Even the trainee dentist can practice the surgery virtually before doing any practical task.

Virtual reality technologies are very important for the *surgery simulations*. The doctor can practice surgery virtually before doing the actual surgery. Even the doctor can perform any surgery remotely. It is possible to make any treatment from anywhere and in time. So it gives a global expansion of healthcare system. Remote presence is one of the main advantages of this virtual reality system. Even the doctor can perform any surgery from their home. Virtual reality technologies do not only help in surgery training purpose but also it helps in pre-surgery planning [6, 41]. Before the surgery the doctors plan the whole procedure with the help of virtual reality and explain the procedure to the patient's relatives with the help of a 3D model. So it is very helpful in *patient education* about the treatment and *communication with patient relatives*.

Virtualization is another aspect of virtual reality technology. The whole system will be virtualized, so the chances of occurrence error are minimized, which reduces the *risk factor* and increases the safety. Virtual reality technologies are also able to create the 3D model of any objects. Therefore it gives a perfect picture regarding the size, shape, and the dimension of any object [4, 14, 45]. The doctor gets much benefits with this *3D model features*. The doctor can virtually *measure the size* of any tumor, which is not possible with only the two-dimensional medical reports.

One of the opportunities of virtual reality is that it is an *interactive technology*. The healthcare professional can directly interact with the patient and with the patient's relatives. So there is a high dependency of the healthcare professionals with the system. *Artificial intelligence* technologies also perform a vital role in the virtual reality environment [4, 8, 43, 48]. The data stored in the *database* is always analyzed with big data analytics and data mining technologies. A 3D model of any object can also be stored in the database.

Implementation of VR or allied technology in the areas of *rehabilitation* is also emerging and very popular. It improves the patient's physical and mental condition and improves the satisfaction label. It helps the patient to get fast recovery from any general orthopedic problem, sports injuries, neurological problem, stroke rehabilitation, or any specific problem. It is also popular for physical improvement as well as cognitive improvement of the patient [9, 33, 35]. It improves memory, attention span, and problem-solving skills of the patient. Figure 2.4 shows the opportunities of VR importance implication in the areas of medical and health-related sector.

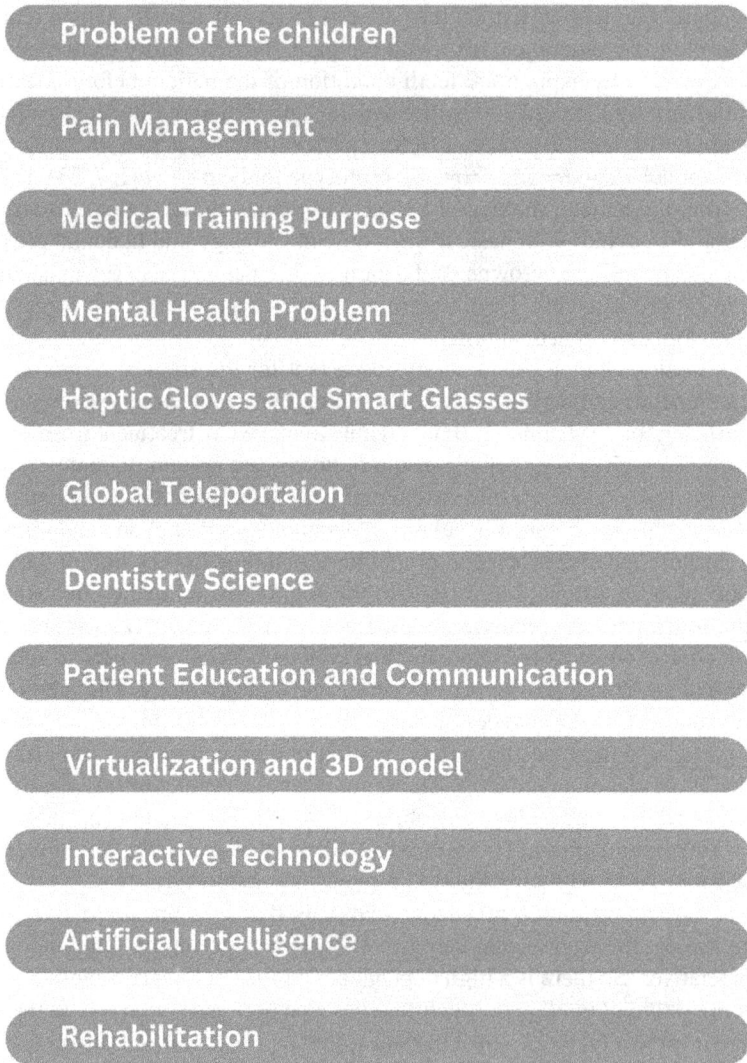

Problem of the children

Pain Management

Medical Training Purpose

Mental Health Problem

Haptic Gloves and Smart Glasses

Global Teleportaion

Dentistry Science

Patient Education and Communication

Virtualization and 3D model

Interactive Technology

Artificial Intelligence

Rehabilitation

FIGURE 2.4   Opportunities of virtual reality and its important implications in the healthcare sector

2.6.1 Benefits of Virtual Reality Importance Implication in Healthcare Sector

Virtual reality (VR) is being used to decrease the operational risk and *increase the outcome* of the healthcare system. By the use of virtual reality technologies in the healthcare system, all the stakeholders are benefited. Patients are one of the important parts of the healthcare system. Patients benefit using virtual reality in the healthcare system because the whole system works together for the betterment of the patient. The using of virtual reality technologies in healthcare system *increases the productivity* and efficiency of the system. As it provides an organized and methodical system so it helps to maintain and *streamline work progress*. After performing any task, the other user will get the updated result. Thus, it provides the *real-time inspection* of any system.

It creates a virtual environment so all the tasks can be performed virtually, which also provides environment. The user can change, modify, or perform any task as they wish because the physical environment will not be affected anymore by this activity. It is doing tasks virtually before doing the actual task so *early detection of the flow* or error or any mistake can easily be noticed. The use of different 3D models and creating a simulation in virtual environment and showing the prototype to the patient help save the *operational cost* of the system. This will also help to enhance the decision-making for both doctors and patient's relatives. It also reduces the *development time* of any customized medical device. As it shows various types of prototype, there is the least chance of unwanted operational cost, so it provides *financial stability* of the system and helps to manage conflicting requirements [1, 9, 18].

Virtual reality is technology so it does not have any geographical constant. It can be accessed from anywhere and anytime. Different countries can jointly perform any surgical or treatment-related work. It provides *cross-geography collaboration* with the countries. As it is performed virtually, it enhance the *security and the privacy* of the system.

Virtual reality technologies create a virtual environment so it provides the learning to the medical students in different types of games. The medical students learn any topic *automatically* with the help of the games. As the learning is performed virtually, so the learning can be performed with *multiple students* simultaneously. Even the learning session can be possible with *virtual instructor*. The learning is so joyful with 3D models, which help to build a clear concept among the medical students [2, 19, 25]. Figure 2.5 shows three major stakeholders and benefits of healthcare segment.

2.7 HEALTH INFORMATICS, INDIA, AND VIRTUAL REALITY

Both in government and private sector, digital healthcare system initiation is considered as worthy and important. In a country like India, there are lot of issues and concerns, such as data susceptibility, lack of IT literacy, implementation loopholes, cyber security issues, excessive server hits, man-in-the-middle attack. In addition to these impediments, deploying Wi-Fi centers as well as hotspots should be considered

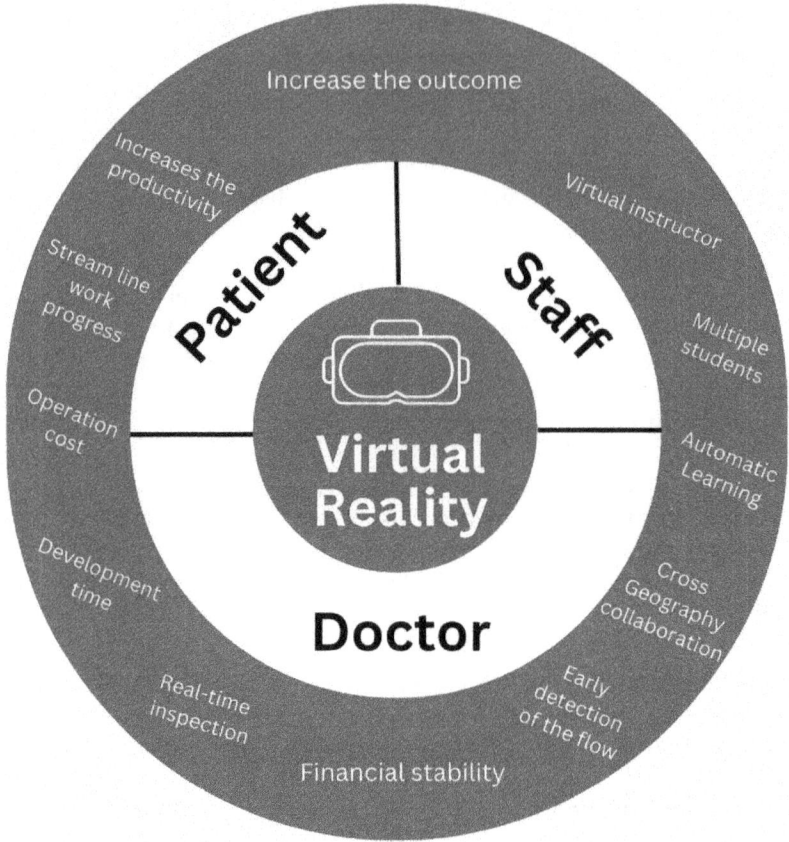

FIGURE 2.5   Three major stakeholders in the healthcare sector and major benefits

a worthy and important issue. Gradually different diseases are increasing, and for managing and curing such diseases, application and integration of digital healthcare informatics is increasing rapidly. There are massive needs of technological implementation of healthcare for medical and healthcare system's developments. World Health Organization (WHO) states various types of noncommunicable diseases, which are basically originated from chronic conditions combining physiological, behavioral, genetic, as well as environmental factors. Further it has shown that 63% of all deaths are basically caused by mortality [20, 22, 49]. Furthermore, another study shows that 80% of such deaths are basically identified in the "low income countries" and "middle-income countries." India is growing but still a developing country, and a population of 1.3 billion, therefore with the immense burden of these noncommunicable disease, and in all such cases, information technology applications play a leading role, but there are some lacunas in designing and developing healthcare systems digitally or digital technological applications in healthcare. As mortality rate has increased drastically for certain noncommunicable diseases all over India between 1990 and 2016, therefore technological implementation is worthy and required in present day context. Further it is also important to note that in the year 2016 about 8.3% of all deaths and 5% of total disability-adjusted is due to the cancer, and that has doubled since the year 1990. As a result, use of proper technology in healthcare is important and at the same time advanced and intelligent healthcare supported systems [12, 20, 22]. Many alarming diseases, such as heart disease, stroke, and specifically diabetes, need proper attention with technology by its side, and such things are a high burden in India. Conventional therapeutic and prophylactic care monitoring may be difficult in certain cases as in India, adequate physical healthcare infrastructure is weak and an important matter to look into. There is also an important concern in trained manpower availability to be used in digital healthcare development and also in the conventional healthcare systems [8, 25, 45]. As face-to-face patient and physicians/medical professionals involvement is a critical challenge in a country like India for complete healthcare development. Thus, IT supported healthcare system may bring improved healthcare centers, also timely diagnosis, and it is partially supported by health informatics to reach its desired goals of the healthcare organizations. In India, Union MEITy (Ministry of Electronics and Information Technology) initiated some of the steps for digitalization of healthcare, and some of them are considered under the Digital India Project. Here are the three vision areas:

• Digital Infrastructure as a Utility to Every Citizen
• Governance and Services on Demand
• Digital Empowerment of Citizens

The program and flagship initiative of "Digital India" is one of the important technology enabled programs dedicated in promoting as well as advancing government services in different areas with transparency and higher and advanced speed, advantages, and benefits from digitalized systems offered via electronic format that is easy as well as convenient to the beneficiaries. The support of various kinds of digital technologies and a good number of mHealth and eHealth interventions have been formulated towards better and excellent healthcare services. Various basic devices such as mobile and smartphone, website and web portals, software and systems, wearable devices, including computer and tablet systems and computers considered as important. Furthermore here adoption of online as well as various offline digital technology platforms are being used in modern healthcare, and use of such systems is called digital health [27, 38, 50]. The WHO promotes the "universal health coverage" in offering high-quality delivery of healthcare in helping in diseases like preventive diseases, diagnostic diseases, therapeutic diseases, and also in palliative care with the use of smartphone and electronic gadgets, portable computing devices, Internet-dependent services, mobile applications, and social media interfaces. There are many studies conducted in digital healthcare in the context of technologies, people, health professionals, infrastructure and governance, etc. [22, 26, 47]. It has noted that various diseases like cardiovascular diseases increasing viz. stroke, osteoarthritis, depression, and chronic obstructive pulmonary, and in this context use of technology plays a leading role in minimizing and control of such diseases. In the context of the following, digital technologies and health informatics considered is important:

- In symptom assessment
- In self healthcare management
- In distress reduction
- In proper health awareness
- In accurate communication with others
- In timely medical service delivery and promotion
- In caring and follow-up systems
- In the healthcare adherence
- In improving aspects and quality of life of the patients

Different digital healthcare technological implementation and initiatives applications has increased in recent years, and such applications are mainly from the healthcare segment in the areas of diagnosing diseases and formulating methodologies towards better healthcare and delivery of the services. mHealth is important to launch overall health system in India for fostering healthcare service delivery. Furthermore, the overhauling of digital healthcare infrastructure, including the penetration of smartphones and tablets in remote areas and urban and rural landscape, with dynamic support from Internet service providers, needs to be prioritized more. The telecom regulatory authority have already developed many steps and systems, and more advanced communication technology needs to make it on the citizens' doorstep [20, 33, 49]. However there is a shortage of the free-of-cost training in mobile app installation and systematic usage by patients and healthcare professionals required in the healthcare organizations, and in this regard proper steps and initiatives are essential from the research institutions, private sector, NGOs, schools, colleges, universities and higher educational institutions, etc. Government funding is important in implementing digital healthcare systems not only for the infrastructure, implementation, technologies, tools but also in developing awareness and in reducing the knowledge gap about patient-centered applications [20, 32, 51, 52]. Proper regulatory initiatives are practically ahead of us, and for an optimal digital healthcare system, we need to eliminate such poor regulations to make a true developed country where there is quality healthcare even in the most different, remotest corner of the country, but also affordable digital navigation and systems, digital devices, and accessible digital platforms.

Virtual reality gives a simulating experience, which is responsible in creating artificial experiences and reality, and for this, there is no need for users to be in the actual places or presence. The use of headsets and headphones is important in using virtual reality systems [9, 11, 42]. Earlier, this was used only in the game and entertainment segment, but virtual reality extended its higher uses in entertainment and game designing and development and gradually healthcare has become a potential user. Fundamental and basic virtual reality (VR) used in healthcare includes the following:

- Medical, healthcare, and allied education and training
- Robotic surgery

- Pain management
- Biosensor management
- Healthcare device management

Various healthcare organizations and institutions are using virtual reality technologies in their systems, operations, and services. Even in India too, such symptoms and scenario can be seen in some of the service providers of healthcare organizations and institutions. And in the future, definitely more applications and integration can be seen [1, 7, 20]. Virtual reality has many significant side effects, such as the following:

- In sickness like dizziness and nausea.
- In healthcare issues like headaches and eye-related issues.
- It is useful in reducing limb control and management.
- For minimizing postural control and management.
- Regarding decreased sense of presence, and so on.

Though there are certain issues in healthcare organizations and management in respect to virtual reality in a country like India, viz. availability of proper funds, availability of proper technologies and systems, availability of skilled manpower, initiatives, and so on. The advancement in latest technologies of IT and computing are a help to reaching and enhancing Healthcare 5.0, for the development of flexible, customized, and personalized healthcare services and mechanism. And ultimately it can enhance quality, responsiveness, and fairness as depicted in Figure 2.6.

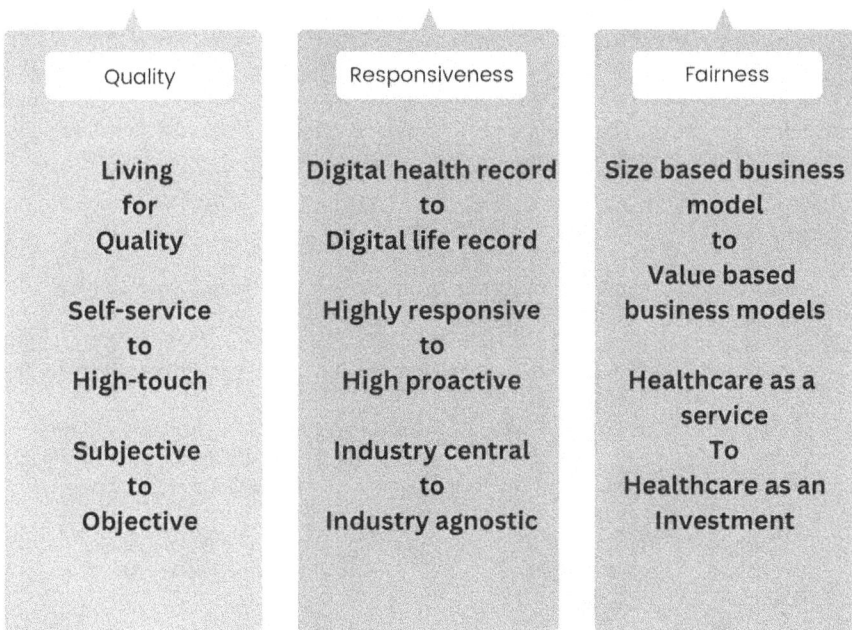

Quality	Responsiveness	Fairness
Living for Quality	Digital health record to Digital life record	Size based business model to Value based business models
Self-service to High-touch	Highly responsive to High proactive	Healthcare as a service To Healthcare as an Investment
Subjective to Objective	Industry central to Industry agnostic	

FIGURE 2.6 Virtual reality and other ICT implications in Healthcare 5.0 development

2.8   SUGGESTIONS WITH CONCLUDING REMARKS

Digital healthcare is a modern healthcare service and has gained immense popularity all over the world, including in India. The traditional healthcare centers and services are changing rapidly and shrinking day by day, and there are certain issues in the accessibility, lack of resources, and poor and non-skilled medical practitioners emanating from the high population to be served by paucity of medicos; digital healthcare remains to be an indispensable option for healthcare providers both in the government and private sector of India. Health information technology, including integration of cloud technologies, various models of Internet of Things, data analytics including machine learning technology, should be used in the national and global healthcare sector in order to offer quality healthcare with proper health information exchange and interoperability. There are many healthcare organizations, such as hospitals, medical practitioners, independent laboratories, radiology centers, pharmacies, which have widely adopted and meaningfully used health informatics (HI). Health informatics as an extension of bioinformatics is the greatest tool in digital healthcare, especially with the union of digital and smart healthcare, information and communication technology, including business administration. All these are helpful for better patient health and medical facilities experience viz. clinical care. Better nursing services, healthy pharmacy management, and improved public health can be aptly determined and subtly delivered on patients' doorsteps just in time. In India there are many ongoing research and practicing projects in designing and developing healthcare system development. And with proper initiative and more steps, sophisticated development is becoming possible.

ACKNOWLEDGMENT

The authors express their sincere thanks to all the other members of Informatics Research Group (Dept. of CIS, Raiganj University, India), specially Mr. Deep Debnath for UXD for some of the contents related support.

REFERENCES

[1] H. A. Aziz, "Virtual reality programs applications in healthcare," *Journal of Health & Medical Informatics*, no. 9(1), pp. 1–3, 2018.
[2] I. Bhattacharya, and A. Ramachandran, "A path analysis study of retention of healthcare professionals in urban India using health information technology," *Human Resources for Health*, no. 13(1), pp. 1–14, 2015.
[3] M. Habes, M. Alghizzawi, S. Ali, A. SalihAlnaser, and S. A. Salloum, "The relation among marketing ads, via digital media and mitigate (COVID-19) pandemic in Jordan," *International Journal of Advanced Science and Technology*, no. 29(7), pp. 12326–12348, 2020.
[4] S. R. Alotaibi, "Applications of artificial intelligence and big data analytics in mHealth: A healthcare system perspective," *Journal of Healthcare Engineering*, no. 1, pp. 1–15, 2020.
[5] A. L. Beam, and I. S Kohane, "Big data and machine learning in health care," *The Journal of the American Medical Association*, no. 319(13), pp. 1317–1318, 2018.

[6] D. Freeman et al., "Virtual reality in the assessment, understanding, and treatment of mental health disorders," *Psychological Medicine*, no. 47(14), pp. 2393–2400, 2017.

[7] M. Javaid, and A. Haleem, "Virtual reality applications toward medical field," *Clinical Epidemiology and Global Health*, no. 8(2), pp. 600–605, 2020.

[8] C. Moro et al., "The effectiveness of virtual and augmented reality in health sciences and medical anatomy," *Anatomical Sciences Education*, no. 10(6), pp. 549–559, 2017.

[9] M. T. Schultheis, and A. A. Rizzo, "The application of virtual reality technology in rehabilitation," *Rehabilitation Psychology*, no. 46(3), pp. 296–311, 2001.

[10] R. Zhaoet al., "Deep learning and its applications to machine health monitoring," *Mechanical Systems and Signal Processing*, no. 115, pp. 213–237, 2019.

[11] A. Rizzo et al., "Virtual reality goes to war: A brief review of the future of military behavioral healthcare," *Journal of Clinical Psychology in Medical Settings*, no. 18(2), pp. 176–187, 2011.

[12] P. K. Paul, A. Bhuimali, and P. S. Aithal, "Allied medical and health science and advanced telecommunications: Emerging utilizations and its need in indian healthcare system," *Current Trends in Biotechnology and Chemical Research*, no. 7(1–2), pp. 27–30, 2017.

[13] N. Karthikeyan, and R. Sukanesh, "Cloud based emergency health care information service in India," *Journal of Medical Systems*, no. 36(6), pp. 4031–4036, 2012.

[14] P. K. Paul, D. Chatterjee, and M. Ghosh, "Medical information science: Emerging domain of information science and technology (IST) for sophisticated health & medical infrastructure building-an overview," *International Scientific Journal of Sport Sciences*, no. 1(2), pp. 97–104, 2012.

[15] H. S. S. Bhambere, B. Abhishek, and H. Sumit, "Rapid digitization of healthcare: A review of COVID-19 impact on our health systems," *International Journal of All Research Education and Scientific Methods*, no. 9, pp. 1457–1459, 2021.

[16] S. Balsari et al., "Reimagining health data exchange: An application programming interface–enabled roadmap for India," *Journal of Medical Internet Research*, no. 20(7), p. e10725, 2018.

[17] R. Agrawal, and S. Prabakaran, "Big data in digital healthcare: Lessons learnt and recommendations for general practice," *Heredity*, no. 124(4), pp. 525–534, 2020.

[18] A. H. Chang et al., "Effectiveness of virtual reality-based training on oral healthcare for disabled elderly persons: A randomized controlled trial," *Journal of Personalized Medicine*, no. 12(2), p. 218, 2022.

[19] P. K. Paul, P. S. Aithal, and A. Bhuimali, "Health information science and its growing popularities in Indian self financed universities: Emphasizing private universities—a study," *International Journal of Scientific Research in Biological Sciences*, no. 5(1), pp. 1–11, 2018.

[20] S. Madon, S. Sahay, and R. Sudan, "E-government policy and health information systems implementation in Andhra Pradesh, India: Need for articulation of linkages between the macro and the micro," *The Information Society*, no. 23(5), pp. 327–344, 2007.

[21] S. K. Mishra, L. Kapoor, and I. P. Singh, "Telemedicine in India: Current scenario and the future," *Telemedicine and eHealth*, no. 15(6), pp. 568–575, 2009.

[22] N. Kapadia-Kundu, T. M. Sullivan, B. Safi, G. Trivedi, and S. Velu, "Understanding health information needs and gaps in the health care system in Uttar Pradesh, India," *Journal of health communication*, no. 17(sup2), pp. 30–45, 2012.

[23] A. Dasgupta, and S. Deb, "Telemedicine: A new horizon in public health in India," *Indian Journal of Community Medicine: Official Publication of Indian Association of Preventive & Social Medicine*, no. 33(1), pp. 3–8, 2008.

[24] S. Sahay, E. Monteiro, and M. Aanestad, "Toward a political perspective of integration in information systems research: The case of health information systems in India," *Information Technology for Development*, no. 15(2), pp. 83–94, 2009.

[25] P. K. Paul, D. Chatterjee, and M. Ghosh, "Neural networks: Emphasizing its application in the world of health and medical sciences," *Journal of Advances in Medicine*, no. 1(2), pp. 93–99, 2012.

[26] P. K. Paul, R. K. Sinha, J. Ganguly, and M. Ghosh, "Health and medical information science and its potentiality in Indian education sector," *Journal of Advances in Medicine*, no. 4(1and2), pp. 21–37, 2015.

[27] S. K. Kar, Saxena, S. K., and R. Kabir, "The relevance of digital mental healthcare during COVID-19: Need for innovations," *Nepal Journal of Epidemiology*, no. 10(4), pp. 928–929, 2020.

[28] S. K. Mishra, I. P. Singh, and R. D. Chand, "Current status of telemedicine network in India and future perspective," *Proceedings of the Asia-Pacific Advanced Network*, no. 32(1), pp. 151–163, 2012.

[29] S. P. Dash, "The impact of IoT in healthcare: Global technological change & the roadmap to a networked architecture in India," *Journal of the Indian Institute of Science*, pp. 1–13, 2020.

[30] E. Jain, "Digital employability skills and training needs for the Indian healthcare industry," in *Opportunities and Challenges in Digital Healthcare Innovation*, pp. 113–130. IGI Global, 2020.

[31] N. A. Behkami, and T. U. Daim, "Research forecasting for health information technology (HIT), using technology intelligence," *Technological Forecasting and Social Change*, no. 79(3), pp. 498–508, 2012.

[32] P. Pandey, and R. Litoriya, "Implementing healthcare services on a large scale: Challenges and remedies based on blockchain technology," *Health Policy and Technology*, no. 9(1), pp. 69–78, 2020.

[33] R. Itumalla, "Information technology and service quality in healthcare: An empirical study of private hospital in India," *International Journal of Innovation, Management and Technology*, no. 3(4), pp. 433–436, 2012.

[34] M. Saab et al., "Nursing students' views of using virtual reality in healthcare: A qualitative study," *Journal of Clinical Nursing*, no. 31(9–10), pp. 1228–1242, 2022.

[35] M. Samadbeik et al., "The applications of virtual reality technology in medical groups teaching," *Journal of Advances in Medical Education & Professionalism*, no. 6(3), pp. 123–129, 2018.

[36] J. L. King et al., "Institutional factors in information technology innovation," *Information Systems Research*, no. 5(2), pp. 139–169, 1994.

[37] A. Kumar, P. Mahajan, D. Mohan, and M. Varghese, "IT—information technology and the human interface: Tractor vibration severity and driver health: A study from rural India," *Journal of Agricultural Engineering Research*, no. 80(4), pp. 313–328, 2001.

[38] P. K. Mony, and C. Nagaraj, "Health information management: An introduction to disease classification and coding," *National Medical Journal of India*, no. 20(6), pp. 307–310, 2007.

[39] W. J. Orlikowski, and D. Robey, "Information technology and the structuring of organizations," *Information Systems Research*, no. 2(2), pp. 143–169, 1991.

[40] D. King et al., "Virtual health education: Scaling practice to transform student learning: Using virtual reality learning environments in healthcare education to bridge the theory/practice gap and improve patient safety," *Nurse Education Today*, no. 71, pp. 7–9, 2018.

[41] H. Mäkinen, E. Haavisto, S. Havola, and J. M. Koivisto, "User experiences of virtual reality technologies for healthcare in learning: An integrative review," *Behaviour & Information Technology*, no. 41(1), pp. 1–17, 2022.

[42] A. Rahouti, R. Lovreglio, S. Datoussaïd, and T. Descamps, "Prototyping and validating a non-immersive virtual reality serious game for healthcare fire safety training," *Fire Technology*, no. 57(6), pp. 3041–3078, 2021.

[43] J. Kasurinen, "Usability issues of virtual reality learning simulator in healthcare and cybersecurity," *Procedia Computer Science*, no. 119, pp. 341–349, 2017.

[44] R. Chatterjee, A. Bandyopadhyay, S. Chakraborty, and S. Dutta, "Digital education: The basics with slant to digital pedagogy-an overview," in Choudhury, A., Biswas, A., Chakraborti, S. (eds) *Digital Learning Based Education. Advanced Technologies and Societal Change*. Singapore: Springer Nature, 2023, pp. 63–80.

[45] K. Kim, "Is virtual reality (VR) becoming an effective application for the market opportunity in health care, manufacturing, and entertainment industry?" *European Scientific Journal*, no. 12(9), pp. 14–22, 2016.

[46] S. Malhotra, S. Chakrabarti, and R. Shah, "A model for digital mental healthcare: Its usefulness and potential for service delivery in low-and middle-income countries," *Indian journal of psychiatry*, no. 61(1), pp. 27–36, 2019.

[47] S. K. Srivastava, "Adoption of electronic health records: A roadmap for India," *Healthcare informatics research*, no. 22(4), pp. 261–269, 2016.

[48] C. Vijai, and W. Wisetsri, "Rise of artificial intelligence in healthcare startups in India," *Advances in Management*, no. 14(1), pp. 48–52, 2021.

[49] T. Kumari, "A study on knowledge and attitude towards digital health of rural population of India-innovations in practice to improve healthcare in the rural population," *International Journal of Emerging Multidisciplinary Research*, no. 3(3), pp. 13–21, 2019.

[50] A. Rana, "The immense potential of M-care in India: Catering better to patients needs in the context of a fragmented healthcare system," *International Journal of Reliable and Quality E-Healthcare (IJRQEH)*, no. 6(4), pp. 1–3, 2017.

[51] R. R. Pai, and S. Alathur, "Assessing awareness and use of mobile phone technology for health and wellness: Insights from India," *Health Policy and Technology*, no. 8(3), pp. 221–227, 2019.

[52] S. Pingle, "Occupational safety and health in India: Now and the future," *Industrial Health*, no. 50(3), pp. 167–171, 2012.

[53] C. L. Aasheim, S. Williams, P. Rutner, and A. Gardiner, "Data analytics vs. data science: A study of similarities and differences in undergraduate programs based on course descriptions," *Journal of Information Systems Education*, no. 26(2), pp. 103–109, 2015.

3 Virtual Reality Applications in Healthcare

A New Age Technology Perspective

Himani Mittal

3.1 INTRODUCTION

Virtual reality (VR) is the interaction of humans within a simulated environment created using computing technology involving primarily computer graphics and artificial intelligence. The word *virtual* means imaginary, and *reality* means truth. In VR, the human can hold virtual objects or animated objects. The 3D environments created using virtual reality are used for many interesting applications, including driving practice for cars and aeroplanes, computer games, and many more. There is another term often confused with VR, known as augmented reality. Augmented reality is the mixing of virtual objects in a real environment, for example, adding stickers on Snapchat. VR is the introduction of humans in a simulated 3D environment with humans experiencing the sound and sight of the 3D scene, creating an illusion that it is a reality. This is possible using the VR Gear (Mittal, 2020). To give the user a sense of immersion, a lot of hardware and software are required. Input devices let the user interact with the virtual world. It can be joysticks, controller wands, data gloves, on-device control buttons, motion trackers, bodysuits, and motion platforms. Other devices include gyroscopes and motion sensors for tracking head, body, and hand positions; a 3D mouse; the wired glove; motion controllers; and optical tracking sensors. Output devices stimulate a sense organ to create the VR environment. These include visual, auditory, or haptic displays, headphones and speakers. Other devices include small HD screens for stereoscopic displays; VR headsets; omni-directional cameras; head-mounted displays, or the CAVE; and haptics and sensor technology. Virtual reality has applications in the military, healthcare, education, scientific visualization, and entertainment. The industry is growing fast, and newer and better applications with advanced hardware are reaching the market. There is demand for VR-based products in the market. However, there are certain concerns related to acceptance of virtual reality as a toll for multiple applications.

DOI: 10.1201/9781003340133-3

VR and augmented reality are often confused. Augmented reality (AR) (Mekni and Lemieux, 2014), on other hand, is the reverse, where the animated/virtual characters are added to real-world images and videos. Augmented reality (AR) is an extension of the real world, where the digital visual elements, sounds, and other sensory stimuli are delivered via technology. No separate hardware or software gears are required to experience augmented reality. However, enhanced graphics algorithms and AI-enabled digital cameras are required to generate augmented reality. The applications of augmented reality are in the field of medicine, military, manufacturing, entertainment, robotics, visualization, education, navigation, tourism, path planning, shopping, construction, designing, and many more. Augmented reality is the mixing of virtual objects in a real environment, for example, adding stickers on Snapchat. VR is the introduction of humans in a simulated 3D environment with humans experiencing the sound and sight of the 3D scene, creating an illusion that it is a reality.

Healthcare services are in ever-increasing demand. Healthcare institutions are trying to match the demand with all the new technological developments. The high expectation of patients concerning the quality of services in the institution has increased due to high-quality services in other areas of life. People are aware that technology can automate a lot of steps for them—that is, online appointments, sharing of reports, videoconferencing, and much more. There are on-demand healthcare services using health tracking apps and search platforms. Such services are relevant for underdeveloped nations, where there is an acute shortage of resources and manpower. This also helps in cost reduction. Another benefit is less waiting time and faster delivery of service. There is awareness in healthcare ecosystem regarding the usefulness of VR tools in the upcoming healthcare technology. It is believed that technology can bring improvements to any process within healthcare operation and delivery.

The new age technology, namely: AI, digital twin, machine learning, IoT, blockchain, and VR can be used to increase the experience of the patients and doctors in the healthcare industry. This chapter reviews several applications of these technologies in healthcare. AI is a system where a machine is given artificial intelligence so that it can do things that humans do better. A lot of algorithms and methods are utilized for the same. Digital twin is creating a hardware/software replica of an entity and studying its behavior and pairing it with the real entity. This helps in the prediction of response to a situation and better designing and fault recovery. Machine learning is using the data to predict and classify the decision-making in a process. IoT is collecting data through sensors and processing it to generate predictions. Big data is also related to data collection and processing. Blockchain is the storage of data securely. The VR technology along with all the new age technology can be used to improve the status of the healthcare industry and create a better experience for the doctors and the patients.

This chapter is organized as follows: Section 3.2 includes the review of general applications of VR. Section 3.3 includes a review of the applications of VR to healthcare, taking into account the new age technology. In Section 3.4 a model for healthcare is proposed based on IoT and blockchain. Section 3.5 includes the conclusions.

3.2   REVIEW OF TRADITIONAL APPLICATIONS OF VIRTUAL REALITY

Virtual reality is already used in a wide variety of applications, and these are reviewed in this section.

3.2.1   MILITARY, NAVIGATION, AND PATH PLANNING

In an article by Baumann (Baumann, 1993), three applications of virtual reality are discussed in the area of the military. First, pilot training through simulations. Second, design special weapons and remotely piloted vehicles. These can be controlled remotely, and the controller can get the real-time environment information through virtual reality and operate the vehicle from a safer place. Third, the design of head-up displays for pilots that combine virtual and real displays. The virtual display includes information such as speed, altitude, and the enemy aircraft that is not seen by the real display can also be shown using camera-captured scenes on the virtual display. In another work by Rizzo et.al. (Rizzo et al., 2011), virtual reality is used for healthcare in the military. The traumatized soldiers who experienced life-changing and deeply traumatizing war situations in Arab countries were cured using virtual reality simulations. The soldiers were put into the virtual scene using VR gear, and the therapist can control their interactions with the environment. In the work by Lele (2013), virtual reality–based simulations are used to give soldiers exposure to warlike situations (as on-the-job real training is possible only when a war occurs); in training to use war equipment, which is otherwise expensive to be given in reality; in creation of advanced synthetic environments that train on reality-based situations; and in simulation training for transport, fighter aircraft, and unmanned vehicle control. He further emphasized that various industrial sectors such as information technology, biomedical engineering, structural design, and training aids technology sector are investing in this technology. In the year 2016, Pallavicini et al. in his work (Pallavicini et al., 2016) has reviewed 14 studies performed to estimate the effectiveness of virtual reality in managing stress among aircrew, including soldiers and pilots. In these separate 14 studies, the personnel included were the control group and trained groups. It is found in all the studies that the use of VR in training individuals leads to fewer stress levels. The survey was conducted following the PRISMA guidelines for selecting studies (Moher et al., 2009). Liu (Liu et al., 2018) summarizes the developments in hardware and software of virtual reality technology and its application in the military field, including virtual training, virtual weapon manufacture, and virtual battlefield exercises training. Ahir (Ahir et al., 2020) states that virtual reality is fast emerging as an interdisciplinary field. He reviewed the work of other authors that use VR for education, military, and sports training, manufacturing, learning, and virtual visits.

3.2.2   HEALTHCARE AND MEDICAL

The role of VR in healthcare is for treatment, training, and assistive technology. All the three uses are reviewed here. Lányi (2006) overviews the use of virtual reality in medical informatics, rehabilitation, and assistive and preventive healthcare. For healthcare staff, VR applications are used to help make diagnoses, for education, further training, and teleconferencing. VR is an information, education tool and rehabilitation tool for patients. Training healthcare professionals using simulations and planning surgery in VR. He reviewed the works of several universities for teaching medicine using virtual reality. Preparation of human body models, teleconferencing, virtual presentations, and so on are used for VR-based training. Mehrer (Mahrer and Gold, 2009) and Bidarra (Bidarra et al., 2013) have discussed the use of VR in creating games that can help in distracting the attention of patients undergoing dental or any other medical procedures. Haniff (Haniff et al., 2014) prescribes the use of VR for mental healthcare. Fertleman (Fertleman et al., 2018) observes in his work that virtual reality is found to be a useful training tool as it can induce behavior change, which other methods cannot bring about. Through virtual reality consultation, a doctor can develop greater self-awareness and modify their future reactions in a better, therapeutic way. Mäkinen (Mäkinen et al., 2022) performed an integrative review of the use of VR in training and the effect of UX design on the user. It points out that three different VR technologies used in the field of healthcare education and practice are haptic device simulators, computer-based simulations, and head-mounted displays (HMDs). The haptic simulators are the most often used, whereas the HMD devices are the least used technology in the field of healthcare. In immersive virtual environments, UX includes ten components, namely, presence, engagement, immersion, flow, usability, skill, emotion, experience consequence, judgement, and technology adoption. Most of the components have been observed in the context of haptic devices and HMD devices, with all ten components observed with the HMD devices. Almost all of the components are rated as positive and reported to enhance skill development, enabling remote access to training, and ultimately, improving patient safety.

3.2.3 Scientific Visualization

In research work by Van Dam (Van Dam et al., 2002), he states the size of datasets generated by experiments through simulation and real monitoring is growing from terabytes to petabytes. The visualization by itself will not solve the problem of understanding truly large datasets that would overwhelm the display capacity and the human visual system. He promotes a human-computer partnership that draws on the strengths of each partner, with algorithmic culling and feature-detection used to identify the small fraction of the data that should be visually examined in detail by the human. IVR is a potent tool to let humans "see" patterns, trends, and anomalies in their data well beyond what they can do with conventional 3D desktop displays.

In research work performed in 1996, Haase (Haase, 1996) mentioned that virtual reality systems must be integrated with scientific visualizations. He commented that systems for scientific visualization offer an intermediate degree of autonomy (semantics), a high degree of interaction (access to parameters), and a very low degree of presence (immersion). On the other hand, VR systems offer a high degree of presence, a lower degree of interaction, and usually very little autonomy. So the integration of both can solve many problems. He has cited a research work by Bryson

(Bryson and Levit, 1992), who developed a virtual tunnel application. This virtual tunnel application was an immersive virtual reality-based system for use in the investigation of simulated airflow by geographically distributed, collaborative teams. The Participants in the virtual tunnel interact with the airflow simulation as if they were in the same room interacting with a model, even if they are spread across the country. It plays two roles, providing an immersive environment for collaborative design, as well as acting as a test bed for developing new methods. In another work cited by Haase, he quotes nano manipulators (Taylor et al., 1993) that manipulate the scientific experiments at the atomic scale through virtual reality. In the work by Haase (Haase et al., 1996), a system is discussed for investigating molecule data. Using combined virtual environment and scientific visualization techniques allows for an immersive exploration of individual molecules as well as for the investigation of docking behavior between two molecules. In the work of Haase (1996), he has designed a system for integrating a scientific visualization system with VR. Both of these systems work on common data, and the object in VR is controlled according to the data available. The visualization system makes use of a very flexible calculator for complex operations on raw data, for example, scaling of time-varying tensor, interpolation in space (using shape functions) and time between given node values; data or the combination of three scalar fields into one vector field; mapping functions of values to color, vector arrows, deformed geometry, etc.; slicing, particle tracing, iso-surfaces in unstructured grids; and comparison of computed and measured values (e.g., the strain on a steel shaft under load). The virtual reality system offers a flexible framework for the design and application of virtual environments. Among other things, it offers an interaction toolkit, collision detection, and sonification. Virtual design employs Vis-A-Vis, the same rendering system which is being used by the visualization system. It can generate appropriate output for VR display devices such as large screen projection, the BOOM or a head-mounted display. To avoid the conversion of graphical data structures, the Vis-A-Vis version of the virtual reality system is used for ISVAS-VR integration. In a research work by Rhyne (1997), the integration of scientific visualization, geographic information systems, and virtual reality is discussed. He says that this is possible by the use of a multidisciplinary approach of geographic information systems, digital cartography, scientific visualization, computational modelling, and videoconferencing to answer the needs of the user through the web-based interface for global positioning systems and mobile computing technologies.

Laviola (2000) makes use of VR with scientific visualization for the study of the flow of fluids. He specifically talks about the input mechanisms used with a VR system. The traditional input devices like the keyboard and mouse are of little use. He speaks about multimodal input devices so that they can give proper inputs. With proper input devices, the user can interact sufficiently with the objects in VR and study the datasets of the flow of fluids appropriately. In another work by Laviola (LaViola et al., 2009), he points out that there was ongoing research in archaeology, biology, computational fluid dynamics (CFD), and geosciences using VR in which huge datasets are used to perform scientific visualizations and combined with VR to make better predictions. He is working on several projects using VR. He was involved in the development of the widget library that facilitated the interaction of the user with VR applications. Another application is a virtual cardiovascular laboratory. After the artery graft surgery in cardiac arrests, VR systems are used to study the fluid flow as there were many failed surgeries. Domain scientists projected the virtual cardiovascular laboratory would quickly verify previously discovered results due to the human-sized visualizations (vessel walls and the data within were scaled up such that they were about eight feet in diameter) that researchers could move inside and carefully study intricate flow features throughout the volume. He has discussed many other applications of scientific visualizations and VR systems.

In work performed by Sua (Sua et al., 2015), a VR system is implemented for scientific visualization and study of the interaction of humans with 3D Objects in VR simulation. Su (Su et al., 2020) has discussed VR applications enabling scientists and engineers to perform advanced data analysis and assessment on their simulated and collected scientific research data. For mechanical engineers, the visualization solutions enabled data analysis and assessment of large simulation of jet fuel primary atomization in complex geometries simulation. In another VR application, VR technology is used to augment the information visualization framework to enable visualization of 3D data in its natural format instead of displaying the 3D data on a 2D display.

3.2.4 ENTERTAINMENT

3.2.4.1 Gaming

Bates (1992) in his work has mentioned that traditional entertainment methods have used different mediums to retain the interest of the user in TV, video, or any interaction. VR-based entertainment has to ensure changes in the traditional methods to change the cognitive elements, presentation, and drama that would retain the interest of the viewer in the entertainment piece. Zyda (2005) in his work discusses the importance of gaming in VR and vice versa. He says that VR has advanced so much because of game designers designing better and more advanced 3D scenes and using immersive technology. The design of serious games where the aim is to entertain and alongside impart a special skill to the player is the aim behind the new age of mobile games and video games. In the work of Cruz-Neira (Cruz-Neira et al., 2018), the role of VR in entertainment, its applications, and the use of VR in serious gaming is discussed. It includes a review of the state-of-the-art available VR applications specifically for gaming.

3.2.4.2 Tourism

A work by Beck (Beck et al., 2019) classified the use of virtual reality in tourism as non-immersive, semi-immersive, and fully immersive, enabling virtual touristic experiences that stimulate the visual sense and potentially additional other senses of the user for planning, management, marketing, information exchange, entertainment, education, accessibility, or heritage preservation, either before, during, or after travel. The non-immersive experience is the use of 3D videos on a regular computer screen. Semi-immersive is the use of 3D videos displayed on wall-sized displays. Fully immersive is with the use of VR headgears and other VR hardware. Rácz and Zilizi (2019) reports a VR application for a virtual tour of Mediterranean tourist destinations. Adachi (Adachi et al., 2020) performed a study on the impact of VR-based promotional videos of destinations in tourism. They found that the videos do not affect the intention to visit, but it helps to create a positive image of the destination and make the visitor more informed.

3.2.4.3 Other Uses in the Entertainment

Apart from gaming, VR can be used for other entertainment purposes. Lai (Lai et al., 2019) discusses the use of VR for the entertainment of the elderly who have limited resources, family conditions, physical conditions, and other factors. They can get better emotional health with the help of VR technology. Nilsson (Nilsson et al., 2018) discusses the use of VR in virtual travel. He discusses the challenges in actually performing a virtual walk. The user must be able to get the correct stimuli from the experience so that it makes the right effect.

3.2.5 Education

In the mentioned applications, we have already seen the use of Virtual Reality for training purposes. Kavanagh (Kavanagh et al., 2017) performed a systematic review of the use of virtual reality in education, as well as two distinct thematic analyses. In the two-stage analysis, the first investigated the applications and motivations for using VR in education, while the second reported the problems in doing so. The studies indicate that VR is used for intrinsic motivation of students and are influenced by effective teaching methods, team playing, and gamification of whole experience. Similarly, a small number of educational areas account for the vast majority of educational virtual reality implementations identified by him. Next, he introduced and compared a multitude of recent virtual reality technologies, discussing their potential to overcome several of the problems identified in the analyses, including cost, user experience, and interactivity. However, these technologies are not without their issues, so he suggests methods to address these issues.

3.3 REVIEW OF NEW AGE TECHNOLOGY IN HEALTHCARE APPLICATIONS AND ROLE OF VR

The new age technology, namely: AI, digital twin, machine learning, IoT, blockchain, and VR can be used to increase the experience of the patients and doctors in the healthcare industry. This section reviews several applications of these technologies in healthcare. AI is a system where a machine is given artificial intelligence so that it can do things that humans do better. A lot of algorithms and methods are utilized for the same. Digital twin is creating a hardware/software replica of an entity and studying its behavior and pairing it with the real entity. This helps in the prediction of response to a situation and better designing and fault recovery. Machine learning is using the data to predict and classify the decision-making in a process. IoT is collecting data through sensors and processing it to generate predictions. Big data is also related to data collection and processing. Blockchain is the storage of data securely. The VR technology along with all the new age technology can be used to improve the status of the healthcare industry, as discussed later.

The application of artificial intelligence (AI) can provide substantial improvements in all areas of healthcare from diagnostics to treatment (Bohr and Memarzadeh, 2020). There is already a large amount of evidence that AI algorithms are performing on par or better than humans in various tasks, for instance, in analyzing medical images or correlating symptoms and biomarkers from electronic medical records (EMRs) with the characterization and prognosis of the disease. Some of the applications are as follows:

- **Precision medicine:** Tailor-made medicines for patients based on their genetic information, test reports, food intake, various medical records, mood swings, and so on. This is possible by applying machine learning algorithms to the patient's data.
- **Genetics-based solutions:** The genetic information of the patients is collected, and from these huge datasets, the patterns are identified in order to create disease markers and much more.
- **Drug discovery and prediction:** Machine learning and pattern recognition methods can be used to study the large datasets of chemistry and estimate the optimum drugs in a given situation. Generation of new chemical structures using deep learning is another application. Assessment of drug-target interactions is possible using AI technology.
- **Medical visualization:** Interpretation of data that appears in the form of either an image or a video is another area where AI can help. Computer vision can be used for disease diagnosis and surgery. Deep learning is used for medical image recognition.
- **Augmented and virtual reality (AR and VR):** These systems can be implemented at the early stages of education for medical students and for training of specific specialty and experienced surgeons.
- **Patients using AR/VR:** Patients who cannot move around due to debilitating conditions can interact with their surroundings with audiovisual cues and utilize their limbs to engage and move within this world.
- **Intelligent personal health records:** Collection of patients health data through wearables. Using NLP to update the health records of patients is another application of AI. It also facilitates integration of multiple records on several EMR platforms.
- **Robotics:** Performing minimally invasive surgery using robotic arms and neuroprosthetics (artificial robotic limbs) for handicapped patients. In all the mentioned applications, VR is utilized for visualization of data and scenarios.
- **Trauma recovery:** Psychological recovery of patients can be facilitated using these technologies.
- **Health Record management:** Managing the patient's health record.

In Björnsson et al. (2020), the authors propose a solution to this challenge that is based on constructing digital twins. These are graphical models with high definition, for individual patients. These models help in determining the effective medicine for the patients. Digital twins (Bruynseels et al., 2018) technology has individual physical artifacts paired with digital models that dynamically reflect the status of those artifacts. When applied to persons, digital twins build on *in silico* representations of an individual that dynamically reflect molecular status, physiological status, and lifestyle over time. The author assumes availability of complete statistics of the person related to bio-physical and lifestyle parameters, which help in development and use of digital twin. This perspective redefines the concept of "normality" or "health" as a set of patterns that are regular *for a particular individual*, against the backdrop of patterns observed in the population. These twins can be utilized for identifying personalized medicines. In the work reported in Croatti et al. (2020), digital twins are utilized for **trauma recovery** of a patient. Healthcare represents an application domain where the introduction of digital twins could be the digital counterpart not only for physical computational assets (e.g., vital signs monitors, diagnostic machinery, surgery rooms, etc.) but also for care processes—from the simplest to the most critical ones, such as trauma management. In his paper, author puts forth and discusses the idea of agent-based digital twins, integrating the digital twin paradigm with agents in a modelling and design framework based on mirror worlds. This application of digital twin requires simulation and visualization using VR.

Alam et al. (2018) proposes the use of IoT-enabled wearables that can be used to monitor sugar, BP, heart rate, pulse rate, and other vitals and creating a cloud-based record of the patient. With the advances in the wearables, biosensors, and other technology, the author says that serious infections will also become diagnosable using IoT-based technologies. Chandy (2019) reviews the work involving IoT to collect and store the medical images such as MRI, ultrasound, and X-ray scans and then digitally processing the same to identify the problems in the patients. Bharadwaj et al. (2021) includes a detailed survey of all the applications of IoT and machine learning in healthcare for monitoring of patients' health.

Blockchain (Alhadhrami et al., 2017) technology provides data security and privacy. It eliminates third party from the financial transactions, thereby simplifying the transactions and yet not endangering the users' security. New structures of blockchain are designed to accommodate the need for this technology in other fields such as eHealth. In his paper the author has discussed the use of blockchain in managing and sharing electronic health and medical records to allow patients, hospitals, clinics, and other medical stakeholder to share data amongst themselves, and increase interoperability. Although the use of blockchain reduces redundancy and provides caregivers with consistent records about their patients, it still comes with few challenges which could infringe patients' privacy or potentially compromise the whole network of stakeholders. Dwivedi (Dwivedi et al., 2019) applied blockchain along with IoT to healthcare, and in his work he discusses the problems faced in maintaining security in the application. McGhin (McGhin et al., 2019) discusses the use of blockchain for patient record maintenance and sharing.

As we can see, the new age technology applications mentioned changed the face of the traditional applications. The same things are being done with the new technology to increase the user experience. The VR technology is used to enhance the user experience and visualize the scientific data.

3.4 MODEL FOR HEALTHCARE BASED ON NEW AGE TECHNOLOGY

In this section a model for the modern healthcare applications is discussed. Figure 3.1 includes the model. The data is collected with wearables and radiology devices for the patients and stored on blockchain-based data stores using IoT. The blockchain-based stores ensure security for the data. IoT enabled collection ensures wide reach and 24/7 availability of the data to all medical record requirements. This data then can be processed using machine learning models to predict the patient's health. It can be used for pattern recognition and simulation, which can be combined with VR to generate interesting 3D images. All the other applications discussed previously can make use of this data.

3.5 CONCLUSIONS

In this chapter, we have seen the definition of AR/VR and the difference between the two. The traditional applications of VR in several fields has been seen, namely, healthcare, medicine, tourism, gaming, military, and so on. All these applications have their roots and can be issued in the healthcare industry in one way or the other. Then we have focused on the applications of the new age technology like digital twin, IoT, machine learning, blockchain to the area of healthcare. Some of the applications discussed are in precision medicine, genetics-based solutions, drug discovery and prediction, medical visualization, augmented and virtual reality (AR and

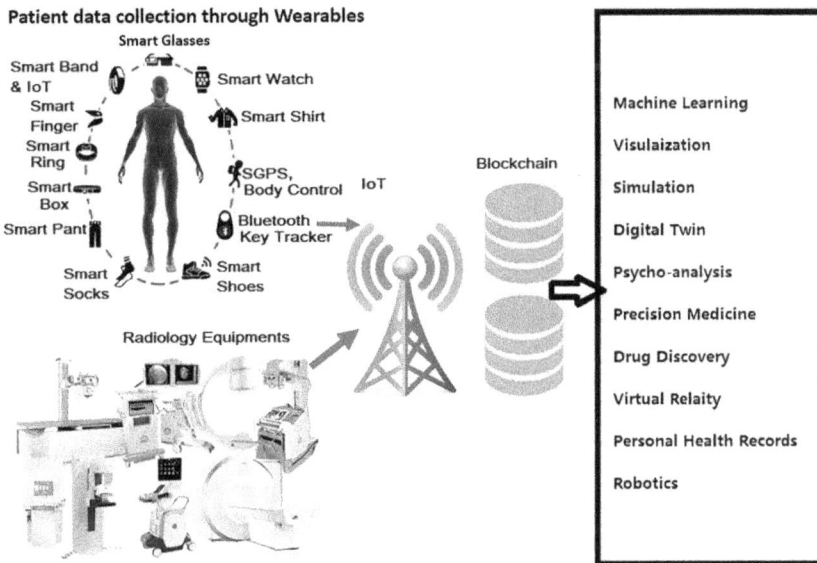

FIGURE 3.1 Model for healthcare

VR), patients using AR/VR, intelligent personal health records, and robotics. As we can see, the new age technology applications have changed the face of the traditional applications. The same things are being done with the new technology to increase the user experience. The VR technology is used to enhance the user experience and visualize the scientific data. The chapter proposes the model for healthcare systems based on IoT and blockchain, which will be really helpful in simplifying and amalgamating the diverse applications of VR, IoT, digital twin, blockchain, and machine learning.

REFERENCES

Adachi, R., Cramer, E. M., & Song, H. (2020). Using virtual reality for tourism marketing: A mediating role of self-presence. *The Social Science Journal*. doi:10.1080/03623319 .2020.1727245.

Ahir, K., Govani, K., Gajera, R., et al. (2020). Application on virtual reality for enhanced education learning, military training and sports. *Augmented Human Research*, 5(7). https:// doi.org/10.1007/s41133-019-0025-2.

Alam, M. M., Malik, H., Khan, M. I., Pardy, T., Kuusik, A., & Le Moullec, Y. (2018). A survey on the roles of communication technologies in IoT-based personalized healthcare applications. *IEEE Access*, 6, 36611–36631.

Alhadhrami, Z., Alghfeli, S., Alghfeli, M., Abedlla, J. A., & Shuaib, K. (2017, November). Introducing blockchains for healthcare. In *2017 International conference on electrical and computing technologies and applications (ICECTA)* (pp. 1–4). Ras Al Khaimah: IEEE.

Bates, J. (1992). Virtual reality, art, and entertainment. *Presence: Teleoperators & Virtual Environments*, 1(1), 133–138.

Baumann, J. (1993). *Military applications of virtual reality*. www. hitl.washington.edu/scivw/ EVE/II.G.Military.html.

Beck, J., Rainoldi, M., & Egger, R. (2019). Virtual reality in tourism: A state-of-the-art review. *Tourism Review*, 74(3), 586–612.

Bharadwaj, H. K., Agarwal, A., Chamola, V., Lakkaniga, N. R., Hassija, V., Guizani, M., & Sikdar, B. (2021). A review on the role of machine learning in enabling IoT based healthcare applications. *IEEE Access*, 9, 38859–38890.

Bidarra, R., Gambon, D., Kooij, R., Nagel, D., Schutjes, M., & Tziouvara, I. (2013). Gaming at the dentist's–serious game design for pain and discomfort distraction. In *Games for health* (pp. 207–215). Wiesbaden: Springer Vieweg.

Björnsson, B., Borrebaeck, C., Elander, N., Gasslander, T., Gawel, D. R., Gustafsson, M., . . . Benson, M. (2020). Digital twins to personalize medicine. *Genome Medicine*, 12(1), 1–4.

Bohr, A., & Memarzadeh, K. (2020). The rise of artificial intelligence in healthcare applications. In *Artificial intelligence in healthcare* (pp. 25–60). New York: Academic Press, Elsevier.

Bruynseels, K., Santoni de Sio, F., & Van den Hoven, J. (2018). Digital twins in health care: Ethical implications of an emerging engineering paradigm. *Frontiers in Genetics*, 31.

Bryson, S., & Levit, C. (1992). The virtual wind tunnel. *IEEE Computer Graphics and Applications*, 12(4), 25–34.

Chandy, A. (2019). A review on IoT based medical imaging technology for healthcare applications. *Journal of Innovative Image Processing (JIIP)*, 1(1), 51–60.

Croatti, A., Gabellini, M., Montagna, S., & Ricci, A. (2020). On the integration of agents and digital twins in healthcare. *Journal of Medical Systems*, 44(9), 1–8.

Cruz-Neira, C., Fernández, M., & Portalés, C. (2018). Virtual reality and games. *Multimodal Technologies and Interaction, 2*(1), 8.

Dwivedi, A. D., Malina, L., Dzurenda, P., & Srivastava, G. (2019, July). Optimized blockchain model for internet of things based healthcare applications. In *2019 42nd International conference on telecommunications and signal processing (TSP)* (pp. 135–139). Budapest: IEEE.

Fertleman, C., Aubugeau-Williams, P., Sher, C., Lim, A-N., Lumley, S., Delacroix, S., & Pan, X. (2018). A discussion of virtual reality as a new tool for training healthcare professionals. *Front Public Health, 6*(44). doi:10.3389/fpubh.2018.00044.

Haase, H. (1996, August). Symbiosis of virtual reality and scientific visualization system. In *Computer graphics forum* (Vol. 15, No. 3, pp. 443–451). Edinburgh, UK: Blackwell Science Ltd.

Haase, H., Strassner, J., & Dai, F. (1996). VR techniques for the investigation of molecule data. *Computers & Graphics, 20*(2), 207–217. doi:10.1016/0097-8493(95)00127-1.

Haniff, D., Chamberlain, A., Moody, L., & De Freitas, S. (2014). Virtual environments for mental health issues: A review. *Journal of Metabolomics and Systems Biology, 3*(1), 1–10.

Kavanagh, S., Luxton-Reilly, A., Wuensche, B., & Plimmer, B. (2017). A systematic review of virtual reality in education. *Themes in Science and Technology Education, 10*(2), 85–119. Retrieved June 21, 2022, from www.learntechlib.org/p/182115/

Lai, X., Lei, X., Chen, X., & Rau, P. L. P. (2019, July). Can virtual reality satisfy the entertainment needs of the elderly? The application of a VR headset in elderly care. In *International conference on human-computer interaction* (pp. 159–172). Cham: Springer.

Lányi, C. S. (2006). Virtual reality in healthcare. In N. Ichalkaranje, A. Ichalkaranje, & L. Jain (Eds.), *Intelligent paradigms for assistive and preventive healthcare. Studies in computational intelligence* (Vol. 19). Berlin and Heidelberg: Springer. https://doi.org/10.1007/11418337_3.

LaViola, J. J. (2000, November). MSVT: A virtual reality-based multimodal scientific visualization tool. In *Proceedings of the third IASTED international conference on computer graphics and imaging* (pp. 1–7). Calgary: ACTA Press.

LaViola, J. J., Forsberg, A. S., Laidlaw, D. H., & Dam, A. V. (2009). Virtual reality-based interactive scientific visualization environments. *Trends in Interactive Visualization*, 225–250.

Lele, A. (2013). Virtual reality and its military utility. *Journal of Ambient Intelligence and Humanized Computing, 4*(1), 17–26.

Liu, X., Zhang, J., Hou, G., & Wang, Z. (2018, July). Virtual reality and its application in military. In *IOP conference series: Earth and environmental science* (Vol. 170, No. 3, p. 032155). London: IOP Publishing.

Mahrer, N. E., & Gold, J. I. (2009). The use of virtual reality for pain control: A review. *Current Pain and Headache Reports, 13*(2), 100–109.

Mäkinen, H., Haavisto, E., Havola, S., & Koivisto, J. M. (2022). User experiences of virtual reality technologies for healthcare in learning: An integrative review. *Behaviour & Information Technology, 41*(1), 1–17.

McGhin, T., Choo, K. K. R., Liu, C. Z., & He, D. (2019). Blockchain in healthcare applications: Research challenges and opportunities. *Journal of Network and Computer Applications, 135*, 62–75.

Mekni, M., & Lemieux, A. (2014). Augmented reality: Applications, challenges and future trends. *Applied Computational Science, 20*, 205–214.

Mittal, H. (2020, July). Virtual reality: An overview. *CSI Communications, 44*(4), 9, ISSN 0970-647X.

Moher, D., Liberati, A., Tetzlaff, J., & Altman, D. G. (2009). Preferred reporting items for systematic reviews and meta-analyses: The PRISMA statement. *PLoS Medicine, 6*(7).

Nilsson, N. C., Serafin, S., Steinicke, F., & Nordahl, R. (2018). Natural walking in virtual reality: A review. *Computers in Entertainment (CIE)*, *16*(2), 1–22.

Pallavicini, F., Argenton, L., Toniazzi, N., Aceti, L., & Mantovani, F. (2016). Virtual reality applications for stress management training in the military. *Aerospace Medicine and Human Performance*, *87*(12), 1021–1030.

Rácz, A., & Zilizi, G. (2019, May). Virtual reality aided tourism. In *2019 Smart city symposium Prague (SCSP)* (pp. 1–5). Prague: IEEE.

Rhyne, T. M. (1997). Going virtual with geographic information and scientific visualization. *Computers & Geosciences*, *23*(4), 489–491.

Rizzo, A., Parsons, T. D., Lange, B., Kenny, P., Buckwalter, J. G., Rothbaum, B., . . . Reger, G. (2011). Virtual reality goes to war: A brief review of the future of military behavioral healthcare. *Journal of Clinical Psychology in Medical Settings*, *18*(2), 176–187.

Su, S., Perry, V., Bravo, L., Kase, S., Roy, H., Cox, K., & Dasari, V. R. (2020). Virtual and augmented reality applications to support data analysis and assessment of science and engineering. *Computing in Science & Engineering*, *22*(3), 27–39.

Sua, S., Chaudhary, A., O'Leary, P., Geveci, B., Sherman, W., Nieto, H., & Francisco-Revilla, L. (2015, March). Virtual reality enabled scientific visualization workflow. In *2015 IEEE 1st workshop on everyday virtual reality (WEVR)* (pp. 29–32). Arles: IEEE.

Taylor, R. M., Robinett, W., Chi, V. L., Brooks, F. P., Wright, W. V., Williams, R. S., & Snyder, E. J. (1993, August). The nanomanipulator: A virtual-reality interface for a scanning tunneling microscope. *Computer Graphics, Proceedings SIGGRAPH, Anaheim*, 127–134.

Van Dam, A., Laidlaw, D. H., & Simpson, R. M. (2002). Experiments in immersive virtual reality for scientific visualization. *Computers & Graphics*, *26*(4), 535–555.

Zyda, M. (2005). From visual simulation to virtual reality to games. *Computer*, *38*(9), 25–32.

4 Applications of Machine Learning in Cancer Diagnosis and Prognosis

*Rakesh Kumar Dhaka, Sampurna Panda,
Babita Panda, and Naeem Hannoon*

4.1 INTRODUCTION

In the battle against cancer, diabetes, Alzheimer's, and other debilitating diseases, bioinformatics has emerged as a key weapon. Mutations and changes in a person's genetic microenvironment are what ultimately lead to cancer. It's challenging to treat cancer because of the cancer microenvironment's extreme complexity. Patients with the same cancer subtype may nonetheless have varying responses to the same treatment. Time and effort are required for clinical trials and the conventional method of drug discovery. Scientists are working hard to develop effective solutions for these challenging illnesses. Cancer analysis has seen an important change throughout the past many decades [1]. Various methods, such as early stage screening, were utilized by scientists in an attempt to detect cancer kinds before they manifest symptoms. In addition, they have developed new methodologies for the recent forecasting of the issue of cancer medication. With the development of recent techniques in the field of medicine, vast amounts of these related input samples have been acquired and made accessible to the medical research association. However, accurately predicting the prognosis of an illness is exciting and difficult problems for clinicians. Consequently, ML approaches have gained demand among medical communities. These algorithms may detect and find patterns and links within complicated datasets, as well as accurately forecast the future results of a particular cancer category. Large amounts of patient data are becoming more readily available as we continue to embrace the digitalization of medical information in the list of patient-provided datasets as well as medical outcomes derived via cutting-edge equipment. One consequence of this information revolution is the enormous challenge of making sense of information. In addition to being a daunting task, making sense of such a massive dataset typically requires the use of manual tools and processes, which can be time-consuming and inefficient. Data-driven methods from computational sciences, sometimes known as data science or data analytics, are urgently needed to aid with data comprehension. These methods can be used to medical data analysis, allowing for the extraction of vital health information that can guide informed decision-making for both patients and doctors. Both private companies and universities are now making sizable bets on the ability of data science tools to aid in the analysis of medical data. Because of

DOI: 10.1201/9781003340133-4

the increasing quantity of medical information, data science will play a crucial role in the near future.

Cancer research has long been made because of the application of machine learning. The field of cancer detection, and diagnosis has been using artificial neural networks (ANNs) and support vector machine (SVMs) for approximately 20 years (K. Kourou 2015) [1]. ML techniques are currently being utilized in a variety of settings, from the detection and classification of tumors using X-ray and CRT images (A. Z. Woldaregay et al. 2019) to the grouping of malignancies using proteomic and genomic (microarray) assays (A. Z. Woldaregay et al. 2019) [2]. Recent data from PubMed indicates that over 1,500 articles have been written on the same topic. But the maximum of these studies focus on applying machine learning techniques to the detection and identification of cancers and other malignances. That is to say, machine learning has mostly been employed as a tool in cancer detection and diagnosis (Y. Yang et al. 2022) [3]. Recent years have seen an uptick in efforts to use machine learning for forecasting of cancer and treatment. Because of this, there isn't a huge amount of published research on the topic of machine learning for cancer forecasting and cure (about 120 articles).

Prediction and prognosis of cancer are aimed at different ends than detection and diagnosis, which have different priorities. There are three main areas of focus in cancer prognosis and prediction: (1) predicting cancer susceptibility (i.e., risk assessment), (2) predicting cancer reoccurrence, and (3) predicting cancer survival. In this scenario, a person is attempting to foretell their cancer diagnosis before the sickness has even manifested itself.

In the latter scenario, the goal is to estimate how likely it is that cancer will return after initially disappearing. The third scenario involves making a prognosis once a diagnosis has been made, whether it is regarding survival chances, tumor growth, or response to treatment. The accuracy of a prognostic forecast in the latter two cases is reliant on the accuracy or quality of the investigation. Nonetheless, a prediction can only be made after a medical diagnosis has been made, and there is more to a prognostic prediction than a mere diagnosis (S. S. Raoof et al. 2020) [4].

Certainly, a cancer prediction is often made by a team of doctors from several fields, taking into account a wide range of characteristics such as the age of the patients and general health, the size and type of cancer, the stage of the tumor, and so on (D. A. Almuhaidib et al. 2018) [5]. In order to make an accurate prediction, the attending physician must typically carefully integrate historical, analytical, and numerical data. This is challenging work for even the most experienced medical professionals. Both doctors and patients face similar difficulties when trying to address the concerns of cancer avoidance and susceptibility forecasting. A person's chance of acquiring cancer can be affected by factors such as their age, genealogy, food, being overweight, high-risk activities (smoking, excessive drinking), and being in contact with environmental toxins like UV radiation etc. (S. Gupta et al. 2021) [6]. Traditional "macro-scale" clinical, environmental, and behavioral characteristics, however, do not typically furnish ample data to establish meaningful forecasting. What is ideally required are highly exact molecular facts regarding either the tumor itself or the patient's genetic makeup (M. Sughasiny et al. 2018) [7].

This type of molecular-scale data on patients or tumors is nowadays easily obtained because of the rapid improvement of genomic (DNA sequencing, microarrays) techniques. Somatic mutations in particular genes (p53, BRCA1, BRCA2), the presence of particular tumor proteins (MUC1, HER2, PSA), and the tumor's chemical surroundings (anoxic, hypoxic) have all been found to be highly effective prognostic or predictive indications (X. Bao et al. 2020) [8]. Multiple molecular biomarker samples have lately been proven to be even more predictive than any one biomarker alone (K. A. Tran et al. 2021) [9]. Combining these genetic arrangements with large-scale clinical input (tumor kind, genetic features, and risk factors) can further strengthen and refine cancer identification and forecasts. The difficulty of making sense of all this data, however, grows in proportion to the number of parameters we monitor.

In the past, to forecast the risks and outcomes of the cancer, we relied on macro-scale knowledge, which kept the number of variants small enough that traditional statistical approaches could be employed. However, with the advent of modern advanced diagnostic and imaging tools, we are now faced with a plethora of genetic, cellular, and clinical factors. Human intuition and conventional statistics are often useless in these circumstances. Instead, we have to rely more on cutting-edge computational methods like machine learning.

There is a growing movement toward customized, predictive medicine, and one component of this is the use of machines (computers) to forecast and prognosticate the course of disease (P. Bhardwaj et al. 2021) [10]. Patients (in terms of style of living and quality-of-life decisions), doctors (in terms of treatment decisions), and health economists/policy planners all stand to benefit from this shift toward predictive medicine (in using high-scale cancer avoidance or cancer analysis policies).

The proliferation of oncological and pharmacogenomics data resources online has stimulated investigation in this area. In order to better treat genetic illnesses, bioinformaticians are turning to machine learning techniques rather than traditional statistical and computational methods. Each and every living thing is composed of cells. The human body has many different types of cells, including blood cells, muscle cells, fat cells, etc. This cellular variation is a product of genes. The role of genes in transmitting hereditary information and in controlling the body's myriad biochemical and cellular activities cannot be overstated. The variation in genotype and phenotype observed among species can be traced back to differences in underlying genes. Genes are the exclusive carriers of hereditary information for phenotypic characteristics. It is important to investigate genetic predispositions to disease in order to effectively combat heritable disorders. New technologies in high-throughput sequencing and computational biology are facilitating the identification of disease-causing biomarkers (genes). The quest for the gene or group of genes responsible for hereditary illnesses is a major focus of many scientists. Microarray technology allows for the precise quantification of a given microenvironment's gene expression profile. Data on gene expression can be supplemented with information on other levels of the genome, transcriptome, and proteome, such as copy number variations, mutations, etc. Identification of anti-cancer medications, therapeutic targets, and biomarkers relies heavily on gene expression and drug response data.

To better understand inherited illnesses, some scientists are investigating potential molecular pathways. The expression value of a gene is the ratio of its expression in two different situations, as determined by DNA microarray hybridization. Gene expression is quantified by measuring the amount of mRNA each gene produces. As a result of environmental factors, its value may shift. Messenger RNA (mRNA) is involved in transmitting genetic instructions for protein production. There is great promise for the use of gene expression data in the life sciences. It may be useful in pinpointing the genetic root of the observed phenomenon. Using distinguishing genomic characteristics, we can locate disease biomarkers. Genomic assays such as MNaseseq, m-RNA, and DNase-seq may be employed as inputs for machine learning systems to predict a wide range of disease-related information.

In these researches, identification and forecasting properties that may be irrelevant of a particular medication or are incorporated to direct cancer therapy, respectively, are considered [11]. Again, we explore the sorts of ML methods now in use, the kinds of input they incorporate, and the overall achievement of each given scheme, as well as their advantages and cons.

The adoption of ML approaches could increase the precision of cancer susceptibility, reoccurrence, and survival predictions. The implementation of ML approaches has resulted in a 15–20% increase in the accuracy of cancer prognosis during the past few years, according to [12].

4.2 STRATEGIES FOR MACHINE LEARNING

It is essential to have solid knowledge regarding machine learning as well as what it is not, before delving into a comprehensive analysis of which methods of machine learning are the most useful in various categories of circumstances. A subfield of artificial intelligence known as machine learning uses different optimization techniques to "learn" from training datasets and then apply that knowledge to the classification of test samples, the identification of new patterns, or the prediction of new trends (A. Sharma et al. 2017) [13]. In the same way that statistics are utilized, machine learning is utilized when it comes to the interpretation of data. When it comes to modeling data or identifying patterns, machine learning techniques, as opposed to statistical ones, may make use of logical constructs such as Boolean operators, absolute conditional logic, conditional probabilities (the probability of A given B), and nontraditional optimization methods. These more recent tactics are strikingly analogous to the way in which we humans learn and organize information. Machine learning, despite the fact that it is still heavily dependent on statistical and probabilistic concepts, is intrinsically more powerful due to the fact that it is able to draw conclusions and make decisions that would be impossible to draw using more traditional statistical methods (A. P. Pawlovsky et al. 2014) [14]. For example, multivariate regression and correlation analysis are at the foundation of a great deal of different statistical methodologies. In general, these methods are extremely effective, yet in order to describe data, they rely on the assumptions of independence and linearity between variables. When dealing with nonlinear relationships between dependent (or conditional) variables, regular statistical approaches frequently fail to deliver accurate results. In situations like these, machine learning often achieves amazing levels of success. Numerous biological systems have parameters that are conditionally dependent on other variables; as a result, these systems are intrinsically nonlinear. This is due to the fact that many fundamental physical systems are linear, with parameters that are, for the most part, unrelated to one another.

There are occasions when machine learning does not function as anticipated. A comprehensive understanding of the current problem as well as knowledge of the limitations of the data is necessary for achieving success with any method. It is also necessary to have solid knowledge regarding the advantages and constraints imposed by the algorithms being employed. Experiments involving machine learning have a good chance of being successful provided they are meticulously designed, the learners are deployed in a suitable manner, and the outcomes are validated in great detail. Obviously, if the data are inaccurate, the results will be inaccurate as well (the old adage "garbage in, garbage out"). In the same way, if there are more predictors than events to be predicted, one can design a chain of redundant learners. This is because there are more predictors than events to be predicted. These learning algorithms have a tendency to keep their performance at a consistent (bad) level over a large diversity of input data sources. The problem of having an excessive number of variables yet insufficient amounts of data is referred to as the "curse of dimensionality" (M. Anitha 2020) [15]. Nonetheless, ML is not the only industry that has been impacted by this plague. In addition to this, a variety of statistical methods are affected. There is no way around raising the number of training examples or reducing the number of variables. Both of these options are necessary (features). It is advised to have a sample-to-feature ratio that is greater than 5:1 (S. C. Bellad et al. 2021) [16]. In order to train an accurate model, it is required to have access to a training set that is both extensive and varied. The examples and data that are used in training should be chosen so that they are representative of the actual content that will eventually be encountered by the learner. When repetition is applied to insufficiently many or samples that are otherwise uninteresting, a phenomenon known as overfitting can develop (D. German et al. 2008) [17]. An individual who has been overworked will, similar to a pupil who is exhausted, fail to comprehend new knowledge and effectively organize it into categories.

Statistics that have been used for a long time can sometimes outperform machine learning in terms of their effectiveness or precision. In the aforementioned situations, it is quite likely that the user's initial assumptions on the dependency and nonlinearity of the data were inaccurate. This is not a flaw with machine learning per such; rather, it demonstrates how important it is to make sure you are utilizing the appropriate technology for the job at hand. Additionally, it is a fact that not all approaches to machine learning are created equal. Different problems require unique solutions, and some strategies are better suited to addressing those problems than others. Some machine learning approaches scale well while others do not; for instance, when it comes to the size of biological domains, certain algorithms scale well, while others do not. In a similar vein, certain methods might not be suitable because they call for data that is not currently available or because the methodology involves assumptions that are not supported by the evidence. The most effective solution to a particular problem is not always obvious at first glance. As a consequence of this, it is absolutely necessary to evaluate several different approaches to machine learning using the same dataset.

Another frequent misconception is the assumption that the trends it unearths are inherently obscured or difficult to recognize. This is a common misconception because machine learning is so pervasive. Instead, it would be easier for a human expert to recognize many patterns or trends in the data if they looked at it in sufficient detail. To put it more succinctly, machine learning cuts down on the amount of time and effort required to identify patterns or develop classification schemes. Keep in mind that after the fact, the significance of any significant finding will likely be readily apparent to even the most casual observer.

It is a subfield of AI where the concept of inference is used for learning from data samples in general. The process of learning is having two parts: (1) from the training data samples, assessment of unknown relations in a system, and (2) utilization of inferred patterns to forecast new system predictions. ML has also been demonstrated to be an important part of biomedical research with numerous uses, in which an appropriate generalization is reached by searching across n-dimensional sets for biological training samples using various approaches: (1) supervised learning and (2) unsupervised learning are the two most prevalent types of ML approaches. A classified collection of data samples is used in supervised learning to evaluate the input data to the intended response. While unsupervised learning approaches do not provide labeled examples and do not consider the response throughout the learning process. Ultimately, based on a learning scheme or model to detect patterns or groups in the incoming data, this approach can be regarded as a classification challenge in supervised learning. Classification is the challenge of categorizing samples into a collection of finite classes via a learning process. Regression and clustering are two other typical ML problems. In the case of regression, a learning algorithm transforms the samples into a variable with real values. Based on this procedure, predictions can be evaluated for each test sample. Clustering is a typical unsupervised learning in which one tries to classify groups to characterize the sample elements. On the basis of this procedure, each test data can be assigned to one of the discovered groups based on their shared characteristics. Figure 4.1 represents machine learning for picture recognition, an example of training on a dataset.

An example of an application of ANNs is the so-called self-organizing map (SOM) approach (A. Basavanhally et al. 2010) [18]. In this technique, the weights of a grid of artificial neurons are adjusted with the help of input vectors that were taken from a training set. The SOM was first developed with the intention of simulating the processes that occur in the human brain. At the beginning of an SOM, a collection of

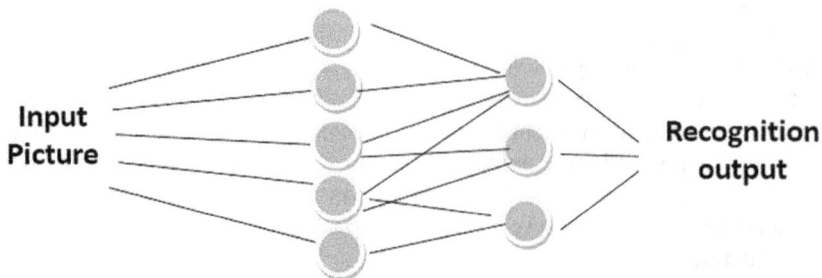

FIGURE 4.1   Machine learning for picture recognition: an example of training on a dataset

virtual neurons, each of which has its own spot on the output map, compete with one another in a so-called "winner-take-all" system (also known as a "competitive system"), in which the node whose weight vector is nearest to the input vector is decided as the winner and has its weights tweaked to bring them into nearer alignment with the inputs. In other words, the node with the weight vector that is nearest to a solitary node is encompassed on all sides by additional nodes. When a node wins, the weights of all of its neighbors are altered in a similar fashion, but to a lower intensity. The farther it is from the winner, the less relative weight it carries in the overall equation. Every single input vector is subjected to this process again and over again for an extremely extended period of time. Winners are subject to change based on the inputs that are used. An SOM that is capable of sorting input into relevant categories and then linking individual output nodes to those categories and patterns is the final product of this process.

An intriguing fact about machine learning algorithms used for cancer forecasting and diagnosis is that almost all of them rely on supervised learning. The majority of these supervised learning algorithms are also grouped with other classifiers that use conditional probabilities or conditional judgments to make their classifications. Key conditional algorithms include the following: There are a number of different methods that can be used to make a prediction: (1) ANNs, (2) decision trees (DT), (3) genetic algorithms, (4) linear discriminant analysis (LDA) techniques, and (5) KNN algorithms (N. G. Maity et al. 2017) [19]. A total of 820 of the 1,585 articles analyzed made use of ANNs. Many classification and pattern recognition problems can be solved by ANNs. McCulloch and Pitts (1943) laid the groundwork for these types of issues, and in the 1980s, Rumelhart et al. (1986). They can execute a variety of statistical operations (such as linear, logistic, and nonlinear regression) and logical functions or inferences as part of the classification process (including AND, OR, XOR, NOT, and IF-THEN). And this is where they shine (G. Chandra et al. 2022) [20]. The original goal of ANN development was to create a system with numerous interconnected neurons and axon junctions, similar to the human brain. Repeated training on classified training samples can either improve or lessen the strength of neural connections, analogous to how biological study modifies the stability of neural connections. Mathematical models of these neural connections can take the form of a wiring diagram or a matrix. It's important to cite this phrase. (Neuron 1 is linked to Neurons 2 and 4, Neuron 2 to Neurons 5, 6, and 8, etc.) This layer of the weight matrix is analogous to the many layers of cortical tissue in the brain. Neural networks often employ many layers (sometimes called hidden layers) to progress their datasets and produce a response (Figure 4.2).

To guarantee that input and output data are compatible with the mathematical framework of each layer, they are generally constructed as a string or vector of numeric. One challenge of working with ANNs is figuring out how to convert the input and output data (a picture, a physical feature, or a forecast) from the actual world into a numerical string. In ANNs, fine-tuning the stability of the neural connections is often performed by a form of optimization known as back-propagation (short for backward propagation of errors—This is a derivative-based technique that checks the previous layer's response against that layer's table. At its most fundamental, a neural network uses its training data's replies to gradually adjust the values

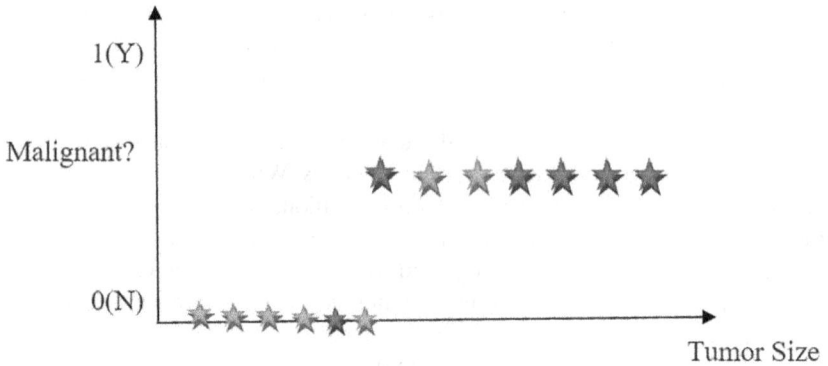

FIGURE 4.2 Classification function in supervised learning

stored in its weight matrices. To be effective, backpropagation requires a differentiable learning or information-transfer function (often a sigmoidal curve). The great majority of ANNs have a multilayered feed-forward structure. This indicates that there is no looping or feedback in their system. To achieve optimal performance, an ANN must be tailored to the specifics of each application through careful consideration of its design and architecture. Poor performance and slow training times can result from selecting a generic ANN design or using a generic input/output scheme. A more tailored architecture will help you avoid these two problems. Another issue is that ANNs have the same limitations as any other "black box" technology. Hardly any insight can be gained into why an ANN failed to act as required or into the strategies it employs for data classification. To rephrase, it takes some effort to understand the reasoning behind a trained ANN.

Decision trees, or DTs, are a simpler alternative to ANNs. To achieve a specific objective, one can create a decision tree, which is a structured graph or flow chart with nodes representing decisions and leaves representing probable outcomes representing branches. The usage of decision trees dates back years, and today they are an integral feature of numerous medical diagnostic techniques. Figure 4.3 is an overarching view of a simple decision tree for making a breast cancer diagnosis.

Typically, decision trees are built after consulting a group of experts, then honed over years of practice, or modified to account for limited resources or lessen the likelihood of harm. In contrast, decision tree learners may automatically build decision trees from a classified set of training samples. If you're training a decision tree to label data, the leaves of the tree will reflect the categories you've decided upon, while the branches will show you who feature conjunctions led you to those categories. When learning a decision tree, the classified data samples are divided into sub-nodes regularly, either using a numerical or logical test, to speed up the learning process (Quinlan 1986). Repeating these steps on each new sub-node yielded is a recursive process that continues until the further subdivision is impossible or a unique classification is obtained. They generate strong classifiers, "learn" quickly, require minimum data preparation, can handle numerical, nominal (named), and categorical data, and are statistically validatable. These are but a few examples of the various uses for

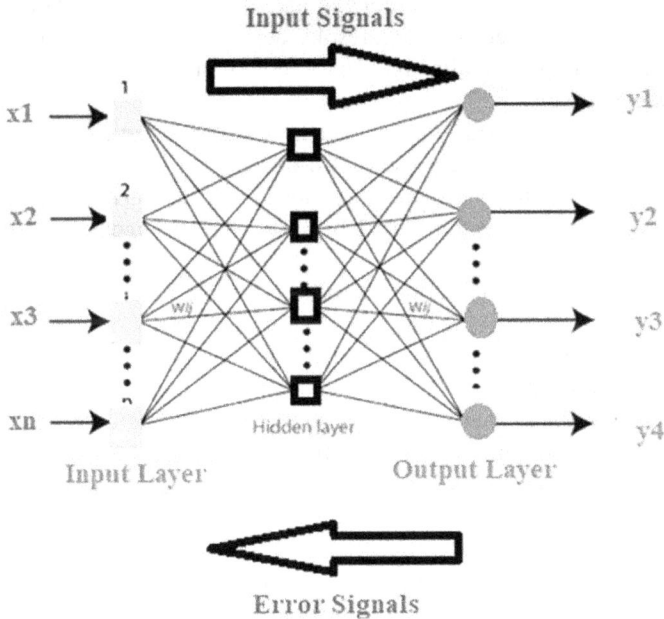

FIGURE 4.3   A representation of the ANN architecture

decision trees. Conversely, when faced with more complex classification tasks, DTs often do not perform as well as ANNs do.

A significant number of academics are currently employing machine learning algorithms in an effort to resolve issues that arise in biological research. The approach of supervised machine learning can be broken down into three distinct stages: learning, training, and testing. During the phase known as "learning," the algorithm for machine learning is built. During the period of training, the machine learning model is provided with huge data in order to develop generalized rules based on the data. During the testing phase, new samples are inputted in order to evaluate how accurately the model predicted the outcome. In contrast, when it comes to unsupervised learning, data samples are offered, but no classifications are ever made available. The threat is to divide up the data samples in such a way that there is the most relevant information possible with the least amount of unnecessary information. The most important step in developing successful treatments for cancer is gaining a deeper comprehension of the intricate workings of the microenvironment in which cancer develops. Even though numerous treatments have been proposed during the course of cancer research, the incurable quality of the disease has not been altered. When applied to this scenario, artificial intelligence (AI) and machine learning present an approach that is dependable, speedy, and effective in the treatment of such serious disorders. One of the effective AI-based tools that are assisting in the field of pathology is called PathAI, for instance. A diagnosis made with the assistance of AI is one that is quicker, more trustworthy, and more accurate. With the assistance of AI, clinical trials can be finished more quickly, and predictions on their success rates can be made with greater precision. Figures 4.2 depicts tumors, denoted by X, and are categorized as benign or malignant. The tumors seen within the circles have been incorrectly classified.

Semi-supervised learning, which is a blend of both supervised and unsupervised learning, is another extensively used form of machine learning (ML) approach. It mixes labeled and unlabeled data to develop a precise learning model. This type of algorithm is typically employed when there are more unclassified datasets than classified datasets.

When employing an ML technique, datasets are the fundamental elements. Each set is characterized by some features, each of which consists of distinct sorts of values. In addition, knowing in prior the precise type of data to be analyzed enables the selection of appropriate tools and methodologies for their study. Some data-related concerns are the data's quality and the pre-processing methods required making them more acceptable for machine learning. Data quality problems consist of the existence of noise, outliers, duplicate data, and skewed or unrepresentative data. Typically, when data quality is enhanced, so is the quality of the subsequent analysis. Concerning making the raw data more acceptable for subsequent investigation, preparation techniques that focus on data modification must also be implemented. There are numerous techniques and tactics for data preparation that target changing the samples to better fit certain ML techniques. Among these methods, (1) dimensionality reduction (2) feature selection, and (3) feature extraction are among the most important. When samples contain many attributes, dimensionality reduction has a variety of advantages. ML algorithms perform better when the dimension is reduced. Moreover, the decrease in dimensionality can reduce appropriate attributes, minimize noise, and build more potent learning systems because less number of attributes are taken into account.

Feature selection is the course of decreasing dimensionality by picking novel attributes that are a subset of the original features. There are three main ways to select features: embedded, filter, and wrapper. In this case, a novel sample of attributes can be derived from the initial sample that encapsulates all the pertinent data in a data sample. The development of new samples of characteristics enables the dimensionality reduction benefits outlined.

The important objective of machine learning algorithms is to generate a system that may be used for classification, forecasting, evaluation, or any other proportionate activity. Classification is an important typical learning action. As explained earlier, this learning technique categorizes the data item into one of the different predefined groups. When developing a classification model using ML techniques, training and generalization mistakes might occur. The former relates to misclassification mistakes on the training samples, whereas the latter refers to the anticipated errors on the testing data. A good classification model should precisely fit the training set and categories in all cases. The phenomenon of model overfitting occurs when the test error rates of a system continue to climb while the training error rates fall. This circumstance is associated with model complication, suggesting that a model's training errors can be reduced if its complication is increased. Connecting the output of one node to the input of another through arrows is presented in Figure 4.3.

Clearly, the optimal complexity of a model which is not prone to overfitting is the one with the lowest generalization error. The bias-variance trade-off is a precise method for evaluating the expected generalization error of a learning system. The bias element of a specific learning algorithm measures the algorithm's error rate. In addition, variance in the learning process is a second error source of overall potential training samples of a given size and all possible test samples. The predicted error of a classification system is the sum of its bias and variance, as determined by the bias-variance trade-off.

DTs adhere to a tree-structured classification method, with nodes representing input variables and leaves representing decision outcomes. DTs are one of the first and most renowned machine learning (ML) classification techniques that have been mostly implemented. The DTs are easy to read and "fast" to learn because of their design. When traversing the classification tree for a new sample, we can make educated guesses regarding its class. The conclusions resulting from their particular architecture provide appropriate argumentation, which makes them an appealing method. Figure 4.4 displays a DT along with its components and regulations.

SVMs are a relatively later use of ML approaches in the area of cancer diagnosis and forecasting. SVMs at the beginning transfer the input variables into a higher-dimensional feature space and locate the hyperplane that divides the data samples into two groups. Maximize the marginal distance between the decision hyperplane and the instances close to the border.

The generated classifier has a high degree of generalizability and can therefore be used to classify new data accurately. It is important to note that SVMs can also provide probabilistic outputs. SVM classifies tumors as benign or malignant based on their size and the age of the patients. The detected hyperplane serves as a dividing line between the two groups. Clearly, the existence of a decision boundary permits the discovery of any misclassifications caused by the approach. Tumors are categorized expending on their volume and the age of the patient. The given arrows represent the misclassified tumors. Predicting and diagnosing cancer using machine learning.

Several ML approaches and feature-selection techniques have been mostly used in the past two decades for disease prognosis and forecasting. To simulate the course of cancer and discover useful features that are subsequently used in a classification scheme, the majority of these studies use machine learning methods. The prognostic

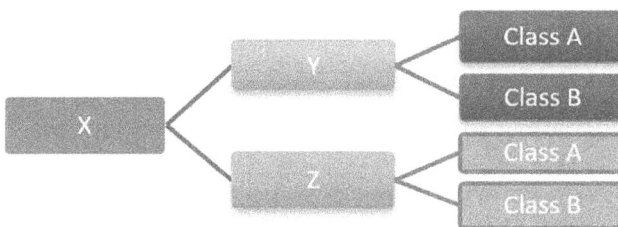

FIGURE 4.4 A representation of a DT showing the tree structure

process is fed information from gene expression profiles, clinical factors, and histological data, all of which are considered impractical in every study. However, prognostic forecasting should take into consideration rather than a simple diagnostic remark when determining a disease's course of treatment. If you're trying to anticipate cancer prognosis/prediction, you are looking for three things: a forecasting of cancer susceptibility, the prediction of cancer recurrence/local control, and an accurate prediction of cancer survival. The likelihood of cancer forming or returning after complete or partial remission is termed as the likelihood of cancer returning. After a cancer diagnosis or therapy, the major objective is to forecast a survival outcome such as disease-specific or total survival. Life expectancy, survival, progression, and treatment sensitivity are all factors that can be used to predict cancer outcomes.

In the past, doctors typically employed histology, clinical, and population-based data to arrive at a realistic cancer prognosis judgment. Integration of factors such as genetic predisposition and environmental exposure to carcinogens have important aspects in forecasting cancer, respectively. Even if traditional statistical methods could be used to forecast using this kind of macro-scale knowledge because of the less number of variables, these kinds of parameters do not furnish enough facts to make sound conclusions. The fast development of genomic, proteomic, and imaging techniques has made it possible to gather new types of molecular data. It has been demonstrated that molecular biomarkers, cellular characteristics, and the expression of specific genes are extremely useful indications for predicting cancer occurrence. High-throughput technologies (HTTs) are now commonplace, resulting in a flood of cancer research data that can be accessed by scientists. Accurately predicting how a patient's sickness will progress is one of the most exciting and complicated challenges that doctors face. As a result, medical researchers increasingly rely on machine learning (ML) approaches. These methods are capable of discovering and identifying trends and links in large data samples, as well as accurately predicting the future course of a particular cancer type. Methods for selecting features for cancer research have also been reported in the literature. Classifying useful traits for reliably identifying illness class is the goal of the computational techniques proposed.

4.3   PREDICTION OF CANCER RECURRENCE

Here we give the most up-to-date and significant publications that have recommended the use of ML approach for predicting cancer recurrence, as determined by our survey. According to the recent research, an investigation into the predictive power of OSCC has been recommended. For this purpose, they proposed a multi-parametric decision support system that may be used to study the evolution of OSCC following complete remission from cancer. For the purpose of predicting a likely relapse of OSCC and thus a subsequent recurrence, they used a variety of data sources (clinical, imaging, and genomic). Relapse was found in 13 of the 86 patients studied; the remaining patients were disease-free in this investigation. With the help of two feature selection algorithms, CFS and wrapper, a specific selection of feature approach was followed. Thus, the researchers could avoid bias when selecting the most informative aspects of their reference heterogeneous datasets. It would therefore be possible to use the selected important variables as input vectors to particular classifiers. There were a total of 65 clinical, imaging, and genomic features in each category prior to the use of feature selection approaches. A total of 8, 6, and 7 pieces of diagnostic imaging and genomic data were employed in the classifiers following the implementation of the CFS algorithm. Clinical characteristics that were most useful for each classification method included smoking, tumor thickness, and the presence of p53 staining, to name a few. When it came to imaging and genomic parameters, the most critical was the extra-tumor spreading, the number of lymph nodes, and the SOD2, TCAM, and OXCT2 genes after the CFS algorithm had been used.

Patients with a disease relapse are separated from those who haven't based on the results of the five classification algorithms in this study. BNs, ANNs, SVMs, DTs, and RF classifiers are among the algorithms used. After each ML approach was completed, an assessment method known as tenfold cross-validation was used to gauge its effectiveness. In addition, the classification scheme's accuracy, sensitivity, and specificity were all evaluated and compared. The authors also used the ROC curve to evaluate their findings. Classification of data without feature selection and classification of data after applying a feature selection technique yielded their prediction outcomes for the classification schemes used. They stated that the BN classifier performed better in discrimination with the direct input of clinical and imaging variables than one that applied a feature selection technique, based on their results (78.6% and 82.8%accuracy, respectively). It was shown that the CFS algorithm in conjunction with the BN classifier was the best performer in genomic-based classification results (91.7% accuracy). The authors integrated the most precise individual predictors (i.e., BN and BN coupled with the CFS) in order to arrive at a consensus conclusion for distinguishing between patients who had an OSCC relapse and those who had not. This method was shown to be more effective than other methods when compared to the literature. Using ML classifiers, the suggested study demonstrated how the integration of heterogeneous sources of data can yield accurate findings when it comes to predicting cancer recurrence rates. The authors also utilized a variety of classification methods to ensure their findings were solid and reliable. A classifier predictor's accuracy can be determined by looking at its performance in comparison to other classifiers. But the study's tiny sample size is a crucial point worth mentioning. Only 86 individuals with clinical, imaging, and genetic characteristics were included in the study. It is important to keep in mind that, despite the positive classification findings, the tiny sample size in comparison with the dimensionality of the data may lead to inaccurate predictions. In the same year, another noteworthy paper suggested the BCRSVM, an SVM-based system for the prediction of breast cancer recurrence. High-risk and low-risk groups can be used to better plan for cancer therapy and follow-up care, according to the scientists. Predicting the recurrence of breast cancer five years after surgery is the focus of their research. SVM, ANN, and Cox-proportional hazard regression were used to create the models and determine which ones were the most accurate. Using accuracy results from all three models, the authors concluded that BCRSVM was the superior model. Only 14 of the 193 available variables in their dataset were chosen by the researchers based on their clinical expertise. There were 733 patients out of 1.541 that were included in this study, which included data on clinical, epidemiological, and pathological characteristics. Finally, a Kaplan-Meier analysis and a Cox regression were used to pick the seven most relevant features.

Cox regression was also used as an input for both the SVM classifiers and the ANN classifiers. Using the hold-out technique, which divides the data sample into training and testing sets, the authors evaluated the models' performance. For a reliable evaluation of the models, accuracy, sensitivity, and specificity were calculated, as in the majority of previous investigations. With an accuracy rate between 84.6% and 72.6%, the authors stated that BCRSVM beat out ANN and Cox regression systems in their study using these criteria. A comparison of BCRSVM's performance with that of other well-established recurrence prediction models indicated that BCRSVM outperformed them all. NMI (normalized mutual information index) was used in this study to determine the relevance of prognostic factors. This study's calculations for each of the three predictive models reveal that the local invasion of the tumor was the most important component in the prediction of breast cancer recurrence. In the event that this work is ever reviewed, it will undoubtedly draw attention to a number of significant shortcomings. Segregation of a large number of patients ($n = 808$) due to a lack of clinical data in the registry had an effect on model performance, as observed by the authors of the study. It's also possible that the authors' selection of 14 factors from a pool of 193 was skewed, as they relied only on their clinical expertise. BCRSVM could also be improved by using additional datasets from other sources in addition to the limitations of the authors' proposed method. The use of SSL learning to predict cancer has grown steadily in the previous few years, as evidenced by our initial list of publications. The most recent study that employs this sort of ML approach for breast cancer recurrence was thought to be interesting, thus we decided to present it. SSL is used to build a graph model that incorporates gene expression data and gene network instructions to predict cancer recurrence in the proposed approach. According to their understanding of biology, the researchers chose gene pairs that show strong biological relationships. The BRCA1, CCND1, STAT1, and CCNB1 genes are part of the sub-gene system found by the suggested technique. In order to build a graph model using just labeled samples, the researchers used a three-part methodology: (1) the identification of gene pairs, (2) the advancement of sample graphs based on informative genes, and (3) graph regularization to discover the labels of unlabeled data. Gene expression profiles from the GEO repository and PPIs obtained from the I2D database were used in this study. More specifically 125, 181, 249, and 112 labeled samples were retrieved from GEO in the five gene expression datasets. There were three sets of samples: (1) recurrence, (2) non-recurrence, and (3) unlabeled and referred to cancers such as breast or colon cancer. The I2D database also provided a set of known, experimental, and anticipated human PPIs, totaling 194.988 interactions. There were 108,544 connections after deleting the duplicated PPIs and interactions that did not contain proteins linked to genes. According to the findings of this study, the gene networks created from the SSL learning method contain many essential genes associated with cancer recurrence. According to the researchers, their strategy is superior to other methods for predicting the return of breast cancer. It was predicted that the suggested strategy outperformed previously known methods that use PPIs to identify useful genes in breast and colon cancer samples by 80.7% and 76.7%, respectively. The experimental results were estimated using a tenfold cross-validation method. This type of machine learning differs significantly from supervised and unsupervised learning approaches in terms of the algorithms they use, but it is evident that it offers greater advantages in terms of dataset collecting and size. Data that has not been tagged is less expensive, and it is also easier to extract. It's not uncommon for label examples to require the expertise of scientists and sophisticated equipment to gather. With the limited labeled samples typically associated with traditional supervised procedures, this work shows that SSL may be an effective alternative to those methods.

4.4 SCOPE OF APPLYING AR/VR IN MEDICAL IMAGING

By 2024, the AR/VR industry might be worth over $150 billion, representing a massive compound annual growth rate of 70.4% (Source: Markets and Markets).

While augmented and virtual reality technologies have undoubtedly revolutionized the gaming and entertainment industries, they also hold great promise for reshaping the healthcare sector by revolutionizing a wide range of traditionally healthcare-related activities and fields.

Despite their infancy, augmented and virtual reality (AR/VR) technologies are already assisting healthcare professionals in making life-or-death choices. It is possible that the use of these technologies might reduce the total cost of medical treatment. If this VR/AR technology pans out, it might radically alter how MRI and CT scans are seen in medical diagnostics. VR/AR technologies have come a long way and have several potential uses in the medical imaging industry.

While administering chemotherapy, tumors may be viewed in real-time with the use of augmented reality and virtual reality technologies. Such augmented and virtual reality imaging tools have the potential to shed light on changes in tumor size, shape, and margin. It can also be used to track how the tumor has changed during the course of treatment. With today's imaging technology, we can only get a two-dimensional picture of a tumor, its position, its laterality (in the case of breast cancer), its distance, and its size. With augmented reality (AR) and virtual reality (VR), this data may be improved by providing contextual elements, such as the orientation of objects, the 3D placement of assumptions, and the distance from neighboring structures. Virtual and augmented reality imaging allows for precise tumor boundary mapping prior to surgery. This will shed light on how a complicated tumor is laid out. It will also be useful during lumpectomies performed to remove tumors, allowing surgeons to confirm that no cancerous tissue was left behind.

4.5 CONCLUSION

In particular, we discovered a few patterns in the machine learning approaches taken, the training data integrated, the endpoint predictions produced, the cancer kinds investigated, and the outcome of these approaches in forecasting cancer susceptibility or occurrences. Despite ANNs' continued dominance, it is understood that many distinct kinds of cancer are being studied using at least three different kinds of machine-learning methodologies. It is also evident that as compared to earlier approaches, the performance or prediction accuracy of most prognoses is enhanced when machine learning approaches are used. While the vast majority of studies are well-designed and adequately verified, it appears that more focus should be placed on experimental design and implementation, particularly in regard to the quantity and quality of biological data. Numerous machine-based classifiers may vastly improve in quality, generality, and reproducibility if experimental design and biological validation were to be enhanced. Collectively, it is clear that the use of machine learning classifiers will become much more widespread in many clinical and medical settings if the quality of studies continues to increase. SVM and ANN classifiers were found to be frequently used among the most commonly applied ML algorithms important to the prediction of cancer patient outcomes. For the past 30 years, ANNs have been employed widely. A more modern technique for cancer prognosis, SVMs have been widely used because of their high accuracy in predicting outcomes. It is important to remember that the best algorithm depends on a variety of factors, including the type of data collected, sample size, time constraints, and expected prediction results.

REFERENCES

[1] K. Kourou, T. P. Exarchos, K. P. Exarchos, M. V. Karamouzis and D. I. Fotiadis, "Machine Learning Applications in Cancer Prognosis and Prediction," *Computational and Structural Biotechnology Journal*, vol. 13, pp. 8–17, 2015, ISSN 2001–0370, https://doi.org/10.1016/j.csbj.2014.11.005.

[2] A. Z. Woldaregay, E. Årsand, S. Walderhaug, D. Albers, L. Mamykina, T. Botsis and G. Hartvigsen, "Data-Driven Modeling and Prediction of Blood Glucose Dynamics: Machine Learning Applications in Type 1 Diabetes," *Artificial Intelligence in Medicine*, vol. 98, pp. 109–134, 2019 Jul, doi: 10.1016/j.artmed.2019.07.007. Epub 2019 Jul 26. PMID: 31383477.

[3] Y. Yang, L. Xu, L. Sun, P. Zhang and S. S. Farid, "Machine Learning Application in Personalised Lung Cancer Recurrence and Survivability Prediction," *Computational and Structural Biotechnology Journal*, vol.20, pp. 1811–1820, 2022 Apr 4, doi: 10.1016/j. csbj.2022.03.035. PMID: 35521553; PMCID: PMC9043969.

[4] S. S. Raoof, M. A. Jabbar and S. A. Fathima, "Lung Cancer Prediction Using Machine Learning: A Comprehensive Approach," *2020 2nd International Conference on Innovative Mechanisms for Industry Applications (ICIMIA)*, 2020, pp. 108–115, doi: 10.1109/ ICIMIA48430.2020.9074947.

[5] D. A. Almuhaidib *et al.*, "Ensemble Learning Method for the Prediction of Breast Cancer Recurrence," *2018 1st International Conference on Computer Applications & Information Security (ICCAIS)*, 2018, pp. 1–6, doi: 10.1109/CAIS.2018.8442017.

[6] S. Gupta, M. Gupta and N. Garg, "ML Assistance in Cancer Detection & Treatment," *2021 International Conference on Computational Intelligence and Computing Applications (ICCICA)*, 2021, pp. 1–5, doi: 10.1109/ICCICA52458.2021.9697314.

[7] M. Sughasiny and J. Rajeshwari, "Application of Machine Learning Techniques, Big Data Analytics in Health Care Sector—A Literature Survey," *2018 2nd International Conference on I-SMAC (IoT in Social, Mobile, Analytics and Cloud) (I-SMAC) I-SMAC (IoT in Social, Mobile, Analytics and Cloud) (I-SMAC), 2018 2nd International Conference on*, 2018, pp. 741–749, doi: 10.1109/I-SMAC.2018.8653654.

[8] X. Bao, R. Shi, T. Zhao and Y. Wang, "Immune Landscape and a Novel Immunotherapy-Related Gene Signature Associated with Clinical Outcome in Early-Stage Lung Adenocarcinoma," *Journal of Molecular Medicine* (Berl), vol. 98, no. 6, pp. 805–818, 2020 Jun, doi: 10.1007/s00109-020-01908-9. Epub 2020 Apr 25. PMID: 32333046; PMCID: PMC7297823.

[9] K. A. Tran, O. Kondrashova, A. Bradley, et al., "Deep Learning in Cancer Diagnosis, Prognosis and Treatment Selection," *Genome Medicine*, vol. 13, p. 152, 2021. https://doi.org/10.1186/s13073-021-00968-x.

[10] P. Bhardwaj, Y. Kumar and G. Bhandari, "AI-Enabled Computational Techniques for Cancer Diagnosis," *2021 IEEE 8th Uttar Pradesh Section International Conference on Electrical, Electronics and Computer Engineering (UPCON)*, 2021, pp. 1–7, doi: 10.1109/UPCON52273.2021.9667624.

[11] S. Hussein, P. Kandel, C. W. Bolan, M. B. Wallace and U. Bagci, "Lung and Pancreatic Tumor Characterization in the Deep Learning Era: Novel Supervised and Unsupervised Learning Approaches," *IEEE Transactions on Medical Imaging*, vol. 38, no. 8, pp. 1777–1787, Aug. 2019, doi: 10.1109/TMI.2019.2894349.

[12] S. Kayikci and T. Khoshgoftaar, "A Stack Based Multimodal Machine Learning Model for Breast Cancer Diagnosis," *2022 International Congress on Human-Computer Interaction, Optimization and Robotic Applications (HORA)*, 2022, pp. 1–5, doi: 10.1109/HORA55278.2022.9800004.

[13] A. Sharma, S. Kulshrestha and S. Daniel, "Machine Learning Approaches for Breast Cancer Diagnosis and Prognosis," *2017 International Conference on Soft Computing and its Engineering Applications (icSoftComp)*, 2017, pp. 1–5, doi: 10.1109/ICSOFTCOMP.2017.8280082.

[14] A. P. Pawlovsky and M. Nagahashi, "A Method to Select a Good Setting for the kNN Algorithm When Using It for Breast Cancer Prognosis," *IEEE-EMBS International Conference on Biomedical and Health Informatics (BHI)*, 2014, pp. 189–192, doi: 10.1109/BHI.2014.6864336.

[15] M. Anitha, S. Gayathri, S. Nickolas and M. S. Bhanu, "Feature Engineering Based Automatic Breast Cancer Prediction," *2020 Second International Conference on Inventive Research in Computing Applications (ICIRCA)*, 2020, pp. 247–256, doi: 10.1109/ICIRCA48905.2020.9182855.

[16] S. C. Bellad *et al.*, "Prostate Cancer Prognosis-a Comparative Approach Using Machine Learning Techniques," *2021 5th International Conference on Intelligent Computing and Control Systems (ICICCS)*, 2021, pp. 1722–1728, doi: 10.1109/ICICCS51141.2021.9432173.

[17] D. German, B. Afsari, A. C. Tan and D. Q. Naiman, "Microarray Classification from Several Two-Gene Expression Comparisons," *2008 Seventh International Conference on Machine Learning and Applications*, 2008, pp. 583–585, doi: 10.1109/ICMLA.2008.152.

[18] A. Basavanhally, S. Doyle and A. Madabhushi, "Predicting Classifier Performance with a Small Training Set: Applications to Computer-Aided Diagnosis and Prognosis," *2010 IEEE International Symposium on Biomedical Imaging: From Nano to Macro*, 2010, pp. 229–232, doi: 10.1109/ISBI.2010.5490373.

[19] N. G. Maity and S. Das, "Machine Learning for Improved Diagnosis and Prognosis in Healthcare," *2017 IEEE Aerospace Conference*, 2017, pp. 1–9, doi: 10.1109/AERO.2017.7943950.

[20] G. Chandra, K. D. Irisha, V. I. Vica, P. A. Suri and M. E. Syahputra, "Systematic Literature Review on Application of Artificial Intelligence in Cancer Detection Using Image Processing," *2022 3rd International Conference on Artificial Intelligence and Data Sciences (AiDAS)*, 2022, pp. 273–277, doi: 10.1109/AiDAS56890.2022.9918734.

5 Secure Remote Monitoring of Diabetes Using IOT and Blockchain

Shobha Tyagi, Deepak Kumar, and Devendra Kumar

5.1 INTRODUCTION

One of the health problems with the greatest rate of growth in the globe is diabetes, which in some countries has epidemic proportions. It is primarily brought on by lifestyle decisions like weight, bad diet, and inactivity. Diabetes causes irregular levels of glucose in the blood, which may also cause a multitude of health problems that damage a person's kidneys, eyesight, and heart. Owing to these reasons, diabetes patients generally monitor their blood glucose levels using SMBG techniques by piercing their fingertips multiple times per day.

According to Anne Marit Longva and Moutaz Haddara [1] IoT technologies may help make diabetic patients' lives easier and better. Monitoring Blood Glucose (BG) levels, exercise, and food are essential for halting the disease's progression. They discovered that various IoT technologies can make it easier for patients and medical staff to keep an eye on these variables without having to make frequent trips to the doctor's office and hence lighten the workload for the typically understaffed medical staff. A few of the current options and services are networked sensors, wearable sensors, smartwatches, and RFID tags. Many advantages of patient security and efficiency are promised to be provided by these technologies. With the use of these solutions, critical problems including patient misidentification, insufficient patient monitoring, subpar patient tracking, and subpar decision-making may be removed [2]. Human error, which is cited as one of the major causes of drug errors, can also be reduced with the help of IoT technologies [3].

A device known as a continuous glucose monitor (CGM) may continuously take measurements of blood glucose all through the day without requiring the patient to be pricked for each measurement, which solves several issues with such techniques. Commercial CGMs that have Internet of Things (IoT) features can monitor patients remotely and alert users to potentially unsafe circumstances. For medical researchers, doctors, and caretakers to communicate accurate, dependable, and secure data,

DOI: 10.1201/9781003340133-5

the system also needs the creation of distributed storage system that acquires, handles, and saves the gathered data [4].

A system that can run smart contracts, automate the procurement of CGM sensors, or compensate users who support the system by providing their data is built using blockchain technology. The use of blockchain technology results in a data structure with built-in security measures. It is based on computer technologies that ensure the integrity of transactions, including as cryptographic methods, decentralization technology, database management, and consensus mechanism ideas. Distributed ledger technology (DLT), or blockchain, organizes the data into blocks. In a cryptographic chain, each block comprises a transaction or group of transactions. The way that each new block is tied to the one before it makes it nearly impossible to tamper with the chain. A consensus mechanism verifies and approves each transaction in the block, ensuring that each transaction is accurate and true. Through user participation over a dispersed peer-to-peer network, blockchain technology benefits from decentralization and distributed systems. There is no single point of failure because only one user can change the transaction record.

This approach would enable the users to crowdsource data and develop cutting-edge mobile health applications for identifying, observing, analyzing, and implementing public health programs that can enhance the treatment of the ailment and raise awareness of diabetes prevalence worldwide.

The COVID-19 pandemic, as per WHO, has resulted in a previously unheard-of global need for home nursing care to handle the 80% of COVID-19 patients with only limited flu-like diagnosis and for the implementation of digital wellness technology to deliver higher health standards. Additionally, the International Diabetes Federation (IDF) claims that the severe acute respiratory syndrome coronavirus may increase the risk of serious illness in older persons and people with chronic conditions like diabetes [5]. Managing diabetics who have a viral infection may be difficult due to variations in BG levels and the possibility of complications from diabetes [6]. If a COVID-19 patient is asymptomatic or has the mild to moderate form of the condition, they may be able to get care at home without the need for hospitalization or other emergency measures. Patients with COVID-19 who have mild, moderate, or asymptotic disease may be able to get care at home without needing to be hospitalized or take additional emergency measures. This necessitates at-home caring, resulting in a rise in the number of unpaid caregivers in the family.

A caregiver, whether paid or unpaid, is someone in the patient's social network who assists them with daily tasks [7]. Caregiving is widely utilized to address limitations brought on by old age, disabilities, illnesses, injuries, and mental disorders. Supporting carers is a crucial issue that has gone unnoticed globally despite the rise in demand for care. In the next 5–7 years, 25% of the world's population will be over 65, according to previously released statistics (United Nations Population Fund, 2021). Additionally, no nursing homes or hospitals are set up to handle the vast and expanding patient population. When it comes to discussing informed judgments about patients in a precise timestamped order, there are several communication problems between caregivers and the care team. Therefore, it is essential to address the difficulties that carers experience [8]. The care staff also faces a range of challenges while managing and keeping track of a large number of patients. Long wait periods and the need to see multiple doctors on the same day to receive comprehensive care are two additional challenges that patients must deal with. Additionally, this process could be distressing for them if they have disabilities.

Healthcare professionals are constantly trying to improve the services they provide. Some patients stand to gain significantly from medicine cost reduction via a pill cutter as they can utilize the savings for diagnostics using virtual reality (VR) and augmented reality (AR). A diabetic person's life is made easier to manage the immediate adjustments following receiving a diabetes diagnosis by incorporating AR and VR devices for surveillance. In order to reduce human error and provide accessible, low-cost healthcare to all people, hospital administrators around the world are eager to introduce AR and VR technologies.

The World Diabetes Federation estimates that 74,194,700 people were living with diabetes in India in 2021, or more than 74 million people. By 2030, this number is likely to increase to 92,973,700 patients, which are approximately 93 million people, as shown in Figure 5.1.

To address the rising epidemic, the IDF has emphasized the importance of developing and implementing multi-sectoral initiatives. Diabetes, as a lifestyle condition with multidimensional causal variables, necessitates multifaceted management. According to the IDF, diabetes accounts for 10% of worldwide health expenditures. All experts agreed that an emphasis on prevention was the way to go. India needs a more effective national diabetes prevention program, which will necessitate collaboration from a variety of sources, including medical education, school health awareness, and urban development.

This chapter describes a creative strategy for developing a patient-centered ecosystem of family care. One e-Home caregiving blockchain-based healthcare application houses all patient-centered data, making it simple for patients, medical professionals, and less-experienced family members to communicate. This is done in order to provide each team member with the psychological, physical, and medical assistance they require in order to monitor the patient's care and guarantee continuity.

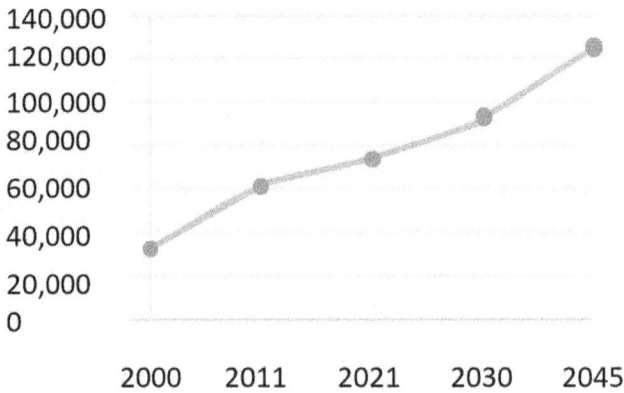

FIGURE 5.1   People with diabetes, in 1,000s, in India

This chapter presents the system design and implementation that incorporates the following elements to the previously mentioned problems:

- A description of a CGM-based Internet of Things (IoT) system that might monitor glucose levels remotely and notify patients and/or their carers of a potentially dangerous condition.
- Utilizing computing gateways to build a system that can immediately inform users in specific areas (such as a nursing home, a hospital, or a patient's home).
- An explanation of a decentralized, blockchain-based mHealth design that does not rely on a single entity.
- The suggestion of an information crowdsourcing system that rewards patients for collaboration.
- Analyzing the suggested architecture to judge how well the blockchain and decentralized storage described work.

5.2 DIABETES AND THE PANDEMIC

People all around the world are afflicted by diabetes, usually referred to as diabetes mellitus (DM). It is characterized by abnormal blood glucose oscillations that affect small blood vessels like the nerves, kidneys, and eyes as well as big blood vessels like the aorta, the coronary arteries, and the arteries in the brain and limbs. The three primary kinds of DM, according to the World Health Organization (WHO) [9], are as follows:

- **Type-1 Diabetes Mellitus (DM1):** is an autoimmune condition that causes noticeably lower insulin levels.
- **Type-2 Diabetes Mellitus (DM2):** this condition results from insulin resistance in peripheral tissues and impaired insulin production in the pancreas.
- **Gestational Diabetes Mellitus (GDM):** pregnant women with higher-than-normal BG levels are impacted by this disorder.

Patients with diabetes are more likely to get a significant disease when exposed to coronavirus 2 causing severe acute respiratory syndrome [10]. The IDF claims that because of changes in BG levels and the onset of diabetes-related complications, the viral infection may be challenging to treat. As a result, the IDF released specific instructions for diabetics who had contracted the virus. The instructions demand that caregivers oversee the patient's diet, including how much food and water they consume, how much medication they have available, and how often they check their blood sugar. Patients should complete this task, especially during the self-quarantine phase, or a family member if the patient is unable to do.

When monitoring or giving treatment for a diabetic patient with COVID-19, all the factors listed in the IDF recommendations should be taken into account. This outlines the ecology of patient-centered family caregiving that was previously mentioned. Figure 5.2 includes these as nutrition, exercise, therapy, and monitoring blood sugar levels. To spread patient-centered home caregiving, each component is

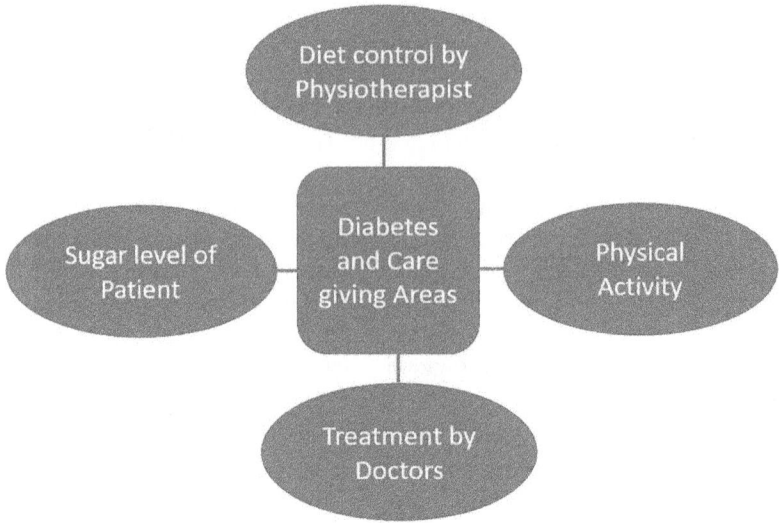

FIGURE 5.2 Diabetes and caregiving scope

supervised by a professional who works with the team. The range of diabetic care is outlined in Figure 5.2.

Applications that help caregiving can be categorized as pHealth and mHealth [11].

mHealth is a general term for the use of mobile devices and other wireless technology in healthcare, mHealth is the most popular application to educate users about various services offered by health care, mHealth is also used for monitoring, treatment support, epidemic outbreak tracking, and chronic disease management.

While this is going on, "pHealth increasingly integrates medical services with public health and epidemiological surveillance, preventative, social and geriatric care, as well as the eating and wellness to provide full care and protection" [12].

In order to treat the 85% of COVID-19 patients with the fewest symptoms of the flu and to increase health standards, the WHO asserts that COVID-19 has resulted in a huge growth of home care demand. The International Diabetes Federation (IDF) also notes that the coronavirus appears to be more dangerous to older persons and those with chronic conditions, such as diabetes, than to healthy individuals. This has created the need to monitor the diseases such as diabetes remotely. Using modern technology such as IoT and blockchain, as discussed next, it is made possible that a patient or the caregiver can share the reports and CGM readings with a doctor remotely from their home, and depending upon the reports, the doctor can prescribe the medicine.

Due to the health problems associated with DM, it's critical to watch out for at-risk populations, including kids, the elderly, and pregnant women. Continuous glucose monitors (CGMs) can address some of the problems with self-monitoring of blood glucose (SMBG) techniques, such as the patient's active participation or his or her caregivers in infection control. CGMs are based on a mobile device with a sensor component that continuously measures blood sugar [13]. Such monitoring has traditionally been carried out by taking blood samples [14]. These assessments help DM patients control their BG levels more precisely, enabling them to make well-informed therapy choices. CGMs may notify patients with low BG levels, which are also referred to as hypoglycemia, and high BG levels, which are also referred to as hyperglycemia, so that they can take the required precautions. Nevertheless, it is important to note that using CGMs has significant drawbacks: CGMs are often costly (some nations are beginning to provide subsidies for their purchases), typically take five to ten minutes to deliver data for glucose concentration [15], some CGMs need daily finger prick calibrations, and their normal lifespan is less (the typical duration is three days to two weeks; however more current CGMs continue to work for up to six months). Despite the existing disadvantages of CGM and the breakthrough of COVID-19 in 2019, the idea of CGM opens the door to the development of Internet of Things (IoT) devices that can issue quick alerts and make autonomous judgments when quick action is required to avert grave consequences [16].

A cloud-based system can therefore be utilized by an IoT CGM to store data and make rule-based decisions (for instance, alerting a physician if a patient's blood glucose level crosses or drops below a particular threshold). Due to the physical distance between the cloud and the patient and the possibility of overloading or cyberattacks, there may be a delay between the choice to act and the communication of the relevant information to the affected individual. In some circumstances, this delay may be too high. These limitations apply to traditional cloud computing architectures. Other approaches that move processing power from the cloud to the network's edge have been successful in situations like these when a quick reaction and little communications overhead are needed [17]. Fog computing is one of these paradigms; it brings communication and cloud computing capabilities close to the sensor devices to reduce latency, distribute storage and computing resources, improve position awareness, and scale networks while enabling connectivity between devices in various physical contexts [18, 19].

In order to expand upon what is already known about DM and to hunt for prospective treatments, physicians and researchers also require data. Since obtaining such medical data is frequently challenging for a variety of reasons, it is imperative to study novel methods for automating data collection on a large scale (for example, absence of access to data and prevailing restrictions, lack of trust of users). One potential method is crowdsourcing, which can tap into an online community's collective knowledge to conduct research, create new products and services with a human-centered focus, and innovate existing ones [20]. Especially in the field of mobile healthcare (mHealth), which utilizes cell phones and wireless communications technologies to increase the accessibility of healthcare treatments, there are few applications for public health crowdsourcing [21].

5.3   IOT AND BLOCKCHAIN

Several businesses are being transformed by the Internet of Things (IoT), which offers previously unimaginable possibilities and opportunities. The healthcare sector is one of those that directly affect people in a significant way. Over the past 40 years, there has been a significant rise in the population with diabetes, and this trend is projected to continue in the upcoming decades.

The Internet of Things (IoT) is a large network of people and objects that are linked together. All of these gadgets collect and exchange data about their surroundings and usage, as seen in Figure 5.3. Sensor-equipped products and goods are connected to an IoT platform, which analyzes data from several devices and integrates it with other sources to deliver the most relevant information with applications made to meet specific requirements [22, 23]. IoT devices are multiplying exponentially. There are currently 20 billion devices linked to the Internet, according to forecasts [24]. Numerous gadgets connect to the Internet each year, storing their data on centralized servers. When handling sensitive and private data, this design poses various concerns about security and privacy. Considering adopting a security framework access control, firewalls, cryptography, intrusion detection systems, redundancy reduction techniques, and standard security precautions are just a few examples of the tools and methods that can be used to support the three essential security components: confidentiality, integrity, and availability [25].

When sensitive and substantial data are handled by smart health systems, data security poses a serious concern. The blockchain, which is already successfully

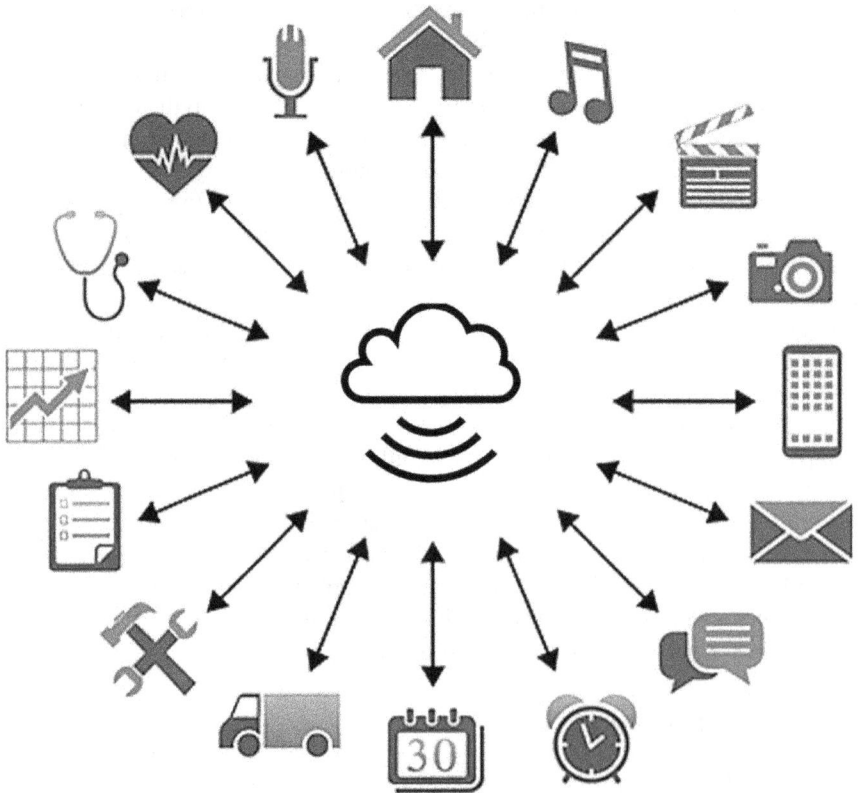

FIGURE 5.3   Internet of Things

protecting cryptocurrency transactions [26], could give further security to the Internet of Things.

The IoT integrity verification and access control have all been addressed by many studies and businesses using blockchain technology in recent years. IoT device management utilizing the Ethereum blockchain is described by the authors in [27]. Electricity usage was monitored via a meter using smart contracts, which were also used to set up energy-use restrictions.

A. Dorri et al. propose a suggestion [28] that protects IoT devices using both public and private blockchains. A private blockchain for smart homes is used to provide regional communication and policy archiving, and it is centrally managed by a miner. Outside of the smart home, transactions are handled on a public blockchain. FairAccess, a solution proposed by the authors in [29]. It is a blockchain-based system for managing IoT access management that uses smart contracts to set policies and issue authorization tokens. Another ongoing project intends to link IoT endpoints with blockchain infrastructure that is low-power and storage-capable [30]. For data routing and integrity checks, they employed the LoRa gateway and Ethereum blockchain.

Blockchain is known as distributed, cryptographic hashed, and immutable ledger of transactions [31]. For instance, to send digital currency to client B, client A needs to start a transaction in the cryptocurrency network. Miners must approve the transaction for the blockchain network to commit it.

The block is entered into the blockchain after being verified by other nodes as genuine. Once the block is appended to the blockchain, the cryptocurrency transferred from A to B is considered complete and legitimate. The consensus mechanism, hash-chained storage, and digital signature are the three main features of Bitcoin blockchain technology.

Blockchain has become a widely used technology that is built using protocols and techniques in distributed systems and cryptography introduced by Bitcoin. Now, numerous uses for the blockchain have been discovered in a variety of fields, including cryptocurrencies, banking, healthcare, advertising, societal applications, non-fungible tokens (NFT), etc. As seen in Table 5.1, blockchain can be roughly divided into public and private categories.

TABLE 5.1
Types of blockchain

	Public	Private
Access	Anyone	Single organization or consortium
Authority	Decentralized	Partially decentralized
Consensus	Permissionless	Permissioned
Data handling	Anyone can read and write	Only an organization or a consortium can read and write
Efficiency	Low	High
Immutability	Full	Partial
Transaction speed	Slow	High

The e-Home caregiving approach is a patient-centered mHealth created for a family caring that uses blockchain technology to address caregiver burnout as it appears in isolation and unpreparedness. By enabling them to continuously monitor and document the care-delivering changes, and general psychological and health status, e-Home caregiving empowers caregivers. The care team's chosen diabetes treatment plan is available to caregivers. The patient's related disease may be treated as part of the treatment plan. Additionally, it offers details on how to manage the time of the nurses and their families as well as the accessibility of authorized individuals. The key benefit is the potential to consistently care for the patient by assembling pertinent caregivers into a blockchain technology-based community [32]. This application lessens the work and financial stress on a single caregiver by connecting the carers who are close to the patient. In this study, effective use of blockchain technology is done. Caretakers may securely communicate with one another using blockchain technology, which eliminates the need for middlemen. Additionally, blockchain technology creates a chain of immutable, trustworthy, and timestamped constituents (changing care continuity) that are distributed across the caregiver network, with each caregiver receiving the same information as a ledger [33].

In accordance with [34], blockchains have four distinct levels of visibility and accessibility, as depicted in Figure 5.4. Only certain people are allowed entry into the permissionless private category. Everyone is allowed access and visibility in the permissionless public category. Only a specific person is allowed access and visibility in the permissioned private category, and visibility is allowed to everyone in the permissioned public category but only specific individuals have access.

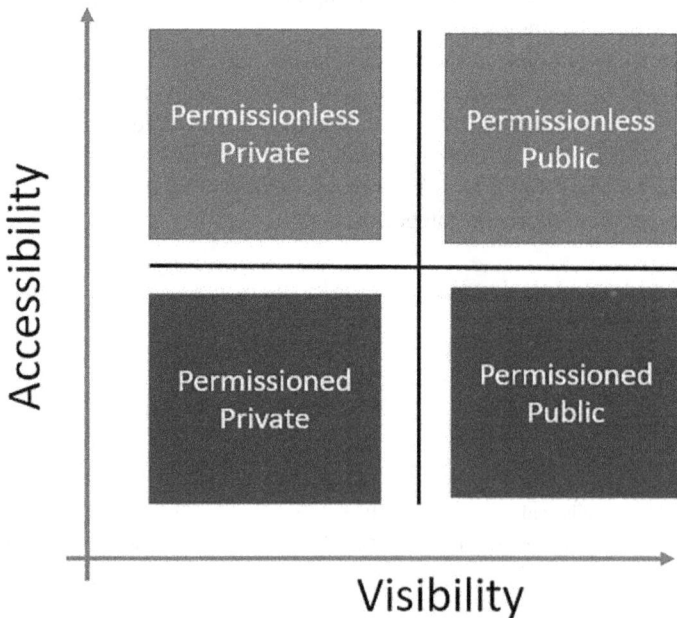

FIGURE 5.4   Blockchain systems visibility and accessibility matrix

For the purposes of this study, private permission is appropriate so that only members of the patient's known care team are allowed to access and read their information. Because Ethereum is open source and allows advanced blockchain versions for applications outside of Bitcoin and financial services, it is used as a blockchain platform [35]. Because the e-Home caregiving ecosystem needs role-based access control, the consensus algorithm used for the blockchain is proof of identity. The private key of the user that is associated with a particular transaction serves as proof of identification. The greatest match for role-based private permission categories is for every recognized user from a blockchain system to be able to construct a block of data that is available to any person on the network (depending on their role). Data integrity and authenticity are guaranteed by the confirmation of identity. The agreement method used by e-Home caregiving allows the comparison of the private keys of authorized carers to an approved identity.

5.4 SYSTEM DESIGN

In this section, system architecture and the data crowdsourcing incentive mechanism are discussed.

5.4.1 SYSTEM ARCHITECTURE

In this section, the functioning of the diabetes monitoring system is discussed. The objective is to build a platform for smart diabetic self-care and monitoring. The benefit of utilizing IoT is that it makes data collection easier and automates data exchange. However, the platform uses blockchain security and smart contracts to guarantee authenticity, consistency, secrecy, and traceability. This would help patients completely control their data. In addition to keeping track of the data that has been accessed, they would be able to define permissions and access rules.

The problem with this combination of IoT with blockchain is that self-care medical equipment has limited storage and processing capabilities. They are therefore difficult to incorporate into a blockchain architecture. Normally, it is not supported for a light client installation to function as a node in the blockchain network. To send data from sensors to the blockchain, some works suggested using a gateway as a node. It is still difficult to safeguard the link between the patient's gadgets and the gateway, though. A malicious third party could, for instance, add devices to convey fraudulent information or harm the gateway. On this level, emphasis is placed on increasing security. The solution is to require each new owner to register the device on the blockchain. This will prevent unauthorized devices from accessing the platform until their owners register them and authorize them. Four components make up the safe remote monitoring architecture: connected gadgets/devices, smart contracts, a blockchain network, and medical personnel.

5.4.1.1 Connected Devices

Two categories of connected devices are distinguished. The first category includes medical equipment, wearables, and sensors that gather data on health, including glucose levels, blood pressure, heart rate, weight, and other crucial indicators for monitoring diabetes. The medical staff receives measurements from these gadgets automatically through a smartphone. A smartphone is the second sort, acting as a link between medical equipment and blockchain technology. It makes use of a mobile application to manage, encrypt, and route data from gadgets to an off-chain database that may be accessed by qualified medical professionals and healthcare staff. By using this application, the patient will be able to communicate with both their equipment and their doctors. By using the application, a patient would be able to add or remove devices and grant or revoke access, and these actions are translated into transactions that will be transferred to and recorded in the blockchain network.

Since the patient is constantly on the go and cannot be at home all the time, the choice of a smartphone as a gateway is not random. A safe system is therefore required that can track him wherever he goes, including at work, home, and even when he travels. Given that the patient is constantly on the go and cannot spend his entire day at home, the choice of a smartphone as a gateway was not made at random.

5.4.1.2   Blockchain Network

Smartphones have enabled the connection of medical devices to a permissioned blockchain. Each patient will use their smartphone to play the role of the light nodes due to the storage capacity limitations of the device. Public health agencies, laboratories, and hospitals will all be full nodes. They'll keep track of data pointers, verify transactions, make blocks, and add these to the blockchain. By recording all data alterations, the blockchain will preserve access control laws, enhance security, and maintain data traceability for each patient. Only a reference to data (a data hash) will be stored on the blockchain, unlike health information, which will be encrypted and kept as a key-value pair off-chain. A peer-to-peer distributed file system keeps the off-chain storage updated. The IPFS will supply the hash that will be stored in the blockchain, and each patient's data will be encrypted and saved there. Patients can decide whether or not to provide access to outside parties. Additionally, they have the option to decide which data should remain public and for whom. All healthcare organizations can access the data while protecting patient privacy thanks to data encryption and the use of distinct IDs to identify each patient (their public key). This serves as their representation on the blockchain and prevents his identification. Doctors should be able to access required data in an emergency, thus every patient may choose the data, encrypt it ahead of time, and then share the secret key via a secret sharing technique. The medical staff should next work with the patient's family members to obtain the decryption key to access this material.

5.4.1.3   Smart Contracts

Smart contracts are generated, converted to byte code, and then implemented on the blockchain network. Sending a transaction to the address of a smart contract will initiate it. Each smart contract has a unique address that serves as its identity. The smart contract will operate autonomously and without help from a third party whenever the predefined criteria are met. By recording each data manipulation, smart contracts will be employed in this project to build a log for traceability. Additionally, it will be used to set policies, authenticate users, allow or revoke access, and register or delete devices.

5.4.1.4   Health Organization and Medical Teams

Researchers, pharmaceutical laboratories, clinics, diabetes management centers, public health groups, and general healthcare practitioners can all be involved. These parties will be connected by a permissioned blockchain so that users can access the data. By doing this, public health organizations will be able to collect information for use in research or statistics, among other things, and doctors will be able to keep an eye on the health of their patients.

5.4.2   Mechanism for Data Crowdsourcing Incentive

Laying the foundation for an ecosystem for mHealth data crowdsourcing that other parties may utilize to increase existing understanding and research on DM is one of the project's objectives. The patients must be encouraged to send the CGM device readings to the decentralized storage nodes in order for anybody with permission to view them, which is necessary to accomplish this goal. The CGM-based IoT system automates this process of data collection as the first incentive step to make it simpler. The user just needs to check their BG levels after the system is configured (i.e., after setting up the required gateways and the mobile application). The remaining procedures (such as data processing, uploading, dissemination, and notifications) can be carried out without user involvement.

The second reward mechanism relates to patients who might not be eager to submit their data through the suggested crowdsourcing platform either publicly or for free. The blockchain makes it possible to establish a private healthcare system where patients are paid for their contributions to the system's mHealth data; the more data they provide, the higher the reward.

The incentive is based on the use of a meta coin, a sort of virtual currency that builds additional transaction logic on top of an already-in-use blockchain. On the Ethereum blockchain, a meta coin named DbtCoin (D) can be developed. Every participant in DbtCoin must create a digital wallet, which performs all the software actions required by a cryptocurrency, primarily involving getting a user's balance and transmitting money from one user account to another.

DbtCoin can be used by users to pay for goods and services, in addition to compensating them for their data. Patients may, for instance, use their DbtCoins to automatically purchase new CGM sensors when their current ones run out.

5.5   SYSTEM IMPLEMENTATION

Various tools required to carry out the aforementioned approach are described in this section.

The usage of a permissioned blockchain is necessary because the blockchain deals with medical data that requires a high degree of safety and privacy control. The nodes that are allowed to take part in the consensus method on this sort of blockchain can be limited. By utilizing authoritative evidence, the consensus is reached (POA). Only the predefined validators (in this case, full nodes) are permitted to add new blocks to the blockchain using this consensus mechanism, keeping the network secure. It is possible to create a speedier blockchain with less computational power and reduced energy consumption. A private Ethereum blockchain is employed in the testing.

To communicate with the blockchain, a decentralized application (DApp) is required. Decentralized applications, or DApps, operate on peer-to-peer networks without a central server. Due to its decentralized structure, it has several aspects that make it incredibly intriguing. Its client-side (front-end) was created using JavaScript, CSS, and HTML. Instead of a backend web server, this side is linked to a blockchain and combined with smart contracts. In this instance, the patient will do several transactions using the application interface (Figure 5.5).

Transactions: Each doctor will create a QR code for each of his patients, which he will then use to add and register each one in the blockchain. The Ethereum address of the doctor and details on the blockchain network will be included in this QR code. The patient will have access to a variety of transactions and activities once he or she has registered in the blockchain, including the capacity to add or delete devices, allow or revoke access to other nodes, make policies, see one's own data, and show particular summaries. These transactions will be started by the DApp and added to the blockchain for traceability. Smart contracts will be launched as a result. His doctor will enter the patient's information and register them in the blockchain.

Device registration: Using an add transaction, the patient will register each new device in the blockchain at this stage. The MAC address of each device will serve as

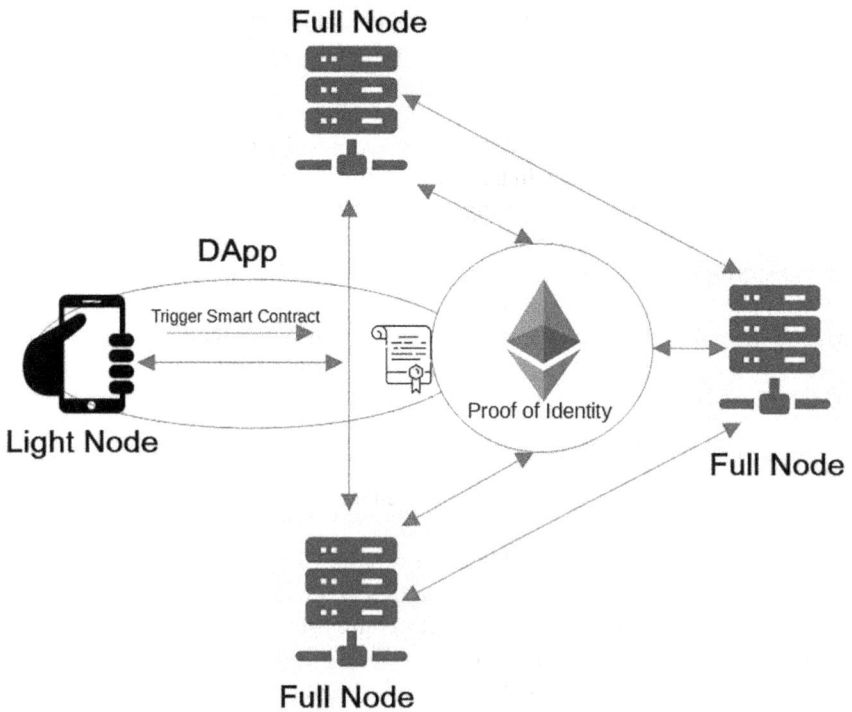

FIGURE 5.5 Blockchain-patient interaction using a decentralized application

its unique identity, and the patient's public Ethereum address will serve as the identity of its owner. Because of this, only the patient can add a device. In this manner, the patient can have complete control over his devices and be shielded from malevolent ones.

Data encryption: Before being stored in the IPFS, the patient will encrypt the data. A smart contract will evaluate a party's eligibility once it sends a transaction through the DApp requesting access to data. The patient will provide the decryption key encrypted by the public key of the permitted party if the party has access authorization. To gain access to the data, the authorized party must decode the message using his private key.

5.6 CONCLUSION

This work addressed the design, development, and evaluation of a mobile crowd-sourced IoT CGM-based system for diabetes care and research. With the help of such a system, blood sugar levels from CGMs that is accessed remotely can be collected. As a result, the technology enables real-time warnings to patients in the event of a critical circumstance.

Monitoring health data, such as BG levels, regularly can help control and manage diabetes, which is a very vital task. The utilization of IoT devices is required to automate that process. Employing a secure system is vital because this information needs to be communicated to a medical team quickly and securely. A system is suggested based on the integration of IoT and blockchain to gather health information and distribute it to medical units for regular smart care.

To safeguard against malicious nodes or devices, attention was given to patient privacy and device security. As proof of identity, consensus algorithm that uses less time and energy was chosen for a faster system. Each system component is currently given a thorough conceptualization. The system is subsequently put into use by offering a proof-of-concept to demonstrate the viability of the technique, to verify its performance, and then, if necessary, to suggest some changes. Future work will also involve the analysis of node activities using artificial intelligence so that the system can quickly spot out-of-the-ordinary node behavior. Advanced and promising technologies such as AR and VR will also be explored and try to incorporated.

REFERENCES

[1] A. M. Longva, and M. Haddara, "How Can IoT Improve the Life-Quality of Diabetes Patients?" *MATEC Web of Conferences*, vol. 292, p. 03016, 2019, doi: 10.1051/matecconf/201929203016.

[2] L. Hu, D. M. Ong, X. Zhu, Q. Liu, and E. Song, "Enabling RFID technology for Healthcare: Application, Architecture, and Challenges," *Telecommunication Systems*, vol. 58, no. 3, pp. 259–271, Oct. 2014, doi: 10.1007/s11235-014-9871-x.

[3] M. Haddara, and A. Staaby, "RFID Applications and Adoptions in Healthcare: A Review on Patient Safety," *Procedia Computer Science*, vol. 138, pp. 80–88, 2018, doi: 10.1016/j.procs.2018.10.012.

[4] K. Azbeg, O. Ouchetto, and S. Jai Andaloussi, "BlockMedCare: A Healthcare System Based on IoT, Blockchain and IPFS for Data Management Security," *Egyptian Informatics Journal*, vol. 23, no. 2, pp. 329–343, Jul. 2022, doi: 10.1016/j.eij.2022.02.004.

[5] A. Hussain, and A. J. M. Boulton, "COVID-19 and Diabetes: International Diabetes Federation Perspectives," *Diabetes Research and Clinical Practice*, vol. 167, p. 108339, Sep. 2020, doi: 10.1016/j.diabres.2020.108339.

[6] T. M. Fernández-Caramés, I. Froiz-Míguez, O. Blanco-Novoa, and P. Fraga-Lamas, "Enabling the Internet of Mobile Crowdsourcing Health Things: A Mobile Fog Computing, Blockchain and IoT Based Continuous Glucose Monitoring System for Diabetes Mellitus Research and Care," *Sensors*, vol. 19, no. 15, p. 3319, Jul. 2019, doi: 10.3390/s19153319.

[7] C. K. Hunt, "Concepts in Caregiver Research," *Journal of Nursing Scholarship*, vol. 35, no. 1, pp. 27–32, Mar. 2003, doi: 10.1111/j.1547-5069.2003.00027.x.

[8] H. A. Alsalamah *et al.*, "eHomeCaregiving: A Diabetes Patient-Centered Blockchain Ecosystem for COVID-19 Caregiving," *Frontiers in Blockchain*, vol. 4, Jun. 2021, doi: 10.3389/fbloc.2021.477012.

[9] "Diabetes," *World Health Organization. Diabetes*, 2 November 2011. https://www.who.int/europe/news-room/fact-sheets/item/diabetes.

[10] A. Hussain, B. Bhowmik, and N. C. do Vale Moreira, "COVID-19 and Diabetes: Knowledge in Progress," *Diabetes Research and Clinical Practice*, vol. 162, p. 108142 Apr. 2020, doi: 10.1016/j.diabres.2020.108142.

[11] T. Fernández-Caramés, and P. Fraga-Lamas, "Design of a Fog Computing, Blockchain and IoT-Based Continuous Glucose Monitoring System for Crowdsourcing mHealth," *5th International Electronic Conference on Sensors and Applications*, Nov. 2018, Published, doi: 10.3390/ecsa-5-05757.

[12] W. Goossen, and B. Blobel, "pHealth 2017," *Proceedings of the 14th International Conference on Wearable Micro and Nano Technologies for Personalized Health,* 14–16 May. 2017, Eindhoven, The Netherlands. IOS Press.

[13] I. Torres, M. G. Baena, M. Cayon, J. Ortego-Rojo, and M. Aguilar-Diosdado, "Use of Sensors in the Treatment and Follow-Up of Patients with Diabetes Mellitus," *Sensors*, vol. 10, no. 8, pp. 7404–7420, Aug. 2010, doi: 10.3390/s100807404.

[14] E. M. Benjamin, "Self-Monitoring of Blood Glucose: The Basics," *Clinical Diabetes*, vol. 20, no. 1, pp. 45–47, Jan. 2002, doi: 10.2337/diaclin.20.1.45.

[15] G. Schmelzeisen-Redeker, M. Schoemaker, H. Kirchsteiger, G. Freckmann, L. Heinemann, and L. del Re, "Time Delay of CGM Sensors," *Journal of Diabetes Science and Technology*, vol. 9, no. 5, pp. 1006–1015, Aug. 2015, doi: 10.1177/1932296815590154.

[16] P. Fraga-Lamas *et al.*, "Enabling Automatic Event Detection for the Pipe Workshop of the Shipyard 4.0," *2017 56th FITCE Congress*, Sep. 2017, Published, doi: 10.1109/fitce.2017.8093002.

[17] E. K. Markakis *et al.*, "EXEGESIS: Extreme Edge Resource Harvesting for a Virtualized Fog Environment," *IEEE Communications Magazine*, vol. 55, no. 7, pp. 173–179, 2017, doi: 10.1109/mcom.2017.1600730.

[18] F. Bonomi, R. Milito, J. Zhu, and S. Addepalli, "Fog Computing and Its Role in the Internet of Things," *Proceedings of the First Edition of the MCC Workshop on Mobile Cloud Computing—MCC '12*, 2012, Published, doi: 10.1145/2342509.2342513.

[19] T. Fernández-Caramés, P. Fraga-Lamas, M. Suárez-Albela, and M. Díaz-Bouza, "A Fog Computing Based Cyber-Physical System for the Automation of Pipe-Related Tasks in the Industry 4.0 Shipyard," *Sensors*, vol. 18, no. 6, p. 1961, Jun. 2018, doi: 10.3390/s18061961.

[20] K. C. Sen, and K. Ghosh, "Designing Effective Crowdsourcing Systems for the Healthcare Industry," *Crowdsourcing*, pp. 257–261, 2019, doi: 10.4018/978-1-5225-8362-2.ch014.

[21] D. C. Brabham, K. M. Ribisl, T. R. Kirchner, and J. M. Bernhardt, "Crowdsourcing Applications for Public Health," *American Journal of Preventive Medicine*, vol. 46, no. 2, pp. 179–187, Feb. 2014, doi: 10.1016/j.amepre.2013.10.016.

[22] G. Alfian, M. Syafrudin, N. L. Fitriyani, M. A. Syaekhoni, and J. Rhee, "Utilizing IoT-Based Sensors and Prediction Model for Health-Care Monitoring System," *Artificial Intelligence and Big Data Analytics for Smart Healthcare*, pp. 63–80, 2021, doi: 10.1016/b978-0-12-822060-3.00009-7.

[23] A. Pati *et al.*, "Diagnose Diabetic Mellitus Illness Based on IoT Smart Architecture," *Wireless Communications and Mobile Computing*, vol. 2022, pp. 1–20, Aug. 2022, doi: 10.1155/2022/7268571.

[24] A. Naseem, R. Habib, T. Naz, M. Atif, M. Arif, and S. Allaoua Chelloug, "Novel Internet of Things Based Approach Toward Diabetes Prediction Using Deep Learning Models," *Frontiers in Public Health*, vol. 10, Aug. 2022, doi: 10.3389/fpubh.2022.914106.

[25] M. Frustaci, P. Pace, G. Aloi, and G. Fortino, "Evaluating Critical Security Issues of the IoT World: Present and Future Challenges," *IEEE Internet of Things Journal*, vol. 5, no. 4, pp. 2483–2495, Aug. 2018, doi: 10.1109/jiot.2017.2767291.

[26] S. Nakamoto, "Bitcoin: A Peer-to-Peer Electronic Cash System," *Bitcoin: A Peer-to-Peer Electronic Cash System*. https://bitcoin.org/en/bitcoin-paper (accessed Oct. 28, 2022).

[27] S. Huh, S. Cho, and S. Kim, "Managing IoT Devices Using Blockchain Platform," *2017 19th International Conference on Advanced Communication Technology (ICACT)*, 2017, Published, doi: 10.23919/icact.2017.7890132.

[28] A. Dorri, S. S. Kanhere, and R. Jurdak, "Towards an Optimized Blockchain for IoT," *Proceedings of the Second International Conference on Internet-of-Things Design and Implementation*, Apr. 2017, Published, doi: 10.1145/3054977.3055003.

[29] A. Ouaddah, A. Abou Elkalam, and A. Ait Ouahman, "FairAccess: A New Blockchain-Based Access Control Framework for the Internet of Things," *Security and Communication Networks*, vol. 9, no. 18, pp. 5943–5964, Dec. 2016, doi: 10.1002/sec.1748.

[30] K. R. Özyılmaz, and A. Yurdakul, "Integrating Low-Power IoT Devices to a Blockchain-Based Infrastructure," *Proceedings of the Thirteenth ACM International Conference on Embedded Software 2017 Companion—EMSOFT '17*, 2017, Published, doi: 10.1145/3125503.3125628.

[31] S. Tyagi, and M. Kathuria, "Role of Zero-Knowledge Proof in Blockchain Security," *2022 International Conference on Machine Learning, Big Data, Cloud and Parallel Computing (COM-IT-CON)*, May 2022, Published, doi: 10.1109/com-it-con54601.2022.9850714.

[32] D. Khan, L. T. Jung, M. A. Hashmani, and M. K. Cheong, "Blockchain Enabled Diabetic Patients' Data Sharing and Real Time Monitoring," *Embedded Systems and Applications*, Mar. 2022, Published, doi: 10.5121/csit.2022.120620.

[33] M. Crawford, "Risk Management Magazine-The Insurance Implications of Blockchain," *The Insurance Implications of Blockchain*. www.rmmagazine.com/articles/article/2017/03/01/-The-Insurance-Implications-of-Blockchain (accessed Oct. 28, 2022).

[34] S. Al-Megren *et al.*, "Blockchain Use Cases in Digital Sectors: A Review of the Literature," *2018 IEEE International Conference on Internet of Things (iThings) and IEEE Green Computing and Communications (GreenCom) and IEEE Cyber, Physical and Social Computing (CPSCom) and IEEE Smart Data (SmartData)*, Jul. 2018, Published, doi: 10.1109/cybermatics_2018.2018.00242.

[35] M. Swan, *Blockchain: Blueprint for a New Economy*. Sebastopol, CA: O'Reilly Media, Inc., 2015, doi: https://dl.acm.org/doi/10.5555/3006358.

6 AR/VR Revolutions in Future Healthcare

Dr. Pawan Whig, Shama Kouser, Ankit Sharma, Ashima Bhatnagar Bhatia, and Rahul Reddy Nadikattu

6.1 INTRODUCTION

Many people think about movies or science fiction whenever we talk about virtual reality. In today's world in which we are talking about Industry 4.0 [1]. With the help of AI and machine learning, a parallel virtual world is created. The advancement and adaptation in technology are so rapid that everyone is addicted to it. After the mobile, VR will either upend our lives in a way that none has, or it's the technical equivalent of attempting to make "fetch" happen. In 2012, when VR first appeared from anonymity at a video game trade show, the poles of that debate were established; they continued through the $3 billion Facebook purchase of headset manufacturer Oculus in 2014, through years of refinement and progress, and well into the first and a half generation of mobile hardware. Somewhere in there, the truth is probable [2]. Yet augmented reality, in any event, marks an unprecedented transition in the way people view the digital world. Computing has always been a controlled experience: Through screens and keyboards, people transfer information back and forth. VR promises to completely do away with the pesky middle sheet. Like the virtual reality (VR) cousin of VR, which is often referred to as mixed reality (MR), not to mention that VR, AR, and MR can both be lumped under the "extended reality" umbrella term XR [3].

6.2 VIRTUAL REALITY

Virtual reality (VR) is a computer-generated universe of scenes and objects that appear to be actual, enabling the user to feel immersed in their surroundings. To view this world, a device known as a virtual reality headset or helmet is used. VR helps one to immerse ourselves in video games as if we were one of the characters, learn how to do heart surgery, or boost the quality of physical fitness to maximize results, as shown in Figure 6.1 [4].

Although this might sound unbelievably modern, it's not as new as we'd assume its origins are. Many people consider that one of the first augmented reality devices was Sensorama, a device with a built-in seat that played 3D movies, gave off smells, and generated vibrations to make the world as vivid as possible. The invention dates

DOI: 10.1201/9781003340133-6

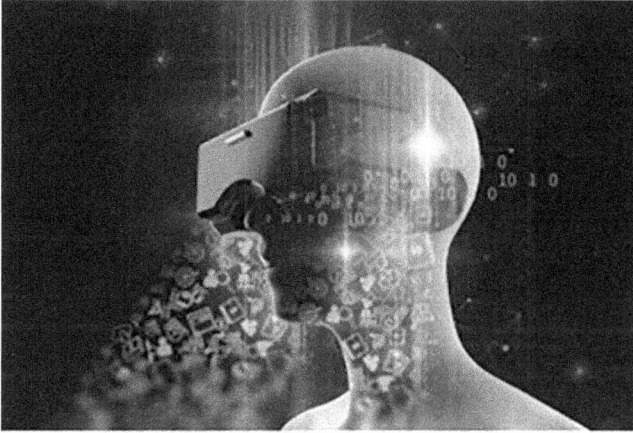

FIGURE 6.1 Virtual reality

to as early as the mid-1950s. Subsequent technological and software developments have taken a progressive transformation of electronics as well as interface design with them over the years that followed [5].

6.3 AUGMENTED REALITY

Augmented reality can be defined as reality, enhanced with digital elements. To showcase the digitally augmented world, the most widely used AR apps these days rely on smartphones: Users can enable the camera on a smartphone, view the world around them on the device, and rely on an AR application to improve the world in any variety of ways:

- Images superimposing
- Adding instructions in real-time
- Insertions of stickers
- Modifying shades

6.4 VIRTUAL ENVIRONMENT

The world in which it takes place is a very critical feature of augmented reality and must be deliberately designed to achieve a compelling experience. For starters, if even the smallest of items are out of place in a virtual reality world, the whole experience will be lost. It must hit at least some level of immersion for it to be persuasive [6]. Immersion is one of virtual reality's main purposes, and it can also be designed with an eye to immersion as a virtual world is engineered. The natural world will also be forgotten as immersion exists.

6.5   VR ENVIRONMENTS TYPES

There are several types of environments for virtual reality, each with its level of immersion and functionality. Any of which are located here:

- Semi-Immersive Augmented Reality CAVE Collaborative Virtual Worlds Immersive Virtual Reality.
- The level of immersion can vary based on the kind of climate. A semi-immersive environment, for instance, does not aspire for full immersion, which allows it to run at much lower costs than the CAVE. Complete commitment, on the other hand, is not feasible, which the CAVE would easily achieve [7].
- Collaborative experiences are a special case in which they can or may not aspire for full immersion, but the primary focus is to communicate with actual persons a simulated experience.

The type of virtual reality experience selected depends solely on the project's budget and priorities. The air force uses a virtual reality flight simulator as a teaching tool, for example. This is one instance of an augmented reality experience that is semi-immersive. A truly interactive experience would not be sufficient. On the other hand, a completely interactive experience would be sufficient for maximum participation and would be a credible tool for the analysis of different ethical problems around virtual reality [8].

6.6   IMMERSION

Immersion is a special sensation related to the realm of virtual reality. Over here, the entire person navigating the three-dimensional realm of augmented reality would only immerse themselves in this world of belief as the real world. It is simply a feeling of user engagement, intelligently built by professionals in the virtual world. This unusual mix is known as telepresence, where the user can immerse and communicate with the simulations as well. This is the theory of Jonathan Steuer, a prominent computer scientist [9]. The consumer, therefore, forgets his real-world scenario, forgets his actual personality, circumstance, and life, and immerses him in a world of fantasy, adventure, and discovery. Inside the realm of virtual reality, he becomes more focused on his newly created persona.

As Jonathan Steuer says, immersion consists of two main components:

- Depth of Data
- Broadness of Data

While a user uses simulations and communications between the user and the simulated world, some data quality is derived from the signals. Such data is known as knowledge depth. Knowledge depth will necessarily include everything and anything, starting with the display device resolution, the nature of the graphics, audio and video performance, etc. Jonathan Steuer also describes knowledge width as a variety of concurrently presented sensory aspects. Whenever it activates all human senses, every simulated world may be designated as providing a broader breadth of knowledge.

The consumer should be fully focused on the new personality and culture that he is discovering. The most studied area in the development of a successful virtual world is the audio and visual effects. These are known as the key variables that can activate all sensory organs of the patient. When it has become the dominating force in relaxing a human being, the sense of touch is given more and more importance. Those systems that allow users to connect by touch are referred to as Baptist Systems [10].

6.7 VIRTUAL REALITY VS. AUGMENTED REALITY

Despite being a technique that emerged decades ago, the augmented reality paradigm is still new to many individuals. Confusing the term virtual reality with augmented reality is still very popular [11]. The biggest distinction between the two is that, with a different headset, VR creates the world in which we immerse ourselves. It is interactive, and all we see is part of a digitally created world through pictures, sounds, etc. In augmented reality (AR), on the other hand, our universe becomes the context through which objects, pictures, and the like are put. All we see is in the real world, and wearing a headset might not be specifically required. Pokémon Go is the clearest and most mainstream example of this notion.

There is, though, a mixture of these realities called blended or mixed reality as well. For example, this hybrid technology makes it possible to see virtual objects in the real world and to create an environment where the tangible and the digital are essentially indistinguishable.

6.8 HISTORY OF VR

It's a bit fuzzier as true VR takes hold of our brains as an all-encompassing simulacrum. As for other scientific breakthroughs, the vision undoubtedly originated with science fiction, primarily the short story *Pygmalion's Spectacles* by Stanley G. Weinbaum in 1935, in which a physicist creates a pair of glasses that will "make it so that you are in the story, you speak to the shadows, and the shadows respond, and the story is all about you and you are in it instead of being on a screen," as shown in Figure 6.2.

6.9 BEGINNING OF VIRTUAL REALITY IN THE '80S AND EARLY '90S

6.9.1 1838

The stereoscope was invented by Charles Wheatstone. He noticed that you'll see a 3D vision if you draw something from two subtly different viewpoints and then see each image from a different lens. The stereoscope gave such a chance to the spectator. For the tools we use today, this gadget paved the way: cinematography, lighting, and others.

6.9.2 1849

David Brewster upgrades the stereoscope and makes a "lenticular stereoscope" in this manner. To create the first portable 3D viewer, he used the effects of his experiments and physical optics.

6.9.3 1901

L. Frank Baum publishes a novel and, for the first time in history, references AR-like technology. *The Master Key: An Electrical Fairy Tale* is a book featuring a young boy who is passionate about electricity and electronics. When the Demon of Electricity was summoned, he gave him a gift—the "character marker," a pair of glasses that exposed the latent character defects of humans.

6.9.4 1929

Ed Link produces the "Link Trainer" flight simulator. Thanks to the use of pumps, valves, and other equipment, this simulator helped pilots to obtain an accurate depiction of how it feels to fly an aircraft. This was a successful effort to introduce a virtual reality prototype.

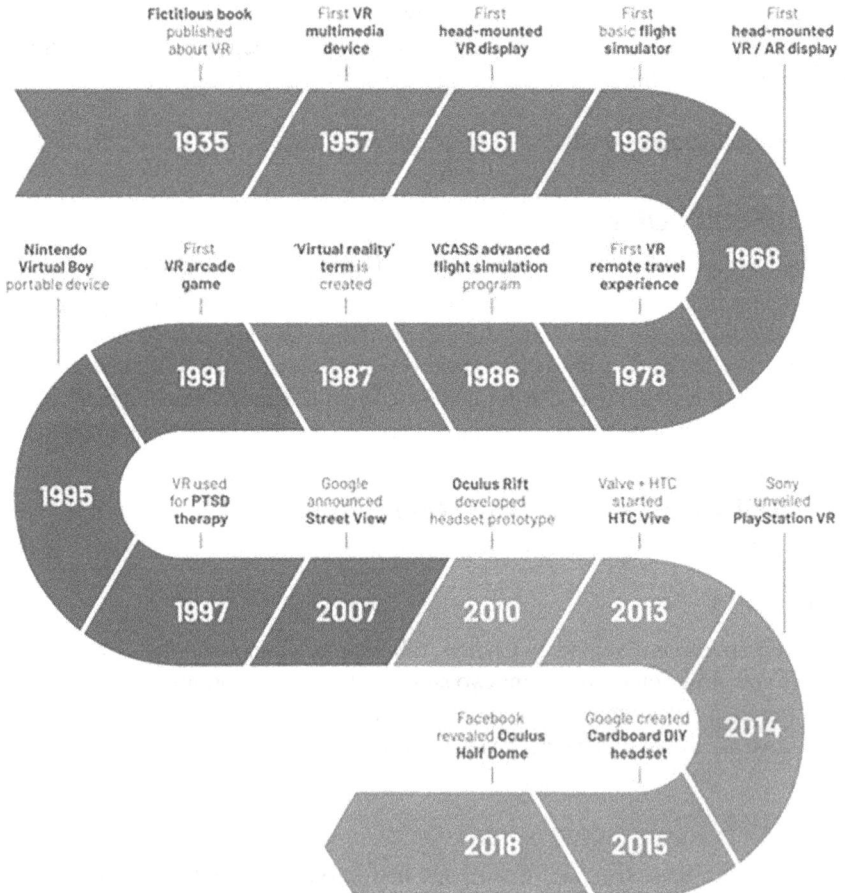

FIGURE 6.2 History of VR

6.9.5 1935

In his novel *Pygmalion's Spectacles*, Stanley G. Weinbaum describes a pair of glasses that allow the user to explore simulated worlds with the assistance of holographic pictures, smell, touch, and taste. Science fiction anticipated, as it always has, what we now have.

6.9.6 1939

The View-Master was created by William Gruber—simple stereoscopic viewers that make you look at two similar cross-eyed images to see a single 3D image. The View-Master was affordable to the consumer market and could be seen in the bedroom of almost any boy.

6.10 VIRTUAL REALITY IN THE '50S AND '60S

6.10.1 1952

Sensorama, the first VR-like device of immersive multimodal technology that included a stereoscopic color monitor, odor emitters, a sound system, and fans, was invented by Morton Heilig. Thanks to the capacity of Sensorama to involve users in a wide-angle stereoscopic image, Morton succeeded in attracting the full attention of the audience.

6.10.2 1960

Morton Heilig is inventing the first head-mounted monitor once again. The customer was given a stereoscopic 3D image and stereo sound by the proprietary Telesphere Mask. Can it share a VR gear resemblance?

6.10.3 1961

The headlight is rendered by Comeau and Bryan. This wearable system monitored the movement of the head and projected each eye on a screen. It had options for magnetic tracking and a remote camera that matched the movement of the head. No computer simulation was done, but the device was partially identical to current VR helmets.

6.10.4 1968

The Sword of Damocles, another VR head-mounted show, was invented by Ivan Sutherland and his pupil, Bob Sproull. Ivan was already known for his successes in the development of computer graphics, and his expertise helped him create this gadget. It showed computer-generated wireframe spaces, and the picture perspective relied on the data for head tracking.

6.10.5 1969

Myron Krueger creates a series of computer-generated worlds. They referred to the individuals within the community that behaved. The technologies developed, for instance, allowed individuals to interact directly with each other. He called "artificial reality" this experience.

6.10.6   1974

Myron Krueger is designing the video place Augmented Reality Lab. From his experimentation with simulated surroundings, his concept was created. The lab was developed by Myron to enable people to interact without gloves in "artificial reality" that would monitor gestures and other equipment. There were all the required hardware components at the video place that allowed the user to be placed in the virtual environment.

6.10.7   1982

On TV, Dan Reitan uses AR. AR gained mass acceptance thanks to this guy, and the following technology is being used even today. To add graphics to a weather broadcast, Dan used space and radar cameras. This digital weather chart was the first time that AR could be used publicly by people.

6.10.8   1987

Thanks to Jaron Lanier, the name "virtual reality" was officially born. He had previously created VPL Testing, and it was the first company to market VR products. Specialized software was also distributed that allowed VR applications to be created. The devices developed at VPL Research were fairly primitive: the EyePhone, the DataGlove for data entry, and even 3D image renderers and stereo sound simulators were just other head-mounted monitors. The DataGlove was later licensed by Mattel to create the Power Glove for Nintendo, but it was not a success.

6.11   VIRTUAL REALITY IN THE '90S AND '00S

6.11.1   1990

The word "augmented reality" was introduced by Tom Caudell. He worked at Boeing and came up with an alternative to the diagrams used to direct staff in the area. He recommended equipping staff with head-mounted wearables that would project the schematics of the aircraft on reusable screens. With the assistance of a computer machine, the displayed photographs may conveniently be edited.

6.11.2   1991

Virtuality Party produces VR arcade machines at video game stores that can be located. The computers had a fast reaction time and equipped players with multiplayer games with stereoscopic vision cameras, game controls, and the ability to collaborate. A bunch of hardware devices were already powered by VR gaming in the '90s, such as VR headsets, graphics rendering subsystems, 3D trackers, and exoskeleton-like wearable parts. This pattern is already underway.

6.11.3 1992

Lawnmower Man, the premiere of the show. The plot was based on a scientist's fictitious story that used VR on a mentally ill patient. This was another case of how VR became a natural part of the film business through the mainstream.

6.11.4 1993

A VR headset is being developed by SEGA. The version was intended to supplement the consoles and arcades of the Sega Genesis and Saturn, but only one arcade was released.

6.11.5 1994

Julie Martin delivers the first-ever "Dancing in Cyberspace" theatrical AR show. Digital artifacts and environments were manipulated by the performers, providing an immersive picture.

6.11.6 1995

Nintendo introduced the patented VR-32 unit, which will later be known as the Virtual Boy. Nintendo reported at the Consumer Electronics Show that their new device would provide players with a beautiful experience of engaging with virtual reality. Virtual Boy was the first home VR system, and they released the first home VR product ever, which was a huge risk for the company.

6.11.7 1996

The first-ever AR device appears with CyberCode 2D markers. It was focused on the 2D barcodes that even low-cost cameras mounted on mobile devices could identify. The device was able to evaluate the tagged object's 2D location and has been a base for a variety of AR applications.

6.11.8 1998

For the NFL game localization, Sportvision applies AR. With the assistance of an AR overlay, the perspective of the spectator was improved. Smoothly drawn on the ground was a yellow first-down marker. It gave a guide to the state of play to the audience.

6.11.9 1999

The first AR wearable equipment for BARS soldiers was published. The Battlefield Augmented Reality System aimed to help soldiers enhance battlefield vision, communications, location-identification of enemies, and overall situational awareness.

AR was used by NASA to guide the X-38 spacecraft. The car was fitted with an AR-powered navigation dashboard.

6.11.10   2000

Released by ARToolKit. This was a groundbreaking library tracking computer that allowed AR applications to be developed. It's open-source and hosted on GitHub right now.

A wearable EyeTap system has been developed. EyeTap perceives the eye of the user as both a display and a camera and, with computer-generated data, enhances the environment the user sees.

6.12   VIRTUAL REALITY TODAY

The world of virtual reality has seen significant strides over the past ten years, mainly from the resulting tech giant battle—Amazon, Apple, Facebook, Google, Microsoft, Sony, and Samsung have developed divisions of VR and AR. However, as it appears to come with a hefty price tag attached, buyers are still on the fence about VR tech [12].

2010: A concept for what would become the Oculus Rift headset for virtual reality was developed by Palmer Luckey.

2014: Shortly after the first shipment of kits went out through the Kickstarter campaign, Facebook acquired Oculus VR for around $3 billion. There was a complaint brought against Facebook and Oculus for stealing business secrets.

2013: Valve Corporation discovered a way for Oculus and other manufacturers to view lag-free VR content and distribute it freely. Along with the HTC Vive headset and controllers, Valve and HTC confirmed their collaboration in 2015 and launched the first version in 2016.

2014: For the video game console PlayStation 4, Sony unveils Project Morpheus, or PlayStation VR.

2016: The final market edition was launched to inspire its users not only to enjoy the game but to "live the game."

2015: Google launched Cardboard, a stereoscopic do-it-yourself viewer where a person holds their phone on their head inside a literal piece of cardboard. It resolved the question of the price tag, but is it just a headset for virtual reality? This is debatable.

2016: The production of augmented reality goods by hundreds of enterprises. Most of the headphones had dynamic binaural audio, but there was also a shortage of haptic interfaces.

2018: Oculus unveiled the Half Dome at the Facebook F8 Developer Conference— a headset with a 140-degree field of view.

6.13   FUTURE OF VR

So from here, where do we go? Virtual reality continues to discover new uses, and you can bet the platform is here to remain with the backing of billion-dollar tech firms. VR Tech is progressing as soon as its compatible hardware is, but for those in the race, it is the best possibility [13].

For customers, the favorable climate on the market side should mean positive news is arriving fast. Pricing will be important to the consumer industry and will make advanced technology a daily commodity of our lives. VR is primarily used as a gaming experience right now, but the prospective potential implementations are fully up to the imagination. Mixed reality environments include a good pathway to complete VR acceptance, or immersive experiences that are part augmented reality and part virtual reality.

6.14 VR S/W

VR is an entirely 3D world built by a blend of hardware and compatible applications. This immerses the user in the 3D environment, allowing them the opportunity to communicate in a seemingly real way with the virtual world [14]. To build an optimal VR user interface, a couple of different steps are needed. The virtual environment is developed by the creators of software and then rendered in a way that users can communicate with developers' created objects. Headsets help create the feeling of being submerged in the 3D world for consumers. Such 3D objects appear to respond to changes in the movement of the user, and the experiences resemble those in the real world.

6.15 WHY VR S/W?

As VR has become more popular, organizations in the workplace are recognizing its importance. This technology will provide consumers in myriad fields with differing benefits. Virtually test a product. VR has the potential to be innovative for companies that market a product, as this tool helps people to imagine what it would be like to buy a product. Until they commit to a purchase, consumers can take a product for a "virtual test drive" VR will take the hands-on experience to the next level to improve schooling. A student or trainee may imagine themselves performing it instead of watching an instructor perform a task. Go one step beyond 3D modeling. Some VR tools allow users in a VR environment to create, sculpt, model, paint, and construct tangible objects. With software like this, users can communicate with 3D objects from any perspective.

6.16 WHO USES VIRTUAL REALITY (VR) SOFTWARE?

In a variety of diverse areas, augmented reality is gradually showing its worth. Only a few examples are the following.

VR is now a widely successful platform of software products for game developers. To create a fully immersive user interface for gamers, developers may use VR software. Many playing the game, as if they are part of the world, will completely engage with the generated characters. Via headphones or handheld devices, users will usually play these games. Within architecture and engineering, 3D modeling is becoming more popular, as this style of design helps users to control the structures they design from any perspective. Users will be fully immersed in the world as they build by designing in VR. These technologies have enhanced the 3D functionality provided by CAD applications, enabling users in a simulated world to plan, control, and work on projects [15].

6.17 KINDS OF VR S/W

Digital reality is still a new technology, but there are still various subcategories of technology evolving. Any subcategories that are prominent in the room are in the next section.

VR visualization: This program type enables users in a simulated world to experience aggregated results. These tools help users to interpret analytics in a manner that helps them to completely appreciate what the knowledge conveys. Businesses may use these tools to capture, store, and review all VR content in a single location via VR content management systems [16].

VR SDK: Software Development Kits for virtual reality (SDK) provides the requisite framework for planning, creating, and testing VR experiences. To construct practically some VR experience, VR SDKs serve as the building blocks.

VR game engine: This app is the secret to building a VR video game environment for developers.

VR sharing platforms: Users can use these resources to communicate in VR from distant locations.

VR simulation simulator: These tools can be used to train staff in a fully immersive environment in almost every industry.

6.18 FEATURES OF VR

For users to create a fully-fledged VR experience, the VR app comes packed with numerous features. In these types of solutions, the following features are usually found but are not necessarily expected to be included.

6.18.1 MANAGEMENT OF CONTENT

Certain tools allow users to directly upload either raw 3D content, which will later be edited into a VR experience, or existing VR content to the website.

6.18.2 INTEGRATION OF HARDWARE

Every VR solution must be combined with a piece of hardware that supports the experience of VR.

6.18.3 COLLABORATION

VR tools allow many users to remotely access the solution at once so that they can interact in real-time.

6.18.4 ANALYTICS

Some VR technologies can offer analytics capabilities to consumers. It will help companies to better understand the behavior of the VR content reaching audiences.

6.18.5 Increased Availability

Large VR names, such as Oculus and HTC, have been working publicly to reduce the cost of their headsets. We would see a greater mass acceptance of VR tools as costs are made more competitive.

VR is still rising as a technology, and the technology needs experienced developers to help get VR to its full potential. More employment in the VR sector.

6.19 PROBLEM WITH VR S/W

Although we should expect VR apps and headphones shortly to become more affordable, pricing is probably the greatest challenge to this technology. Consumers have had only a few VR experiences, with VR apps and applications also costing a great deal of money. As a result, they are reluctant to see instances of need that relate to their jobs and everyday lives [17, 18].

6.20 VARIOUS VR S/W AND SERVICES

With virtual reality, VR also goes hand in hand with (AR). A 3D-generated object is taken by AR software and stitched smoothly into the real world. In another form of technology known as mixed reality (MR), VR and AR have started to merge, enabling users to see virtual objects in real-world environments, while anchoring objects to a point in real space.

6.21 VR HARDWARE

Virtual reality has provided an escape since its early inception. Donating a headset will transport you, full of wonder and curiosity, to a whole new world. Or it will encourage you to visit an environment too unsafe for human life. Or it can also only present you with the real world in a different way. And the hardware is making the goal of unfettered escapism a fact now that we have progressed beyond the age of cumbersome goggles and awkward helmets [19–25].

A quick summary of each unit, ranked in terms of price and complexity, is mentioned next.

6.21.1 Google Cardboard

A wide variety of new smartphones are compliant with Cardboard VR.

The greatest advantage of Google Cardboard, as shown in Figure 6.3.

- Low cost
- Strong support for hardware
- Portability
- Wireless
- Lightweight
- Available in $5–$20

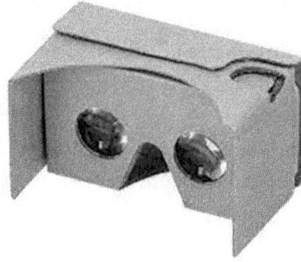

FIGURE 6.3   Google Cardboard

6.21.2   DAYDREAM

The Daydream is designed with fabric material. Daydream VR is a virtual reality platform developed by Google that allows users to experience virtual reality using a smartphone and a Daydream View headset. The platform was introduced in 2016 and is designed to be accessible, affordable, and easy to use.

Daydream VR offers a variety of virtual reality experiences, including games, educational apps, and immersive videos. The Daydream View headset is comfortable and lightweight, making it easy to wear for extended periods of time. The headset also includes a wireless controller that can be used to navigate and interact with virtual environments.

To use Daydream VR, a user must have a compatible smartphone that is equipped with a high-quality display and the necessary sensors for tracking head movements. Once the phone is placed into the Daydream View headset, the user can launch the Daydream app and select from a variety of virtual reality experiences.

Daydream VR provides an accessible and affordable way for users to experience virtual reality and explore immersive digital environments.

Features

- Motion controller with a trackpad
- Excellent optics
- Available for $79

6.21.3   GEAR VR

It only uses a Samsung smartphone, some of the same circuits from the Oculus Rift PC solution Gear VR is a virtual reality headset developed by Samsung in collaboration with Oculus. The headset was first released in 2015 and is designed to work with Samsung smartphones, including the Galaxy S and Note series.

Gear VR provides an immersive virtual reality experience by displaying 3D images and videos in front of the user's eyes, and tracking the user's head movements to adjust the perspective accordingly. The headset is lightweight and comfortable to wear, and includes a touchpad and buttons on the side for navigation and interaction.

To use Gear VR, a user must have a compatible Samsung smartphone and the Gear VR app installed. The phone is inserted into the front of the headset, and the user can launch the app to access a variety of virtual reality experiences, including games, videos, and educational apps.

Gear VR also includes a variety of features to enhance the user's experience, such as a built-in accelerometer, gyroscope, and proximity sensor. The headset can also be used with a wireless gamepad for more advanced gaming experiences.

Gear VR provides an affordable and accessible way for users to experience virtual reality using their Samsung smartphone and offers a variety of virtual reality experiences for users to explore. However, it should be noted that Samsung and Oculus have since stopped supporting the Gear VR platform, so it may not receive any new updates or releases in the future.

In contrast to Google Cardboard, this results in even more sensitive and superior monitoring, while it still just measures rotation.

Available in the price range of $90–$100.

6.21.4 OCULUS RIFT

The Rift uses a PC and external cameras to allow a complete VR experience for the user, and it is available with positional tracking. In their HMDs, the Samsung partnership enables Oculus to use Samsung displays, as shown in Figure 6.4.

Features

- Oculus no longer allows the user to stay seated
- User has to travel within an area of 3 m × 3 m
- Connected to the PC by cable
- A one-button clicker
- Available in the range of $399 to $800

6.22 VR APPLICATIONS

6.22.1 INDUSTRY 4.0

Industry 4.0 is only possible due to virtual reality development. Virtual reality saves a lot of time and money for the Industry 4.0. The products can be reviewed before

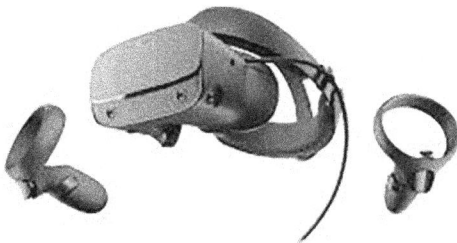

FIGURE 6.4 Oculus Rift

their final productions and thereby reducing lots of difficulties and saving money in product design cycles [26–30].

6.22.2 MEDICAL AND HOSPITALS

Universal healthcare is a vital area where VR is used. Healthcare providers are also using digital templates to prepare themselves to work on human bodies, and VR has also been used as pain control for burn injuries. VR can also be used as a treatment for mental health disorders. Apart from those previously cited, a lot of research is going on to make VR Hospitals in the future for the treatment of diseases in remote locations.

6.22.3 SIGHTSEEING

Imagine getting a chance to test your vacation before you buy it. This is precisely what the future might bring. The industry with the application of VR is taking the first steps to encourage you to visit hotels, restaurants, and tourist landmarks on guided virtual tours.

6.22.4 BUILDING PLANNING AND DESIGNING

VR is increasingly transforming the way architects design their work and play with it. VR makes it easy to see how it will feel, not just what a building or room will look like. They can experience the room for homeowners until it is physically designed and make real-time improvements, saving time and resources for the client and the architect.

6.22.5 GAMING

With Poker VR, you can now play VR multiplayer poker. It's like playing in a true casino where you can speak to other players and read their body language. They already have a prize pool of prizes worth $5,000 in total [31–35].

6.22.6 KNOWLEDGE AND DEVELOPMENT

VR applications with Web VR and collaboration with enterprises and with School LMS (learning management system). This makes schooling more available, and easier, and boosts retention levels of learning [36–39].

6.22.7 EMPLOYMENT

To test graduates for their 2017 admissions, Lloyds Banking Group has implemented a VR exercise. In the future, simulated worlds could replace test days and interviews on their own, saving both the boss and the prospective candidate expense and time.

6.22.8 Theater and Fun

In the entertainment industry, VR is used to improve encounters with 360 films (You-Tube examples) and to maximize the personal bond with them and/or the characters. For starters, Disney Movies VR brings the user to red carpet events and a *The Jungle Book* cast interview.

How media material is rendered may also be revolutionized by VR. The flip side is also the easiest way to create shows that can be watched live and within virtual reality itself via conventional platforms such as Twitter, Twitch, or Facebook.

6.22.9 Teaching and Learning

By empowering students to learn in an interactive, experience-based manner, VR could revolutionize education. University has applications that encourage users to discover the human brain, take a tour of Ancient Rome, and board the Titanic. With their "Engage" piece, Immersive VR Education is creating a VR classroom/meeting room space where people can learn from lecturers around the world.

6.22.10 Sports

With many VR businesses specializing in viewing live sporting matches, the way we watch sports is now evolving. You will watch the NBA, NFL, and other VR events, for instance. Companies like Live Like VR enable broadcasters and sports teams on mobile VR to offer live sports streaming experiences.

6.22.11 Graphic Arts and Enterprise

You don't just build life-size artwork with VR—you can be inside it. You will walk into the photo and come out on the other side. Tiltbrush is the most well-known program for making art in VR and what some individuals have managed to paint in it is incredible. With MasterpieceVR, you can render immersive 3D models and sculptures as well.

6.22.12 Seminars and Discussion

Since VR digitally encourages participants to be in locations, it offers an incentive for organizers to invite more people into in-person activities. For starters, via a virtual reality app linked to the inexpensive Google Cardboard headset, Paul McCartney released a 360-degree concert recording.

6.22.13 Aid and Encouragement

The capacity to elicit emotion is one of the greatest aspects of VR's emergence. For charities, this makes it particularly useful since it can be used to improve awareness of a situation.

When they are engaged in a situation they would either not be able to react to or come close to feeling, people are more likely to be inspired to action. In 2015, for example, Unicef used the film *Clouds Over Sidra* to double its contributions to the Syrian Refugee Crisis's work.

6.22.14 ADVERTISING

Marketing is becoming more and more about how firms make consumers feel, so a logical extension is to use VR.

6.22.15 LIFESTYLE

In VR, there are many real-life hobbies available, and the immersive environment makes them all the more interesting and accessible. If you're a lover of cultural events, you should visit museums like London's Natural History Museum, or if you're more of a thrill-seeker, China has also opened a VR theme park.

6.22.16 MILITARY AND DEFENSE

Military and defense is one of the important sectors which use AR and VR software from many firms to prepare workers with visual, auditory, and physical stimulation in simulated situations.

The technologies also encourage police forces to intensify the realistic experiences of trainees with people inside interactive training settings.

6.22.17 JOURNALISM AND COMMERCIAL

With the advancement in VR nowadays instead of just listening to the news, you will feel stories as though you were standing opposite the reporter where the story is happening. This is one of the applications of VR.

6.23 FUTURE OF AR/VR IN HEALTHCARE

Over the next six years, the Indian AR and VR industry is predicted to increase at a CAGR of 76% (2017 to 2022). The Indian healthcare business has quickly adapted to a slew of cutting-edge digital technologies.

Technological breakthroughs have reshaped the whole landscape of the Indian healthcare business in recent years. Technology advancements and current technologies such as virtual reality and augmented reality have been highly important for their quick expansion and have contributed to the achievement of certain goals that were envisioned as the future of the healthcare business.

The healthcare business has several applications for virtual reality. VR in medicine is revolutionizing the sector by introducing intriguing methods. VR healthcare solutions are pushing the boundaries of science fiction, and the line between fiction and reality is gradually blurring as a result of this application's very beneficial influence. Some of the major causes that are transforming the healthcare sector and opening up new options for improving various medical treatment approaches are highlighted in the next section.

6.23.1 MANAGEMENT OF PAIN

When a patient is engaged in virtual reality, the areas of the brain responsible for pain, the somatosensory cortex, and the insula, become less active. Virtual reality pain treatment reduces pain and can even help individuals withstand uncomfortable medical procedures in this way.

6.23.2 THERAPY

Physicians and medical experts are using virtual reality to treat patients who have phobias. Patients are forced to confront their concerns in virtual reality–controlled surroundings, which trains them to overcome their fears. Virtual simulation is also being used in clinics and hospitals in India to assist people to cope with terrible occurrences in the past. They are designed to encounter genuine situations within immersive surroundings to help patients cope with worries.

6.23.3 COGNITIVE RETRAINING

Doctors frequently utilize virtual reality chronic pain therapy to see patients executing complicated real-world tasks after they have suffered from a chronic stroke or brain injury. Certain duties are reproduced within the virtual world via virtual reality, allowing patients to recover quickly. Cognihab's stroke and cancer rehabilitation suits were developed in collaboration with AIIMS, one of India's premier healthcare facilities, to provide an all-in-one rehabilitation solution. Doctors frequently utilize virtual reality to watch patients execute complicated real-world tasks after they have suffered from a chronic stroke or brain injury. Certain duties are reproduced within the virtual world via virtual reality, allowing patients to recover quickly.

6.23.4 REHABILITATION OF THE PHYSICAL

Virtual reality is benefiting patients suffering from phantom limb discomfort tremendously in the Indian healthcare industry. Virtual reality has made caretakers' jobs simpler by allowing patients to accomplish tasks with their missing limbs, relieving pain and stress.

6.23.5 MEDICAL TREATMENT METHODS THAT ARE BETTER

Virtual reality not only improves doctors' capacity to identify issues but also allows medical students to gain firsthand experience in an immersive setting by enhancing the actual world in a three-dimensional paradigm. Medical simulation methods are artificial representations of virtual environments portraying real-world circumstances that allow healthcare personnel to safely practice, learn, and test their medical abilities. It has become crucial for our culture since it is capable of decreasing human mistakes and allowing learners to produce more precise results. As a result, it has been widely adopted by Indian hospitals to improve medical personnel's ability to manage patients with severe ailments such as cancer, speech disorders, spinal injuries, and multiple sclerosis.

6.24 CASE STUDY

The use of technology has significantly improved communication, training, therapy, and study in healthcare. In the following years, the application of AR/VR in healthcare will be prevalent in terms of intraoperative surgery, healthcare professional training, physiotherapy, improved diagnostics, anatomy, visualization, and much more. Virtual reality technology may be utilized to capture some of the greatest procedures performed by top physicians, which can then be shown to trainees for this first experience. Nowadays many novel applications of AR/VR are in the developing stage, which would make a voluntary change in the healthcare sector. Some of them are discussed in this case study.

6.24.1 VR App

The first well name in this healthcare business has developed a new cough medicine product that doctors would recommend to their patients. Because of the extensive use of an earlier medication, it was a little difficult to place the product in the doctor's mind. We created a software program for both marketing and end users. Users may learn about mucus formation and how the syrup cleaned excess mucus caused by pneumonia by using the VR app. That viewer could enjoy comprehensive narrative narration with flawless video audio sync, putting their fears to rest. This made it easier for the user to remember and increased sales.

6.24.2 Skill App

A game-based app was created for a reputable pharmaceutical company's workers and clients to utilize. The company has invested significant money in developing materials for its workers and consultants to aid in sales and marketing. However, the information was either underused or not used at all. The difficulty was to persuade them to read the information, yet forcing the user to read was not producing the desired results for a variety of reasons. The game-based application was created to enhance this. The program assisted the user in learning and updating himself in a fun way. We also instilled a healthy competitive environment among staff by using leaderboards. As a result of all of this, content consumption has skyrocketed. The software is based on the notion of ninjas.

6.24.3 Pill Production App

An AI-based 3D simulation training process, evaluation, and virtual classroom for a prominent pharmaceutical business that needed to teach its staff in the tablet production process (VC). Employees may complete all safety protocols, as well as the whole tablet production process, in two modes: training and testing. During the test, the system AI will generate random progressing scenarios for the learner to analyze and score. The program used these principles to eliminate mistakes and enforce excellent hygiene at the point of manufacture. Our technology was able to track employees' performance and activities. This accomplished such milestones thanks to our dedicated staff of UI/UX designers, engineers, and project managers.

6.25 SURGICAL TRAINING APP

The reduced training booklets and films are what modern surgical training is all about, which normally lasts one day. This would be a fairly brief cadaver training technique. The training experience would start to fade after a few days. After many months, practitioners are transferred to real operating rooms, where they become extremely apprehensive, and patients distrust inexperienced surgeons. However, with this program, surgeons may gaze around the environment using their headsets, and the hand controllers allow them to grasp things and equipment in the correct order and operate on a patient's organ with exact motions. Drilling and hammering are used in orthopedic procedures and are replicated using haptics.

6.26 CONCLUSION

In conclusion, the advent of augmented reality (AR) and virtual reality (VR) technologies has brought about significant changes in the healthcare industry, with numerous benefits ranging from improved diagnosis and treatment to enhanced patient experiences. This book chapter has explored the various ways in which AR and VR are revolutionizing healthcare, including in surgical planning and training, medical education, therapy and rehabilitation, and patient engagement.

AR and VR technologies have demonstrated great potential in improving the precision and accuracy of medical procedures, reducing the risk of complications and errors, and shortening recovery times. They have also been shown to enhance medical education by providing immersive and interactive training experiences for healthcare professionals, enabling them to better understand complex anatomical structures and disease processes.

Furthermore, AR and VR have proven to be effective tools in therapy and rehabilitation, particularly in cases of neurological and musculoskeletal disorders. They offer a safe and controlled environment for patients to practice and improve their motor skills, cognitive function, and emotional well-being.

In addition to their clinical applications, AR and VR technologies are transforming the patient experience by providing engaging and personalized healthcare services. Patients can now use AR and VR technologies to learn more about their medical conditions, track their treatment progress, and connect with healthcare professionals remotely, making healthcare more accessible and convenient.

Despite the promising potential of AR and VR in healthcare, there are still challenges that need to be addressed, including the high costs of implementation, ethical considerations, and regulatory frameworks. However, with continued investment and development, AR and VR have the potential to revolutionize the healthcare industry and transform the way we approach diagnosis, treatment, and patient care.

REFERENCES

[1] Y. Alkali, I. Routray, and P. Whig. 2022. "Strategy for reliable, efficient and secure IoT using artificial intelligence." IUP Journal of Computer Sciences, vol. 16, no. 2.

[2] M. Anand, A. Velu, and P. Whig. 2022. "Prediction of loan behaviour with machine learning models for secure banking." Journal of Computer Science and Engineering (JCSE), vol. 3, no. 1, pp. 1–13.

[3] G. Chopra, and P. Whig. 2022. "Smart agriculture system using AI." International Journal of Sustainable Development in Computing Science, vol. 4, no. 1.

[4] N. Jiwani, K. Gupta, and P. Whig. 2021. "Novel healthcare framework for cardiac arrest with the application of AI using ANN." In 2021 5th International Conference on Information Systems and Computer Networks (ISCON), 1–5. IEEE.

[5] H. Jupalle, S. Kouser, A. B. Bhatia, N. Alam, R. R. Nadikattu, and P. Whig. 2022. "Automation of human behaviors and its prediction using machine learning." Microsystem Technologies, pp. 1–9.

[6] Y. Khera, P. Whig, and A. Velu. 2021a. "Efficient effective and secured electronic billing system using AI." Vivekananda Journal of Research, vol. 10, pp. 53–60.

[7] A. Rupani, P. Whig, G. Sujediya, and P. Vyas. 2017. "A robust technique for image processing based on interfacing of raspberry-Pi and FPGA using IoT." 2017 International Conference on Computer, Communications and Electronics (Comptelix), 350–53. IEEE.

[8] A. Sharma, A. Kumar, and P. Whig. 2015. "On the performance of CDTA based novel analog inverse low pass filter using 0.35 μm CMOS parameter." International Journal of Science, Technology & Management, vol. 4, no. 1, pp. 594–601.

[9] U. Tomar, N. Chakroborty, H. Sharma, and P. Whig. 2021. AI-based smart agriculture system." Transactions on Latest Trends in Artificial Intelligence, vol. 2, no. 2.

[10] P. Whig. 2019. "Exploration of viral diseases mortality risk using machine learning." International Journal of Machine Learning for Sustainable Development, vol. 1, no. 1, pp. 11–20.

[11] P. Whig, and S. N. Ahmad. 2012. "DVCC based readout circuitry for water quality monitoring system." International Journal of Computer Applications, vol. 49, no. 22, pp. 1–7.

[12] P. Whig, S. Kouser, A. Velu, and R. Reddy Nadikattu. 2022. "Fog-IoT-assisted-based smart agriculture application." In Demystifying Federated Learning for Blockchain and Industrial Internet of Things, 74–93. IGI Global.

[13] L. de Marchi Perelli, A. Marzani, and N. Speciale. 2012. "Acoustic emission localization in plates with dispersion and reverberations using sparse PZT sensors in passive mode." Smart Materials and Structures, vol. 21, no. 2, Article ID 025010.

[14] E. D. Niri, A. Farhidzadeh, and S. Salamone. 2013. "Non linear Kalmann filtering for acoustic emission source localization in anisotropic panels." Ultrasonics, vol. 5, no. 2, pp. 1–10.

[15] A. Liverani, and A. Ceruttii. 2010. "Interactive GT code management for mechanical part similarity search and cost prediction." Computer-Aided Design and Applications, vol. 7, no. 1, pp. 1–15.

[16] P. Whig, R. R. Nadikattu, and A. Velu. 2022. "COVID-19 pandemic analysis using application of AI." Healthcare Monitoring and Data Analysis Using IoT: Technologies and Applications, p. 1.

[17] P. Whig, A. Velu, and R. R. Naddikatu. 2022. "The economic impact of AI-enabled blockchain in 6G-based industry." In AI and Blockchain Technology in 6G Wireless Network, 205–224. Springer, Singapore.

[18] A. Liverani, A. Ceruttii, and G. Caligiana. 2013. "Tablet-based 3D sketching and curve reverse modeling." International Journal of Computer Aided Engineering and Technology, vol. 5, no. 2–3.

[19] S. Debernardis, M. Fiorentino, M. Gattullo, G. Monno, and A. E. Uva, "Text readability in head-worn displays: Color and style optimization in video vs. optical see-through devices." IEEE Transactions on Visualization and Computer Graphics, no. 99, p. 1, 2013.

[20] P. Whig, A. Velu, and R. R. Nadikattu. 2022. "Blockchain platform to resolve security issues in IoT and smart networks." In AI-Enabled Agile Internet of Things for Sustainable FinTech Ecosystems, 46–65. IGI Global, Hershey, PA.

[21] P. Whig, A. Velu, and R. Ready. 2022. "Demystifying federated learning in artificial intelligence with human-computer interaction." In Demystifying Federated Learning for Blockchain and Industrial Internet of Things, 94–122. IGI Global, Hershey, PA.

[22] P. Whig, A. Velu, and P. Sharma. 2022. "Demystifying federated learning for blockchain: A case study." In Demystifying Federated Learning for Blockchain and Industrial Internet of Things, 143–65. IGI Global, Hershey, PA.

[23] R. T. Azuma. 1997. "A survey of augmented reality." Presence, vol. 6, no. 4, pp. 355–385.

[24] R. Azuma, Y. Baillot, R. Behringer, S. Feiner, S. Julier, and B. MacIntyre. 2001. "Recent advances in augmented reality." IEEE Computer Graphics and Applications, vol. 21, no. 6, pp. 34–47.

[25] D. Krevelen, and R. Poleman. 2010. "A survey of augmented reality technologies, applications and limitations." The International Journal of Virtual Reality, vol. 9, no. 2, pp. 1–20.

[26] X. Wang, M. J. Kim, P. E. Love, and S. C. Kang. 2013. "Augmented reality in the built environment: Classification and implications for future research." Automation in Construction, vol. 32, pp. 1–13.

[27] H. L. Chi, S. C. Kang, and X. Wang. 2013. "Research trends and opportunities of augmented reality applications in architecture, engineering, and construction," Automation in Construction, vol. 33, pp. 116–122.

[28] S. Benbelkacem, M. Belhocine, A. Bellarbi, N. Zenati-Henda, and M. Tadjine. 2013. "Augmented reality for photovoltaic pumping systems maintenance tasks." Renewable Energy, vol. 55, pp. 428–437.

[29] J. M. Antonio, S. R. J. Luis, and S. P. Faustino. 2013. "Augmented and virtual reality techniques for footwear." Computers in Industry, vol. 15, pp. 115–125.

[30] A. Farhidzadeh, E. Dehghan-Niri, A. Moustafa, S. Salamone, and A. Whittaker. 2012. "Damage assessment of reinforced concrete structures using fractal analysis of residual crack patterns." Experimental Mechanics, vol. 12, pp. 1–13.

[31] B. Koo, H. Choi, and T. Shon. 2009. "Viva: Win monitoring framework based on 3D visualization and augmented reality in mobile devices." In Ambient Assistive Health and Wellness Management in the Heart of the City, M. Mokhtari, I. Khalil, J. Bauchet, D. Zhang, and C. Nugent, Eds., vol. 5597 of Lecture Notes in Computer Science, 158–165. Springer, Berlin, Germany.

[32] J. L. Rose. 1999. Ultrasonic Guided Waves in Solid Media. Cambridge University Press, New York, NY.

[33] R. Seydel and F.-K. Chang. 2001. "Impact identification of stiffened composite panels: I. System development." Smart Materials and Structures, vol. 10, no. 2, pp. 354–369.

[34] B. Wang, J. Takatsubo, Y. Akimune, and H. Tsuda. 2005. "Development of a remote impact damage identification system." Structural Control and Health Monitoring, vol. 12, no. 3–4, pp. 301–314.

[35] Z. Su, L. Ye, and Y. Lu. 2006. "Guided Lamb waves for identification of damage in composite structures: A review." Journal of Sound and Vibration, vol. 295, no. 3–5, pp. 753–780.

[36] T. Kundu, S. Das, and K. V. Jata. 2007. "Point of impact prediction in isotropic and anisotropic plates from the acoustic emission data." Journal of the Acoustical Society of America, vol. 122, no. 4, pp. 2057–2066.

[37] T. Kundu, S. Das, and K. V. Jata. 2009. "Detection of the point of impact on a stiffened plate by the acoustic emission technique." Smart Materials and Structures, vol. 18, no. 3, Article ID 035006.

[38] F. Ciampa, and M. Meo. 2010. "Acoustic emission source localization and velocity determination of the fundamental mode A0 using wavelet analysis and a newton-based optimization technique." Smart Materials and Structures, vol. 19, no. 4, Article ID 045027.

[39] S. Salamone, I. Bartoli, P. di Leo et al. 2010. "High-velocity impact location on aircraft panels using macro-fiber composite piezoelectric rosettes." Journal of Intelligent Material Systems and Structures, vol. 21, no. 9, pp. 887–896.

7 Implications of Augmented Reality Applications for Vehicle-to-Everything (V2X)

Faiza Rashid Ammar Al Harthi,
Abderezak Touzene, Nasser Alzeidi, and
Faiza Al Salti

7.1 INTRODUCTION

Mobile networks have considerably evolved since the deployment of the first generation (1G) cellular networks in 1980. With the deployment of 5G, mobile broadband communication is expected to target a 20 Gbps peak data rate, extending the network in terms of size and coverage. It also permits more real-time, data-intensive, task-oriented applications demanding high reliability and ultra-low latency as mobile applications. Additionally, 5G has differentiated itself from previous iterations of mobile technologies due to its intent of addressing the needs of vertical industries focused on manufacturing, utilities, public services, energy, automotive, and healthcare. The International Mobile Telecommunications (IMT) for 2020 and beyond, which was defined by the ITU-R Recommendation ITU-R M.2083–0 in 2015 [1], recommended three usage scenarios, as shown in Figure 7.1:

- **eMBB (enhanced Mobile Broadband):** Provides high data rates of up to 10 Gbps as well as high density in terms of connectivity of 1 million devices/km^2 to allow media distribution, online gaming, and virtual and augmented reality.
- **URLLC (Ultra-Reliable Low Latency Communications):** Provides high-speed connectivity with relatively zero latency (1ms) resulting in responsive, reliable and ubiquitous networks that allow devices to move seamlessly between different network access technologies. It can provide connectivity to mission-critical services such as e-surgery, industrial complexity operation (M2M), and Vehicle-to-Everything (V2X) communications.

DOI: 10.1201/9781003340133-7

Enhanced mobile broadband

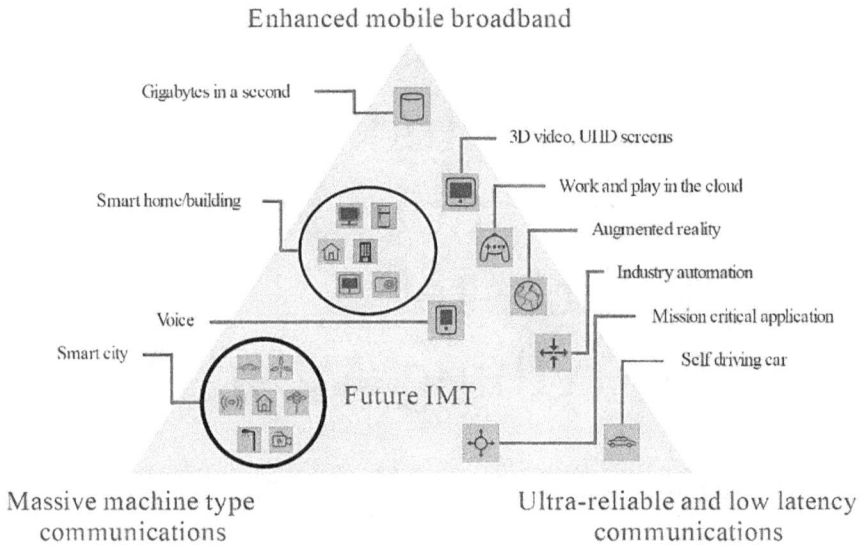

FIGURE 7.1 Usage scenarios of IMT for 2020 and beyond [1]

- **mMTC (massive Machine Type Communications):** Provides a backbone for scalable and energy efficient networks that could support a huge number of Internet of Things (IoT) devices and use cases.

5G technology is expected to shift mobile communications from solely connecting people to something that supports human-centric, machine-to-machine communications capable of scaling and catering to a vast number of use cases and applications [2].

The implementation of digital networks ushered in a transformation that brought about emergent use cases for various users and vertical markets. The introduction of machine type communication (MTC) in 4G long term evolution (LTE) allows data communications between MTC devices and servers or between MTC devices, which has resulted in the realization of Internet of Things (IoT). IoT paved the way for the creation of intelligent objects that utilize network connections. These objects can range from electrical appliances found in homes to devices used for remote driving. IoT's functions are entirely based on the data gathered by sensors that are embedded in every device. These types of devices are expected to exponentially increase, collecting volumes of structured and unstructured data that are shared, analyzed and distributed to users in numerous ways and for many purposes [3].

IoT has continually evolved and formed different types of ecosystems. Although different in many ways, these ecosystems pose common requirements on 5G networks [4]:

- **Energy efficiency:** IoT devices have limited power source, processing, and storage capabilities. Inefficient transmission of data and control packets could lessen the life devices of or could take a huge toll on the usability and performance of devices.

- **High availability:** Operations such as Handover (HO) and data offloading could cause link failures and data loss.
- **Mobility:** Devices must be able to communicate with other devices using different types of access technologies, at any location and at any time.
- **Connection density:** Devices must be able to connect to any network regardless of the huge number of devices and heterogeneous systems.

The evolution of IoT from the basic device-to-device (D2D) connectivity to the use case specific Vehicle-to-Everything (V2X) is one of the factors that drove the 5G mobile network to significant advancements compared to the incremental improvements provided by previous generations. Beyond speed improvement, 5G is expected to unleash a massive 5G IoT ecosystem where networks can serve communication needs for billions of connected devices, with the right trade-offs between speed, latency, and cost. V2X is a type of communication between transport vehicles (V2V), pedestrians (V2P), infrastructure (V2I), and networks (V2N), which requires the features of the 5G network. V2X use cases/applications enable vehicles to connect and exchange data with other vehicles, traffic lights, parking spaces, nearby people, and services to coordinate traffic flow and environmental safety. The usage of vehicles for public transportation, emergency vehicles, business operations, and other types of human activities have raised concerns and challenges on safety, efficiency, and comfort. According to the World Health Organization's (WHO) June 2021 Key Facts, about 1.3 million people die due to road traffic crashes. Annually, more than half of road traffic deaths involve vulnerable road users. The United Nations General Assembly targets a 50% reduction globally in deaths and injuries from crashes by 2030 [5].

Augmented reality (AR) is an immersive technology that can greatly enhance the implementation of V2X in terms of information processing and public safety. AR allows the enhancement of a real object existing in a natural environment using digital technology by overlaying information and digital objects. AR can transform the way users and devices work by turning information into immersive experience. It can produce mixed reality representations of a vehicle's environment that can enhance drivers'/passengers' deep sensing and situational awareness. It can also be used to provide improved real-time hazard alerts and simulate traffic scenarios and pedestrian behavior. These benefits are because, basically, this technology fosters visual learning that aids faster knowledge acquisition, resulting in better work performance and reduction of errors [6].

The implementation of this technology, however, requires an in-depth analysis of how it will effectively mesh with enabling technologies (5G, positioning, AI, etc.), deployment (centralized, distributed), and use cases/applications. This chapter discusses the implications of augmented reality in V2X, taking into consideration the challenges and future directions concerning enabling technologies and other components involved in its implementation.

The chapter is structured as follows: Section 7.2 presents the network digital transformation. Section 7.3 briefly introduces the Internet of Things. Section 7.4 delves into Vehicle-to-Everything. Section 7.5 focuses on augmented reality. Section 7.6 outlines the integration of AR in V2X. Section 7.7 discusses the implications of AR in V2X. Finally, Section 7.8 presents the conclusion.

7.2   NETWORK DIGITAL TRANSFORMATION

Mobile wireless networks have evolved throughout the years, shifting merely from facilitating voice calls to enabling users to connect virtually to everything (Table 7.1). The usage of mobile networks has shown an exponential rise, which prompts operators and service providers to redesign the network infrastructure, allowing user equipment (UEs) with diverse capabilities, technologies, requirements, and use cases to be assured of coverage while enhancing infrastructure capacity, reuse, and efficiency [7]. According to the Cisco Annual Internet Report (2018–2023), the total number of mobile subscribers around the world will be growing from 5.1 billion (which is 66% of the global population in 2018) to 5.7 billion (which is 71% of the population in 2023) [8].

5G Networks, which are currently the latest network infrastructure, were born out of the explosive growth of heterogeneous data from the exponential growth of mobile devices. This mobile network generation's goal is to have a unified control of fixed and cellular ecosystems, be faster and smart to support diverse users and emerging technologies, and ensure lower latency for mission-critical commercial and industrial applications. 5G's innovation is based on a new radio frequency (RF) spectrum that utilizes millimeter waves, boosting signals through massive MIMO technologies. Using this technique, combined with beamforming signals and heterogeneous deployments, 5G is able to adapt to various challenges and changes in the network environment. 5G's initial deployment enabled the realization and deployment of emerging technologies that ushered in the so-called fourth Industrial Revolution (IR4). 5G is expected to bring quality of service (QoS) and quality of experience (QoE) to various applications and usage scenarios as its implementation steadily reach its targets and its development progresses due to increasing user demand [9].

Figure 7.2 clearly illustrates that 5G is anticipated to support massive system requirements, less latency, and about 1 million devices/km². Notable key technologies were developed and deployed to enable 5G to realize its promise [10]. Some of which are as follows:

- **Massive MIMO:** This technology emphasizes the use of numerous antenna elements for signal processing. The use of multiple antennae delivers array gain by concentrating energy in a chosen direction and providing spatial multiplexing gain by transporting independent data streams to each antenna. This results in an increase in the number of users or overall data rate.
- **Software-defined Networking (SDN):** This technology results in a software-centric network where network operators quickly deploy services for various use cases by dynamically allocating virtualized access and core network functions. Network slicing, which is a primary feature, allows the creation of virtual networks over a shared physical infrastructure, optimized for a particular purpose. This capability greatly improves an operator's operational expenditure (OPEX) and capital expenditure (CAPEX). This method has also brought about the usage of the Cloud Radio Access Network (C-RAN).

TABLE 7.1
Mobile Telecommunications Generations

Generations	1G	2G	3G	4G	5G
Deployment Year	1980s	1990s	2000s	2010s	2020s
Frequency	30Hz	1.8 GHz	1.6–2 GHz	2–8 GHz	3–300 GHz
Multiplexing	FDMA	TDMA, CDMA	CDMA	OFDMA	OFDM
Bandwidth	2 Kbps	64 Kbps	2 Mbps	200 Mbps to 1 Gbps	1 Gbps and higher
Delay	NA	629 ms	212 ms	60–98 ms	<1 ms
Applications	Voice	Voice, SMS	Video conference, Location-based services, www, IPV4	Download Movies, www, IPV4	www, IPv6, Vertical Industries

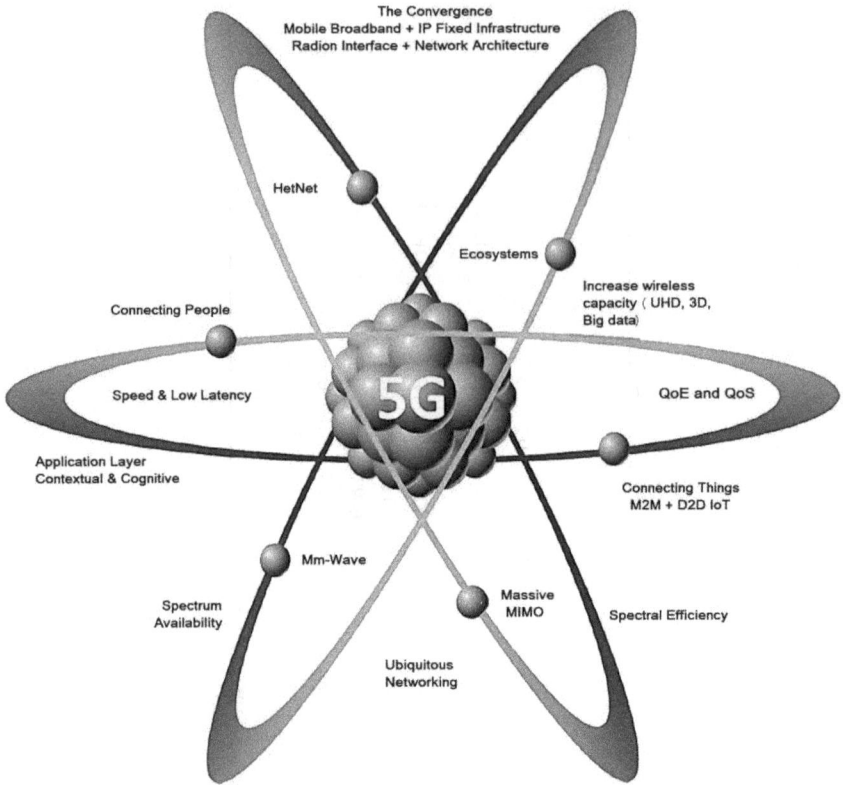

FIGURE 7.2   5G ecosystem and key performance indicators [9]

- **Non-orthogonal Multiple Access (NOMA):** Allows supporting multiple users to use a single resource which can result in system throughput improvement. In systems utilizing NOMA, users can share one spectral band, with each user having a different power allocation.
- **Mobile Edge Computing (MEC):** 5G employs a method where core and data network functions are moved towards the network edge (antenna location) resulting in reduced end-to-end user latency. The closer is the computing capability to the network's edge; the lesser is the application processing delay.

As of April 2021, 162 5G networks have been commercially released in 68 countries and regions around the world. The benefits being offered by this network such as robust network connectivity, lower latency, and higher bandwidth are expected to launch more than a thousand vertical industry applications. A prediction by GSMA (Global System for Mobile Communications Association) states that a massive boost in the number of 5G connections will be experienced globally, from 200 million in 2020 to 1.8 billion 2025 [11].

As depicted in Figure 7.2, there are two business drivers supporting the business models/use cases presented by ITU for 5G. These are the ability to transport voluminous data more rapidly than the previous generations for content delivery and the reduction of response times (latency), which is beneficial for mission-critical applications. The current state of global 5G network deployment is still in the early stages, but efforts have been made to make 5G commercially available. The eMBB use case, which was identified by 3GPP to be in its SMARTER (Study on New Services and Markets Technology Enablers) project, is supported by the deployment of the 3GPP's Radio Access Network (RAN) Non-Standalone (NSA) 5G NR variant (3GPP Release-15 5G NR NSA standard). eMBB has been identified to support 360° video streaming, virtual reality, and augmented reality applications [12].

5G's notable improvements resulted in the use of two high-frequency bands: RF-1: sub-6 GHz (3.5–7GHz) and RF-2: mmWave (>24 GHz). Although using low-frequency bands allows a much wider range of signal propagation, the bandwidth channel is narrow, and the latency is high. Using higher frequencies, on the other hand, allows for much wider bandwidths and ultra-low latencies, but shorter signal propagation range (see Figure 7.3).

By 2021, the sub-6 GHz has become the leading commercialized 5G frequency with mmWave having only a small percentage in the deployment [12]. The slow rollout of mmWave is because once a frequency increases, the range of propagation decreases, resulting in the shrinkage of cell sizes. In such a case, more base stations need to be installed to cover a wider area (network densification), which results in an increase in capital expenditure (CAPEX). Cells would have a typical coverage area radius of 20–150 meters. For a 20-meter cell radius, 800 base stations are required per km^2. This not only results in costly installations but also in delays for acquiring permissions [13].

The current global rollout of 5G presents different deployment statuses according to IDTechEx. An excerpt from its 5G Technology, Market and Forecasts 2022–2032 shows the status of the United States of America (USA) and China, two countries

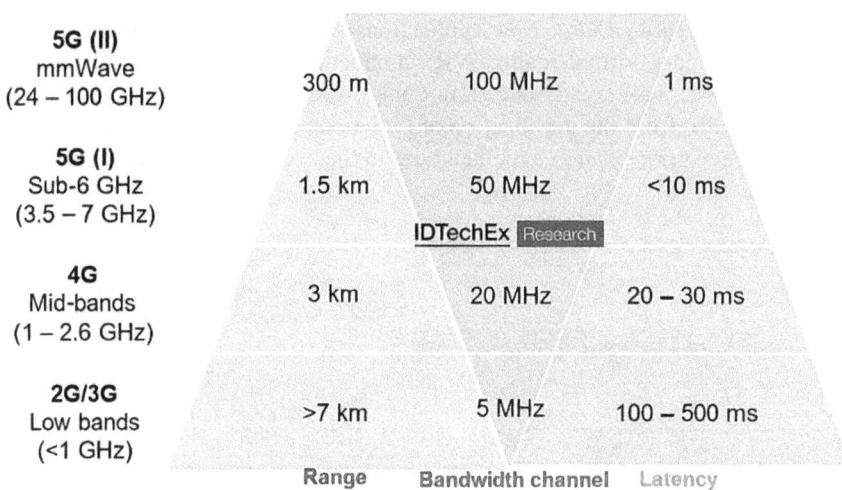

	Range	Bandwidth channel	Latency
5G (II) mmWave (24 – 100 GHz)	300 m	100 MHz	1 ms
5G (I) Sub-6 GHz (3.5 – 7 GHz)	1.5 km	50 MHz	<10 ms
4G Mid-bands (1 – 2.6 GHz)	3 km	20 MHz	20 – 30 ms
2G/3G Low bands (<1 GHz)	>7 km	5 MHz	100 – 500 ms

IDTechEx Research

FIGURE 7.3 Spectrum outlook from 2G to 5G [12]

representing 5G regions in terms of government and telecommunications operators' strategy.

The US government's FCC has significantly released the mmWave spectrum much earlier than other countries, followed by the sub-6GHz in early 2021. Since the US does not have leading US-based 5G equipment suppliers, FCC has supported Open RAN development. Telecom operators have their respective share of the 5G spectrum with Verizon having the majority of mmWave investments [14]. T-Mobile has concentrated on low and mid-band coverage using the 2.5 GHz frequency. AT&T and Verizon planned to deploy the mid-band services in 2021, targeting 100 million people coverage by 2022.

China's Ministry of Industry and Information Technology issued the 5G application action plan for 2021–2023 in April 2021 with identified KPIs: 40% increase in user penetration, more than 50% rise in 5G network access traffic, and a 35% push in big enterprise penetration. The 2022 Winter Olympics was targeted as the rollout event test bed for the mmWave spectrum. Chinese telecom operators worked together for the construction of a collective network infrastructure with China Telecom and China Unicom together building 460,000 base stations by May 2021 [15].

From 3GPP Release 15, 5G has continually improved to target use cases such as eMBB, massive IoT and new vertical industries by providing superior performance in both capacity and coverage. 3GPP Release 18 introduces 5G Advanced, building on Releases 15, 16, and 17. Aside from the need to support new verticals/use cases, 5G Advanced will be used as the first stage for and the bridge to 6G. Figure 7.4 depicts the timeline from the first 5G release to the 6G evolution ushered in by 5G Advanced. 5G Advanced will bring about significant enhancements in network performance focusing on the following areas [16]:

- **Intelligent network automation:** Employing AI/ML solutions to insert intelligence in network operations and enhance the RAN can significantly improve network performance.
- **Extended reality (XR):** New applications such as extended reality (XR), which includes virtual reality (VR), augmented reality (AR), and mixed reality (MR), will greatly benefit not only from high data rate communication but also from the introduction of Low Latency Low Loss (L4S), allowing latency prioritization over data rates in the event of traffic congestion.

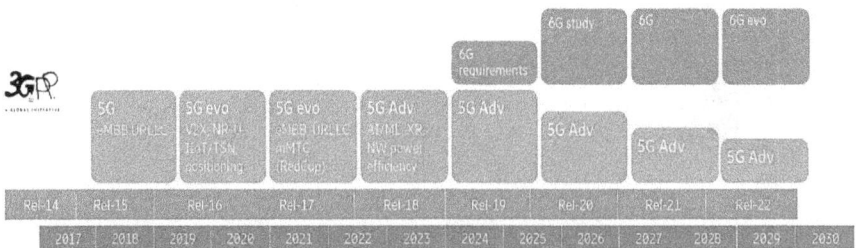

FIGURE 7.4 Ericsson's view of the 5G Advanced and 6G timeline of 3GPP [16]

- **Reduced Capability (RedCap) NR Devices:** RedCap devices are focused on the broadband IoT use cases. The focus of this development is on the reduction of modem costs, design relaxation, leaner procedures, and support for extended discontinuous reception (eDRX), allowing long power down periods and power saving.
- **Network Energy Savings:** Traffic load balancing and sleep mode for gNB will be focused on massive MIMO micro and macro settings to enhance network energy saving schemes.
- **Deterministic Networking for IoT:** 5G Advance will feature support for use cases where there are heavy requirements for bounded low latency, low delay variation, and extremely low loss.

It is argued that the main theme of network 2030 (Figure 7.5) should be "Fully Connected, Fully Intelligent" [17, 18]. This can be interpreted further to encompass intelligently prompt actions. Triple Is is defined as: Intelligent autonomous network infrastructure that supports intelligent operations to produce intelligent decisions based on human prospective. This makes the deployment of 6G wireless networks more conceivable. The 6G network is expected to be the most cutting-edge form of communication that will provide more opportunities for vertical businesses and use cases and bring with it new prospects. In addition to the mobile network conventional method for communication by using base stations, 6G will permit more advanced communication via terrestrial as well as many non-terrestrial communication networks, such as satellites, unmanned aerial vehicle (UAV) communication, and visible light communications [19, 20].

It is anticipated that the market for 6G technology would make significant advancements possible in the fields of imaging, presence technology, and location awareness in conjunction with artificial intelligence [21]. With biosensors and smart broadband-connected hardware, we can monitor our health in real time and store massive amounts of data in the cloud. Our quality of life and ability to care for ourselves will improve. Human-machine interactions can be improved by holographic communication.

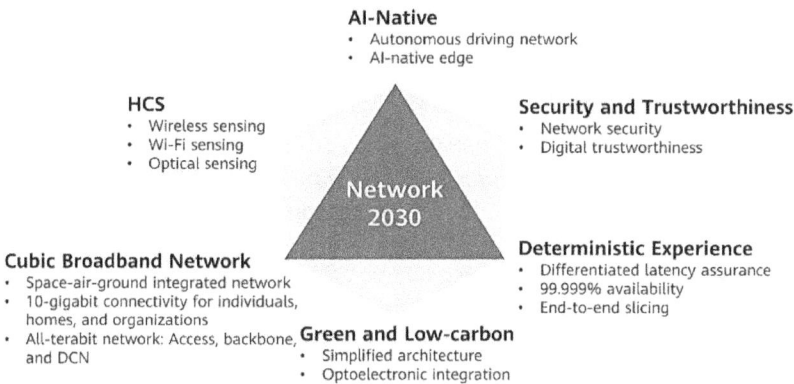

FIGURE 7.5 Huawei Communication Network 2030 [17]

Information exchanges between vehicles can make travel much safer, reduce road congestion, and maintain the eco-environment [18]. Moreover, 6G will extend the boundaries and make use cases such as ER, AR, VR, and advanced V2X more real.

7.3   INTERNET OF THINGS

In the world of mobile networks, the device-to-device (D2D) model allows direct link communication between devices in close proximity. This paradigm is said to realize the ultra-low latency benefits promised by 5G due to the shorter signal instead of having to connect directly to a base station and ultimately to the network core. The Internet has extended human communications and interaction to an unprecedented level. The continuing advancements in technology have evolved communications from solely human-centric to now, machine-centric. Machine-to-machine (M2M) communications, using D2D, allows "smart" devices to interact by establishing connections with each other and exchanging data. M2M brought about the Internet of Things (IoT) evolution. IoT's identity has evolved from the time the term was coined in the 1990s. This is due to the merging of diverse technologies. IoT refers to objects possessing virtual identities, capable of operating on smart spaces through interfaces that allow social and environmental communications [22].

In today's world, IoT has presented itself as an innovation that integrates smart systems, applications and communications frameworks, and intelligent devices. Its notable applications are categorized in wearables, utilities, monitoring, smart environments, security, transportation, and industrial Internet. IoT devices are usually connected using wireless technologies to ease deployment, eliminate physical connectivity costs, and enable mobility [23].

5G is identified as the paramount enabling technology for IoT connectivity. It is able to meet the demand for ultra-dense networks and has the potential to be utilized for low-power wide-area (LPWA) technologies as well as long-distance communication [24]. The future success of large-scale IoT implementations such as those in transportation and Industrial IoT depends on how 5G advancements address the challenges inherent in this technology. These include the following [23]: low power mode, coverage enhancements, URLLC, Massive IoT, and Small Data Burst. IoT devices should be demonstrated to work with various platforms, to facilitate data offloading from congested networks, and to extend network coverage.

The market demand for IoT is higher for such sectors as health IoT, Internet of Vehicles (IoV), and industrial IoT. According to the Cisco report (Internet of Things– Connected Means Informed), by 2030 the number of connected IoT devices will have hugely increased to reach approximately 500 billion devices [25]. The registered IoV itself will reach more than 400 million [26]. Sensors range from normal operations such as monitoring engines and high-speed alerts to traffic congestion sensors and navigation sensors. These are some examples of IoT devices that are involved in improving ITS operations and increasing the degree of automation. You can imagine from now onwards that on your busiest schedule day, your car will check your groceries and collect them for you, drop your children off at school, and bring them home at the end of the day. It can also sense your body temperature, monitor your blood pressure and heart rate, and subsequently, schedule an appointment with your doctor.

7.4 VEHICLE-TO-EVERYTHING NETWORKS

The integration of IoT in industry fosters the rehabilitation of cities to construct a new auto society. A well-known application of M2M is vehicle-to-vehicle (V2V) communications. D2D links are used in this deployment for sharing and offloading data between close-proximity vehicles [27]. This type of use case has evolved considerably due to extensive research and development and has been renamed as V2X (Vehicle-to-Everything), to include not only inter-vehicle communications but also between vehicles and road environment, non-vehicular objects, and network infrastructure.

Intelligent transport system (ITS) refers to the integration of electronics, communications, and automation technologies in vehicles, user systems, and infrastructure for a safe and efficient transport system [28]. In the USA, the Federal Communications Commission (FCC) allocated "75 megahertz of spectrum at 5.850–5.925 GHz to the mobile service for use by Dedicated Short Range Communications (DSRC) systems operating in the Intelligent Transportation System (ITS) radio service" [29]. In the European Union, the European Commission requested the European Standards Organization to develop and adopt standards for the ITS legal framework [28]. The ITS aims at deploying services that improve road safety, reduce traffic congestion, help curb air pollution levels, and conserve the use of fossil fuels [26]. V2X applications are categorized mainly for safety, non-safety, and infotainment purposes. In connection to the aims of ITS, V2X can help reduce accidents and risks to drivers, passengers, and road users (safety) and improve traffic management (non-safety).

Nowadays, V2X communication is a collective term that is used to cover vehicle-to-vehicle (V2V), vehicle-to-infrastructure (V2I), vehicle-to-pedestrian (V2P), and vehicle-to-network (V2N) communications (Figure 7.6). This paradigm, which is deployed with vehicle-sensing instruments and other types of smart technologies, enhances safety mechanisms, optimizes traffic management, and provides improved vehicle users' infotainment. This is attained through various use cases such as intelligent warning, discovery, and advisory systems. These use cases are enabled by a process of message exchanges among vehicles, infrastructures, and pedestrians using wireless connectivity technologies such as dedicated short range communications (DSRC) and Cellular-V2X (C-V2X) [30].

As previously mentioned, V2X is currently based on two radio access technologies, which are DSRC (Wi-Fi, IEEE802.11p) and C-V2X (Cellular). DSRC operates in the 5.9 GHz frequency while C-V2X can operate in both 5.9 GHz and cell operator's unlicensed frequencies. The use of C-V2X has been cited as more advantageous in terms of performance by providing improved link budget, high interference resilience, and better line of non-line-of-sight capacities [30].

For effective implementation of the general use cases presented in Figure 7.6, various regional authorities around the world such as the European Telecommunications Standards Institute (ETSI) and European Conference of Postal and Telecommunications Administrations (CEPT), Institute of Electrical and Electronics Engineers (IEEE) in US, and Telecommunications Technology Association (TTA) in South Korea came up with diverse types of use cases and performance requirements. The Fifth Generation Communication Automotive Research and Innovation (5GCAR), an

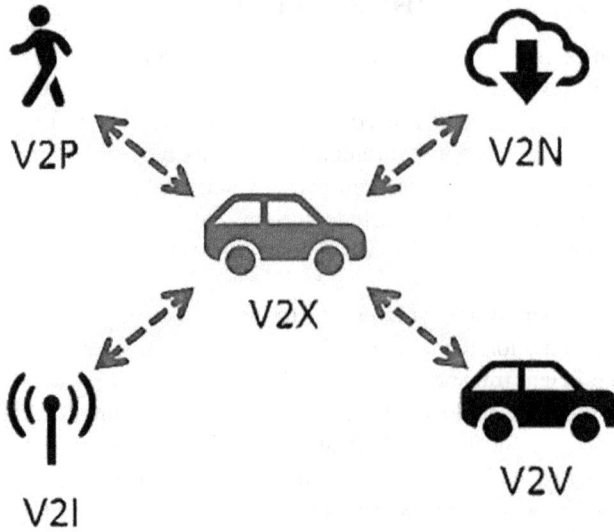

FIGURE 7.6 V2X communications use cases [31]

H2020 5G PPP Phase 2 project funded by the European Commission, proposed five use case classes, which are summarized in the next section with stringent requirements and key performance indicators (KPIs) listed [32]:

- **Vehicle Platooning:** This use case features vehicle group formation using virtual connections. Information is exchanged among the vehicles in the group while traveling together. This enables cooperative automated driving for partial or full automated platooning. This use case requires at least 30 cooperative awareness messages per second, 100 km/h speed, at least 1 meter distance between vehicles, 100 Hz message transmission frequency, 50–1,200 bytes message size, and a 90% reliability rate. For information sharing, the data rates required are 2.7 Mbps between user equipment (UE) and 2.5 Mbps between UE and roadside unit (RSU); 6,500 bytes and 6,000 bytes is the required periodic broadcast/multicast message payload capacity between UEs and between UE and RSU, respectively; 50 messages/sec/UE should be the maximum frequency of exchange and 20 ms end-to-end message exchange latency between UEs or between UE and RSU is required.
- **Remote Driving:** This use case provides the ability to remotely drive a vehicle either by humans or by applications. This capability is necessary in cases of dangerous road conditions, especially if a driver is not advisable to be present in the vehicle. Humans can perform remote driving using broadcasted images and commands executed in real-time. The use case must support speeds of up to 250 km/hour with communications uplink speed of up to 1 Mbps, downlink speed of up to 25 Mbps, a 5 ms end-to-end latency between servers and UEs, and 99.99% uplink and downlink reliability rate.

- **Extended Sensors:** This use case enables raw or processed data exchange collected from sensors, live video feeds, RSUs, pedestrians, and V2X servers. It helps augment the sensing capabilities of UEs, thereby increasing environmental awareness. This use case requires data rates between 10 to 1000 Mbps, 3 to 1,000 ms latency, a payload byte of at least 1,600, and at least 90% reliability rate.
- **Advanced Driving:** This use case permits a high level of automation for automated driving while allowing longer vehicle distances. UEs and RSUs use data from their sensors and from nearby UEs and RSUs to coordinate trajectories and exchange driving intensions, which are beneficial for safe travel, collision evasion, and traffic efficiency. This use case requires >10 ms latency, 99.99% reliability rate, 10 Mbps throughput, and up to 2 KB message size for safe driving maneuvers. Generally, 300–1,200 bytes, 10–100 message exchange/second, 3–100 ms latency, and 90%–99.99% reliability range is required.

In 2021, the Society of Automotive Engineers (SAE) proposed the level for autonomy driving. The levels are categorized from (Level 0–non-driving automation) to (Level 5–full driving automation) [33]. The description of the different levels is illustrated in Figure 7.7.

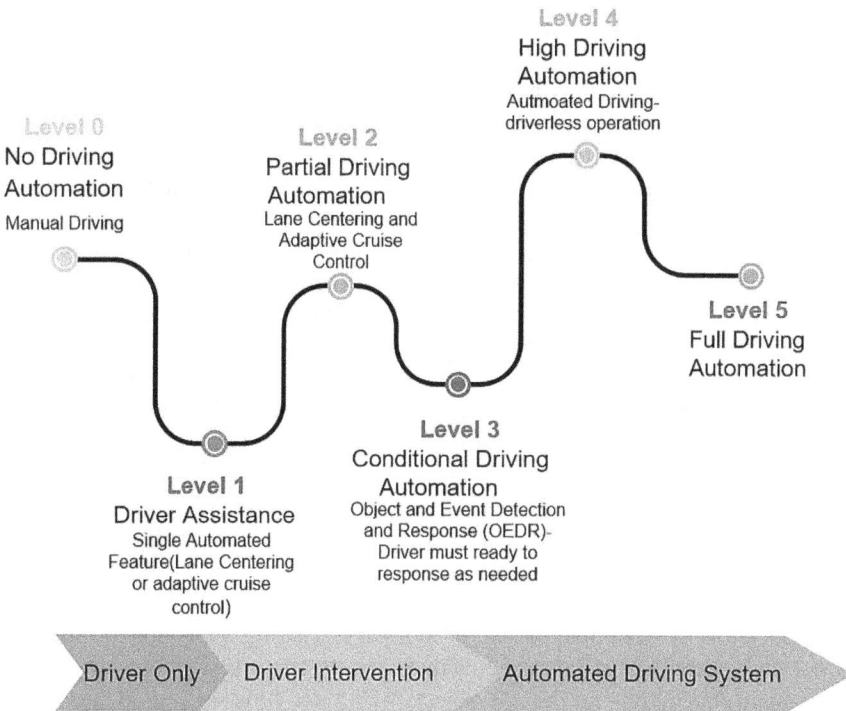

FIGURE 7.7   SAE levels of driving automation

The deployment of 5G-V2x is still in its earliest stages. On average and to 2021, there are approximately 14 different C-V2X vehicle models that have been released to the market, China being the country that has made the most progress in this area. The investment in this technology should focus on the later stage to establish a fully digitalized road infrastructure to ensure cooperative and seamless connectivity [34]. There are still more challenges that need to be addressed by standardization organizations and researchers to reach the goal for fully automated driving. We believe that the integration of emerging technologies in V2X such as augmented reality can make a distinctive improvement and will be a top research area along with tracking and position accuracy.

7.5   AUGMENTED REALITY

Digital transformation has brought about enhancements in the way people present information for various consumption purposes. Mobile networks and portable devices have created a huge demand for the information presented by multimedia applications. AR is considered to be the eighth mass media compared to mobile as the seventh in terms of content storage and consumption. Due to this, network traffic has and will continue to greatly increase, particularly from heavy demands on live streaming content and AR objects posting useful information in different formats (images, video, sound, etc.) throughout the entire urban environment for different types of applications. Among these multimedia applications, virtual and augmented reality (VR and AR) applications are expected, not only to be on the list of data-intensive applications, but also to be some of the tools that will be heavily integrated in various sectors, such as education, healthcare, transportation, tourism, museums, and business, to name a few. For example, the integration of AR in automobile industries has the potential to reduce the time and cost for inspection and maintenance processes. This is especially so when AR aids the designer during the prototyping phase, allowing for the elimination of faults before mass production. Market leaders are increasingly relying on AR as a promotional tool, which is gradually replacing traditional showrooms, allowing their customers to have an interactive view of the new vehicle model by using their mobile and without the need for leaving their home [35].

It has been previously predicted that the VR market will hit 65 billion dollars and that AR will hit around 114 billion dollars by 2021, as per ABI Research [36].

AR is a technology that enhances the real world by superimposing digital objects and information over a user's view. This greatly improves a user's perception of an environment by providing in-depth analysis, essential details, and augmented knowledge from various related sources. Compared to virtual reality (VR), which focuses on virtually simulating the real world, AR combines and aligns real and virtual objects and environments and allows real-time interaction specified by the user application. An example of AR in tourism is visiting a city for the first time and not understanding the language of that specific country. Through his/her goggles or smartphone, moving the AR objects will guide him/her to find specific targets, such as restaurants, ATM bank machines, etc., using a translation service of the highlighted posts and receiving sound direction through earphones to reach the destination. For example, a restaurant AR object may post menus, offers, and other information that could be consulted before arriving at the real restaurant. AR falls under the mixed reality (MR) spectrum since the focus is on mixing virtual with real to produce an augmented environment, as presented in Figure 7.8 [37].

A basic AR system is composed of input components such as sensors and other multimedia devices. The inputs undergo a series of processing steps, after which the outputs in the form of virtual contents are superimposed to present an augmented view of the real world through devices such as smartphones, video displays, and AR headsets. The output devices can be capable of processing the inputs or have the outputs streamed from AR application servers (Figure 7.9).

A variety of AR platforms exist based on particular applications, but the processing steps are quite general [38]:

- **Tracking:** This determines the current space positioning information to aid in the alignment of generated virtual contents and the physical, real-world object in a scene. Tracking can be sensor-based (acoustic, optical, mechanical, magnetic) or vision-based (marker-based, marker-less). In vision-based tracking, markers provide patterns for recognition that can trigger an action.

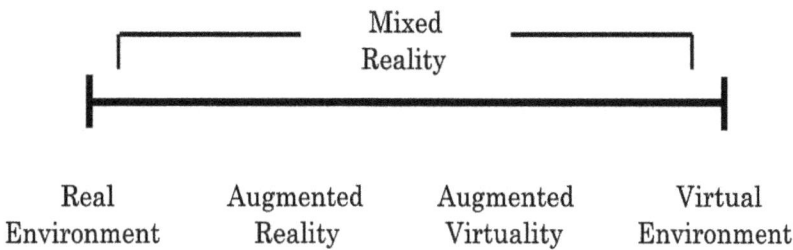

FIGURE 7.8   Milgram and Kishino Reality-Virtuality Continuum (Milgram et al., 1994) [37]

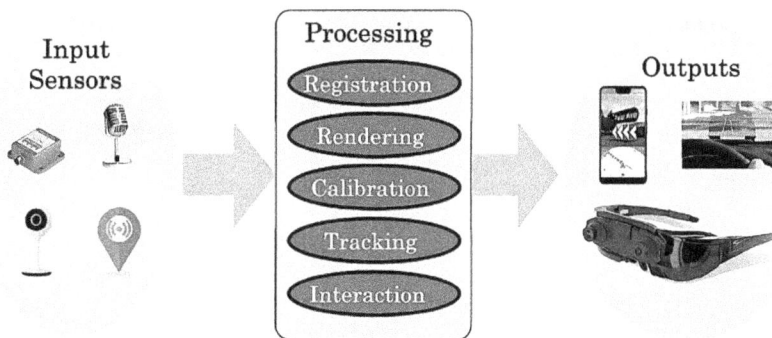

FIGURE 7.9   Basic AR system components [38]

- **Rendering:** Rendering outputs digital contents based on the trigger. This type of action is computationally intensive and requires real-time response that requires rendering to be done by powerful application and content servers instead of the output devices. The transmission of the rendered output, however, is affected by the performance quality of the enabling network technology being used.
- **Registration and Calibration:** These steps involve the precise alignment of rendered objects with the real world.
- **Interaction:** This step refers to how users operate the AR contents. The interaction experience depends on the AR use case/application and the capabilities of the output device used. The level of interaction can range from non-interaction to real-time interaction, as shown in Figure 7.10.

Currently, AR technology is used in a variety of applications, such as healthcare, manufacturing, entertainment and games, military and national defense, robotics, education, business, culture and tourism, museum, etc. The usage is generally challenged by technical requirements (AR and enabling technologies) such as limited contents, lack of public awareness, lack of regulations and standardization, and rendering/visualization issues [38]. On the other hand, AR technology has made its way to notable vertical use cases such as mobile augmented reality (MAR), automotive and intelligent transport systems, and retail industry among others.

AR and VR are rapidly emerging "immersive" technologies that assist the retail industry in enhancing a customer's assessment of various merchandise, view of store environments, and shopping experiences by enabling virtual interaction with items. In contrast to VR, which tends to block the sensations generated by the real world, AR permits enhanced and more realistic experiences within the physical environment [39].

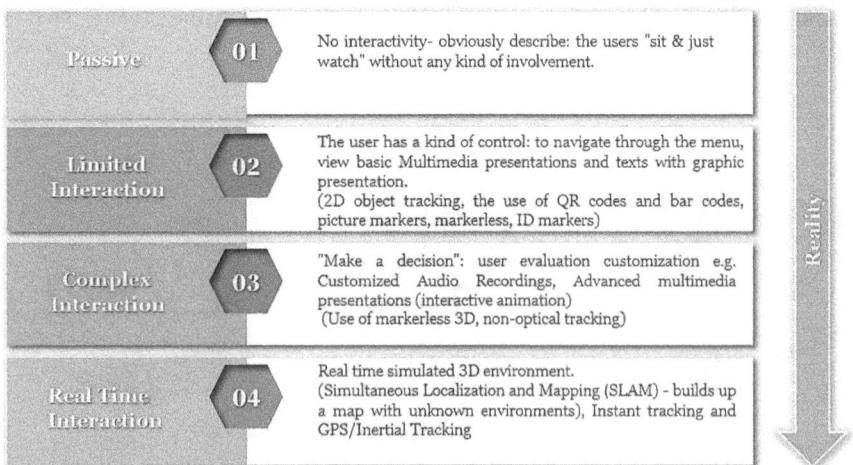

FIGURE 7.10   AR level of interactivity

7.6   AR INTEGRATION IN V2X

AR is an innovative, immersive technology primarily based on computer graphics rendered onto real-world objects. In various industries such as automotive, AR was tapped as a marketing tool to provide an immersive experience to customers by giving them the key features of a vehicle, the customizations that are available to fit their requirements, and the kind of accessories they can buy to improve a car's looks, among others. AR helps make the car purchase experience more informative, immersive, and enjoyable. AR has also been used in the automotive industry for workshop activities such as inspection and maintenance work [35].

The V2X ecosystem is a part of ITS that is primarily focused on improving road safety and efficient traffic management. Various technologies have been integrated in V2X that have made the automotive industry a part of the worldwide digital transformation.

For V2X, AR primarily offers assistive capabilities to adapt human and machine perception on the changing conditions within the driving environment. AR is being integrated in V2X as an enabling technology to increase road safety, provide navigational assistance, enhance driver and passenger experience, and assist other road users using external human-machine interfaces (HMIs). AR has the potential to improve user experience and raise technology awareness, which can be used in establishing trust and acceptance in automated vehicles [40].

AR integration in V2X is further explained in the following application areas [41–43]:

- **Driving Assistance and Safety:** In this area, AR provides driver assistance and increases safety by providing visual cues rendered in the road environment to enhance awareness and attention. AR can also initiate human response by providing alerts for emergency behaviors, bad road conditions, and unfavorable weather patterns. Overall, AR will be able to provide the driver with better situational awareness.
- **Navigation:** In vehicles with low-level automation, AR can be used for navigation aids that not only provide proper guidance but also reduce unwanted distractions. Instead of relying on traditional road signs, drivers will benefit from augmented instructions that are fixed in the outside environment.
- **Human-Machine Interface:** AR fosters the development and use of output devices such as windshield displays (WSDs) and heads-up displays (HUDs) that enhance the visual fidelity of the driving environment. AR can also provide information such as driving conditions, behavior, and intent externally to vulnerable road users such as pedestrians and cyclists.
- **Traveller Guide:** Unlike a GPS, AR can provide the driver with guidance throughout the journey by displaying information about the road ahead in a more dynamic display. This is quite efficient and safe as the information is projected as required, and the driver does not employ hands to give instructions.
- **Passenger Experience:** AR can provide in-vehicle passenger instructions or easy-to-understand guidance, and infotainment, particularly in public

transportation systems, to aid in work-related functionalities and improve comfort. AR is based on real-world environment objects and stored real and generated information and objects combined to create a single perception. Objects and/or data in the form of simulations, location, sound, and visuals all contribute to the creation of the user experience. The quality of the processing and the timely dissemination of the AR contents directly affect the value of the user experience. Aside from the basic AR system components illustrated in Figure 7.9, the integration of AR in V2X depends on additional interconnected diverse components.

- **Applications:** This component refers to the use case representation and interface layer that allows users to interact with the AR system. This includes navigation, warning systems, and other types of contents rendered on the output devices. The wake-up app is an example of an AR warning system [44]. This mobile application makes use of face recognition technology to monitor the driver's eye and hand movements in order to determine whether or not the driver is dozing off behind the wheel.
- **Social Interaction:** The integration of AR into the fully automated system (Level 5) allows projecting family and friends as avatars, reducing driver social isolation.
- **Services:** This component refers to access to network and other connectivity infrastructure, storage, and computing services. This includes wireless and mobile networks, cloud and edge computing services, and application servers.
- **Middleware:** This component represents a collection of software that provides the connection between the hardware, services, and application components.

7.7   IMPLICATIONS OF AR IN V2X

AR's unique features enhance people's experiences through the presentation of information that augments an otherwise ordinary environment. In today's information-centric society, AR creates a situation where human interactions are based on directing attention to points of interest, thereby generating a strong, effective connection to the task at hand. This focused, assistive functionality proves to be an essential aspect in sustaining and ensuring control, especially in dynamic use cases where safety and reliability are of primary concern. V2X is an application area where AR can be integrated to provide navigational assistance, situational awareness, and enhanced human-machine connection to considerably decrease user distractions and increase safety.

7.7.1   Benefits

The integration of AR in V2X is not merely confined to the enhancement of passenger infotainment. It is meant to deliver the following benefits [45, 46]:

- AR provides graphics that augment information in the real world. AR can enhance the real world by superimposing graphic elements on to trigger objects. It annotates the real world with useful information. This greatly helps drivers become aware of current and changing road and environmental conditions that necessitate an alternate or corrective course of action while driving. AR significantly enhances a driver's connection to the task at hand, resulting in lesser distractions.

- It enhances a driver's vision by detecting barely noticeable objects and increases their visibility using overlaid images. In the event of low visibility, particularly at night or due to unfavorable road and weather conditions, AR assists in seeing through by overlaying images on objects. This technique may enhance visibility.
- It presents virtual signs for navigation that greatly aid novice drivers and foreign drivers who are not familiar with the local language. AR can be used to produce guides or markers that help less experienced drivers and foreigners such as tourists to traverse the local geography without a map. AR rendered information can be presented in a preferred language to help those who do not understand the language used in traffic signs.
- It can highlight detected threats and display vehicle trajectory. Through object detection and augmentation, AR can help drivers be aware of dangers along the vehicle's path, resulting in more careful driving.
- It creates a captivating and immersive user experience. AR's use of graphics-based information presentation immerses users by lessening the complexities of driving due to its assistive nature. Drivers will feel adequately capable, and passengers will have a sense of safety, thus enjoying the ride. Because of this benefit, AR can be used to build trust and confidence in autonomous driving.

7.7.2 CONSEQUENCES

Enhancing V2X through the use of AR could pose several unfavorable outcomes [45, 46]:

- AR tends to put some strain on a driver's cognitive load. In manned vehicles, the use of AR can result in frequent "cognitive capture." Poorly designed AR graphics tend to capture the attention of the driver, which could distract driving and lead to increased danger or road traffic accidents.
- AR output devices tend to trigger motion sickness. Due to sensory conflict arising from the discrepancy between a user's head movements and AR's visual display, motion sickness may be experienced.
- AR tends to create safety issues for pedestrians. Vehicles that provide information through external interfaces such as visual displays, as well as applications in a road user's device, tend to capture attention and distract from the road. This could compromise the safety of users such as pedestrians and cyclists.
- AR tends to increase a driver's risk level. Getting used to the safety benefit brought about by AR in V2X can push a driver's or autonomous vehicle owner's risk envelope further. A vehicle operator who has high trust and confidence in assistive technologies like AR would tend to rely on the technology rather than drive carefully, relying on his/her own judgment.

However, despite the presented consequences, AR would still provide an enhanced experience that could greatly change the way V2X provides road and traffic safety and service reliability. Properly designed AR contents, with highly effective human-machine interfaces, can help reduce or eliminate cognitive overload. Ergonomically designed AR devices that are properly integrated into the driving instrumentations and devices can prevent sensory conflict and motion sickness. AR contents delivered through external interfaces should only be limited to low-traffic areas. AR contents should provide precautionary messages to remind drivers not to rely entirely on AR but rather to place primary trust in their own driving skills.

7.7.3 Implications

- AR for V2X will require contents with high visual fidelity. Graphics content is one of the elements necessary for AR. Production of graphics objects that will augment the real world must be developed with a high level of quality to achieve the discriminability which is necessary to elicit the required driver actions, highlight threats, make driving conditions recognizable, and provide the right context. Rendering high-quality content will necessitate considerable computing capabilities. For V2X devices with limited processing power, processing of graphics content must be offloaded to application servers and streamed when required.
- V2X use cases that use AR require 5G network connectivity. Due to the heavy computing requirements for graphics processing in AR, computational work and data storage will be moved away from the V2X devices. Access to these contents will then be enabled through streaming using fast wireless mobile connections. The eMBB feature of 5G provides a viable service for the transmission of high-quality graphics contents. Fog nodes and mobile edge computing (MEC) can also be employed to perform graphics content processing near the network edge for faster transmission. AR post processing is recommended to be done near the edge using high-speed connectivity, high data rate, and low latency.
- For V2X applications, AR needs to be deployed with a wide range of interaction modalities, such as gesture recognition and speech recognition. AR enabled vehicles to necessitate an array of interaction interfaces that are designed with the goal of combining multiple modalities to act on any situational context. Speech-enabled interaction, success or error feedback, context awareness, and gaze-based interface should be considered. The design of the interface should also take into consideration avoidance of straining the driver's cognitive load. AR interfaces should not be so eye-catching or difficult to use that it takes a driver's attention from the road [41].
- Traditional AR output should be redefined for V2X. VR contents are usually displayed using VR headsets. In the case of AR for V2X, display devices come in the form of WSDs and AR HUDs. These devices should be designed in such a way that they will not cause the driver visual overload and/or

distractions. WSDs/AR HUDs should present the right balance of objects presented in a scene, otherwise, the driver will be overwhelmed by the available information that may lead to stress and loss of situational awareness. In [47], the author claims that AR contact lenses might be the solution of the future, with the potential to deliver contextual information about the surrounding environment to the driver.

- AR for V2X should consider creating designs for different people. AR equipped V2X is considered a new type of technology. At the design stage, technology products are usually engineered for the young, experienced, or technology-proficient segment. V2X will be used by people of all age groups. The AR elements and interfaces should be designed with inclusiveness in mind. Developing and testing a multimodal interface must involve users that represent each group [41].

7.8   CHALLENGES

The success of integrating and implementing AR in V2X rests on overcoming the following technological challenges and solutions in order to enhance usability, obtain user satisfaction, and achieve the set goals and objectives of ITS [44, 48–51]:

- **Content Caching:** Caching improves the speed of data transmission from storage to application. Caching contents at the intermediate locations (base stations, network edge, and other devices) will result in a more responsive system, which is a stringent requirement for AR. Reactive caching can be implemented to serve requests, while proactive caching can be used to anticipate the user's next request.
- **Processing Location:** Computationally intensive AR tasks can be migrated to other locations, especially if V2X devices have limited computational abilities. MEC will enable devices to access Fog/Cloud infrastructures on demand, while distributed computing will enable the sharing of computational load.
- **Short-Range Wireless Communications:** Network congestion is one of the main concerns when it comes to V2X connections. By using short-range wireless communications such as D2D and proximity services (ProSe), network congestion can be alleviated.
- **Multimedia:** The introduction of high-definition cameras has created enhanced video and other multimedia data. Today's media requires more computational power for processing and usage and bigger storage capacities to store. This poses a challenge especially in the implementation of graphics-dependent applications like AR in V2X.
- **Context Information:** Optimizing a technological implementation has been one of the concerns of technology adopters. To maximize the use of AR in V2X, context information must be extracted and must be dwelt upon to provide meaningful experience. This is not easy to achieve since behavioral, emotional, and inherent information must be taken into consideration but are not easy to obtain.

- **Performance Trade-offs:** For a given set of constraints, which one should be prioritized to give a more meaningful and immersive AR experience in V2X? AR is a computationally heavy application that processes complex sets of data, requiring fast network connectivity with high reliability rate. The right balance of prioritization must be applied in order to achieve acceptable results for the AR implementation. One of the key technologies in 5G is network slicing. This technology concept provides the flexibility of having a logical dedicated slice level for different use cases.
- **Frequent Changes in Connection:** The stability and availability of network connections is a prime challenge for AR technologies, especially when it is integrated with critical use cases such as V2X. An optimal solution that ensures seamless connectivity is the main goal for 5G networks in order to prove the availability with low latency.
- **Security:** AR contents are usually developed and rendered by third-party providers/vendors and applications. Contents can be rendered unreliable if the generation and transmission of AR contents are done by unauthenticated and unauthorized providers. Without stringent authentication and authorization mechanisms, attackers can insert their own contents, allowing them to give incorrect information. This could cause serious risks and damage, eventually compromising V2X safety.

7.9 CONCLUSION

The application of AR in V2X will create a fundamental change in the transport industry, particularly in terms of safety and operational efficiency. The success of integration relies on the upcoming advancements not only for AR and V2X, but also for their enabling technologies as well. For the improvement of the AR elements for V2X, research must be undertaken on the utilization of context information for specifying the types of AR devices, users, use cases, and interface modalities. Studies should be conducted on applications that focus on driving analytics, improving calibration and registration for effective display adjustments, counteracting motion sickness, and optimizing content caching for a more responsive AR implementation. Standards that are solely focused on the implementation and/or integration of AR in V2X must be enacted in order to attain a level of reliability and quality of service. AR's graphics content must conform to an acceptable resolution, color accuracy, typography, elements layout, and types of information representation. AR-assisted vehicles must be equipped with reliable, high-speed network connectivity components to ensure that information is processed and provided to the drivers in real time. Information security standards need to be ratified as well in order to ensure that AR devices are not prone to attacks that can impair functionalities or be used as vectors for attacking other users and vehicles. AR integration in driving must imply a certain limitation that prevents drivers from relying entirely on AR rather than their driving skills and experience. Implementation will continually encounter issues and challenges, but disruptive technologies and solutions will present themselves as viable solutions.

REFERENCES

[1] "M.2083: IMT Vision—Framework and Overall Objectives of the Future Development of IMT for 2020 and Beyond", *Itu.int*, 2015. [Online]. Available: www.itu.int/rec/ R-REC-M.2083 [Accessed: 10-Jul-2022].

[2] S. Asif, *5G Mobile Communications Concepts and Technologies*. Boca Raton, FL: CRC Press, Taylor & Francis, 2019.

[3] H. Fattah, *LTE Cellular Narrowband Internet of Things (NB-IoT)*. Boca Raton, FL: CRC Press, 2021.

[4] Focus Group on Technologies for Network 2030, "Network 2030 Architecture Framework," *ITU*, Jun-2020. [Online]. Available: https://www.itu.int/en/ITU-T/focusgroups/net2030/ Documents/Network_2030_Architecture-framework.pdf [Accessed: 10-Jul-2022].

[5] "Road Traffic Injuries", World Health Organization, 21-Jun-2021. [Online]. Available: www.who.int/news-room/fact-sheets/detail/road-traffic-injuries.

[6] J. Chen and G. Fragomeni, *Virtual, Augmented and Mixed Reality*. Switzerland, AG: Springer Nature, 2020, pp. 154–170.

[7] E. Gures, I. Shayea, A. Alhammadi, M. Ergen and H. Mohamad, "A Comprehensive Survey on Mobility Management in 5G Heterogeneous Networks: Architectures, Challenges and Solutions", *IEEE Access*, vol. 8, pp. 195883–195913, 2020. Available: 10.1109/access.2020.3030762.

[8] "Cisco Annual Internet Report (2018–2023) White Paper," 10-Jul-2022. [Online]. Available: www.cisco.com/c/en/us/solutions/collateral/executive-perspectives/annual- internet-report/white-paper-c11-741490.html.

[9] R. Prasad and P. S. Rufino Henrique, "6G: The Road to the Future Wireless Technologies 2030," In Paulo Sergio Rufino Henrique, Ramjee Prasad. (eds) *6G The Road to the Future Wireless Technologies 2030*, River Publishers, Aalborg, Denmark, 2021, pp. i–xxvi.

[10] M. Vaezi, Z. Ding and H. Poor, "*Multiple Access Techniques for 5G Wireless Networks and Beyond*," Springer, Berlin, Heidelberg, Germany, 2019.

[11] "5G-Advanced Technology Evolution from a Network Perspective White Paper Release," *Huawei*, 2021. [Online]. Available: www-file.huawei.com/-/media/CORP2020/pdf/ event/1/5G_Advanced_Technology_Evolution_from_a_Network_Perspective_2021_ en.pdf [Accessed: 10-Jul-2022].

[12] I. P. Chochliouros et al., "5G Promotive Actions Based upon Enhanced Mobile Broadband (EMBB) Communication Trials between the EU and China," *2020 5th South-East Europe Design Automation, Computer Engineering, Computer Networks and Social Media Conference (SEEDA-CECNSM)*, Corfu, Greece, 2020, pp. 1–10. Available: 10.1109/SEEDA-CECNSM49515.2020.9221805.

[13] D. Chang, "5G: A Summary of 2021 and What to Expect Going Forward", *IDTechEx*, 2021. [Online]. Available: www.idtechex.com/en/research-article/5g-a-summary-of- 2021-and-what-to-expect-going-forward/25315 [Accessed: 16-Jul-2022].

[14] "What Is 5G Technology", Verizon Business. [Online]. Available: www.verizon.com/ business/resources/5g/what-is-5g-technology/ [Accessed: 24-Sept-2022].

[15] D. Chang and D. Edmondson, "5G Technology, Market and Forecasts 2022–2032", *IDTechEx*, 2021. [Online]. Available: www.idtechex.com/en/research-report/5g-tech- nology-market-and-forecasts-2022-2032/835 [Accessed: 16-Jul-2022].

[16] "5G Advanced: Evolution Towards 6G", *ericsson.com*, 2022. [Online]. Available: www.ericsson.com/en/reports-and-papers/white-papers/5g-advanced-evolution- towards-6g#:~:text=In%20addition%2C%20the%20need%20for,thus%20bridge%20 5G%20with%206G [Accessed: 16-Jul-2022].

[17] "Communications Network 2030", *Huawei*. [Online]. https://www-file.huawei.com/-/ media/corp2020/pdf/giv/industry-reports/communications_network_2030_en.pdf [Accessed: 16-Jul-2022].

[18] "Extended Reality Market Size & Share I Industry Report, 2021–2026 I Marketsand-Markets™", *Marketsandmarkets.com*, 2021. [Online]. Available: www.marketsand markets.com/Market-Reports/extended-reality-market-147143592.html [Accessed: 15-Jul-2022].

[19] S. G. Ansari, "Toward Automated Assessment of User Experience in Extended Reality," *2020 IEEE 13th International Conference on Software Testing, Validation and Verification (ICST)*, Porto, Portugal, 2020, pp. 430–432. Available: 10.1109/ICST46399.2020.00056.

[20] V. Hui, T. Estrina, G. Zhou and A. Huang, "Applications of Extended Reality Technologies Within Design Pedagogy: A Case Study in Architectural Science", *International Journal for Digital Society*, vol. 12, no. 2, pp. 1710–1720, 2021. Available: 10.20533/ijds.2040.2570.2021.0214.

[21] S. Doolani et al., "A Review of Extended Reality (XR) Technologies for Manufacturing Training", *Technologies*, vol. 8, no. 4, p. 77, 2020. Available: 10.3390/technologies8040077 [Accessed: 16-Jul-2022].

[22] K. Salih, T. Rashid, D. Radovanovic and N. Bacanin, "A Comprehensive Survey on the Internet of Things with the Industrial Marketplace", *Sensors*, vol. 22, no. 3, p. 730, 2022. Available: 10.3390/s22030730 [Accessed: 16-Jul-2022].

[23] H. Sun, C. Wang and B. Ahmad, *From Internet of Things to Smart Cities Enabling Technologies*. Boca Raton, FL: CRC Press, 2018, pp. 4–28.

[24] L. Chettri and R. Bera, "A Comprehensive Survey on Internet of Things (IoT) Toward 5G Wireless Systems," *IEEE Internet of Things Journal*, vol. 7, no. 1, pp. 16–32, Jan-2020. Available: 10.1109/JIOT.2019.2948888.

[25] "At-a-Glance Connected Means Informed", *Emarsonindia.com*. [Online]. Available: https://emarsonindia.com/wp-content/uploads/2020/02/Internet-of-Things.pdf [Accessed: 21-Oct-2022].

[26] X. Krasniqi and E. Hajrizi, "Use of IoT Technology to Drive the Automotive Industry from Connected to Full Autonomous Vehicles", *IFAC-PapersOnLine*, vol. 49, no. 29, pp. 269–274, 2016.

[27] U. Kar and D. Sanyal, "An Overview of Device-to-Device Communication in Cellular Networks", *ICT Express*, vol. 4, no. 4, pp. 203–208, 2018. Available: 10.1016/j.icte.2017.08.002 [Accessed: 16-Jul-2022].

[28] "ITS Standards—Intelligent Transport Systems", *Itsstandards.eu*. [Online]. Available: www.itsstandards.eu/ [Accessed: 17-Jul-2022].

[29] *Docs.fcc.gov*, 1999. [Online]. Available: https://docs.fcc.gov/public/attachments/FCC-99-305A1.pdf [Accessed: 17-Jul-2022].

[30] S. Gyawali, S. Xu, Y. Qian and R. Hu, "Challenges and Solutions for Cellular Based V2X Communications", *IEEE Communications Surveys & Tutorials*, vol. 23, no. 1, pp. 222–255, 2021. Available: 10.1109/comst.2020.3029723 [Accessed: 18-Jul-2022].

[31] F. Al Harthi and A. Touzen, "Hybrid Cell Selection Mechanism for V2X Handover," *Inventive Computation and Information Technologies. Lecture Notes in Networks and Systems*, vol. 563, pp. 641–655, Springer, Singapore. Available: 10.1007/978-981-19-7402-1_45.

[32] A. Alalewi, I. Dayoub and S. Cherkaoui, "t-V2X Use Cases and Enabling Technologies: A Comprehensive Survey", *IEEE Access*, vol. 9, pp. 107710–107737, 2021. Available: 10.1109/access.2021.3100472 [Accessed: 18-Jul-2022].

[33] SAE, "Taxonomy and Definitions for Terms Related to Driving Automation Systems for On-Road Motor Vehicles," *SAE International*, Apr-2021. Available: https://www.sae.org/standards/content/j3016_202104/ [Accessed: 20-Jul-2022].

[34] "5GAA Shares Latest C-V2X Developments at ITS World Congress (Hamburg)—5G Automotive Association", *5gaa.org*. [Online]. Available: https://5gaa.org/news/5gaa-shares-latest-c-v2x-developments-at-its-world-congress-hamburg-5g-will-have-the-most-revolutionary-impact-by-reducing-accidents-and-saving-millions-of-lives/ [Accessed: 22-Oct-2022].

[35] A. Z. A. Halim, "Applications of Augmented Reality for Inspection and Maintenance Process in Automotive Industry," *Journal of Fundamental and Applied Sciences*, vol. 10, no. 3S, pp. 412–421, Feb-2018. Available: 10.4314/jfas.v10i3s.35.

[36] M. Mahbub and B. Barua, "Optimal Coverage and Bandwidth-Aware Transmission Planning for Augmented Reality/Virtual Reality," *2021 International Conference on Information Technology (ICIT)*, Amman, Jordan, 2021, pp. 612–615. Available: 10.1109/ICIT52682.2021.9491124.

[37] P. Sirohi, A. Agarwal and P. Maheshwari, "A Survey on Augmented Virtual Reality: Applications and Future Directions," *2020 Seventh International Conference on Information Technology Trends (ITT)*, Abu Dhabi, United Arab Emirates, 2020, pp. 99–106. Available: 10.1109/ITT51279.2020.9320869.

[38] Y. Siriwardhana, P. Porambage, M. Liyanage and M. Ylianttila, "A Survey on Mobile Augmented Reality with 5G Mobile Edge Computing: Architectures, Applications, and Technical Aspects", *IEEE Communications Surveys & Tutorials*, vol. 23, no. 2, pp. 1160–1192, 2021. Available: 10.1109/comst.2021.3061981 [Accessed: 19-Jul-2022].

[39] M. C. tom Dieck and T. Jung, Eds., *Augmented Reality and Virtual Reality: The Power of AR and VR for Business*, Progress in IS, Springer, 2019. Available: 10.1007/978-3-030-06246-0.

[40] P. Wintersberger, A.-K. Frison, A. Riener and T. von Sawitzky, "Fostering User Acceptance and Trust in Fully Automated Vehicles: Evaluating the Potential of Augmented Reality", *Presence* (Camb.), vol. 27, no. 1, pp. 46–62, 2018.

[41] A. Riegler, A. Riener and C. Holzmann, "Augmented Reality for Future Mobility: Insights from a Literature Review and HCI Workshop", *i-com*, vol. 20, no. 3, pp. 295–318, 2021. Available: 10.1515/icom-2021–0029 [Accessed: 20-Jul-2022].

[42] L. Paule, "Advances in Mobility Using Virtual and Augmented Reality", *Laval Virtual*, 20-Sep-2021. [Online]. Available: https://blog.laval-virtual.com/en/advances-in-mobility-using-virtual-and-augmented-reality/ [Accessed: 20-Oct-2022].

[43] Infopulse, "How Does Augmented Reality Affect the Automotive Industry Today?" *Medium*, 24-Mar-2019. [Online]. Available: https://medium.com/@infopulse global_9037/how-does-augmented-reality-affect-the-automotive-industry-today-274d6408ecfc [Accessed: 24-Oct-2022].

[44] P. Zhou, W. Zhang, T. Braud, P. Hui and J. Kangasharju, "Enhanced Augmented Reality Applications in Vehicle-to-Edge Networks," *2019 22nd Conference on Innovation in Clouds, Internet and Networks and Workshops (ICIN)*, Paris, France, 2019, pp. 167–174. Available: 10.1109/ICIN.2019.8685872.

[45] K. Chang and T. Seder, "Automotive Augmented Reality: User Experience and Enabling Technology", *Information Display*, vol. 38, no. 1, pp. 12–18, 2022. Available: 10.1002/msid.1272 [Accessed: 20-Jul-2022].

[46] A. Dirin and T. Laine, "User Experience in Mobile Augmented Reality: Emotions, Challenges, Opportunities and Best Practices", *Computers*, vol. 7, no. 2, p. 33, 2018.

[47] A. Winkler, "These AR Contact Lenses Could Help Us Enter the Metaverse", *Big Think*, 30-Oct-2021. [Online]. Available: https://bigthink.com/the-future/augmented-reality-metaverse/ [Accessed: 24-Oct-2022].

[48] E. Bastug, M. Bennis, M. Medard and M. Debbah, "Toward Interconnected Virtual Reality: Opportunities, Challenges, and Enablers", *IEEE Communications Magazine*, vol. 55, no. 6, pp. 110–117, 2017. Available: 10.1109/mcom.2017.1601089.

[49] E. O'Connell, D. Moore and T. Newe, "Challenges Associated with Implementing 5G in Manufacturing," *Telecom*, vol. 1, no. 1, pp. 48–67, 2020.

[50] P. Zhou et al., "5G MEC Computation Handoff for Mobile Augmented Reality," *arXiv [cs.NI]*, 2021.

[51] "What Are the Security and Privacy Risks of VR and AR", *www.kaspersky.com*, 30-Mar-2022. [Online]. Available: www.kaspersky.com/resource-center/threats/security-and-privacy-risks-of-ar-and-vr [Accessed: 24-Oct-2022].

8 Development of a Road Map for Primary Healthcare Integrating AR-based Technology
Lessons Learned and the Way Forward

Khar Thoe Ng, Ying Li Thong, Nelson Cyril, Kamalambal Durairaj, Shah Jahan Assanarkutty, and Sivaranjini Sinniah

8.1 INTRODUCTION

8.1.1 PRIMARY HEALTHCARE: OPERATIONAL DEFINITION AND JUSTIFICATION OF TECHNOLOGY INTEGRATION

Primary healthcare (PHC) is an essential part of healthcare made accessible and affordable by all with practical, scientifically and socially acceptable methods. The fundamental assumption/truth/supposition of PHC is that all people all over the world warrant the right care and health needs in their respective community throughout their lifetime physically, psychologically, or mentally and socially. Among the PHC's whole-of-society approaches include disease prevention, treatment, health promotion, palliative care, and rehabilitation through multisectoral policy and action. The communities, families, and individuals are empowered to take charge of their own health. In brief, there are five types of PHC, that is, curative, preventive, promotive, rehabilitative, and supportive. The principles of PHC are accessibility, appropriate technology, health promotion, intersectoral cooperation, and participation by public [1–3].

Health education integrating technological tools, for example, augmented reality (AR) has been the concern in educational settings in recent years. As discussed, an essential component of PHC, that is, appropriate technology is very pertinent, especially in the advent of digital era in which the importance of improved knowledge should be highlighted with ongoing capacity building based on the design and delivery of healthcare services. Health promotion involves the following eight basic

144 DOI: 10.1201/9781003340133-8

requirements or essential components of PHC: (1) appropriate treatment of common diseases and injuries; (2) health education on prevailing health problems as well as how to prevent and control them; (3) immunization against major infections; (4) maternal and child healthcare; (5) nutrition, including food supply; (6) prevention and control of local endemic diseases; (7) provision of essential drugs; as well as (8) safe water supply and sanitation. All these eight basic components are incorporated in the 2030 sustainable development goals (SDGs) no. 2 to no. 5 [1, 4]. Health education for the community with health problems (e.g., common endemic and infectious diseases) and preventive measures (e.g., immunization) is now an essential basic component of PHC.

8.1.2 Road Map Development for Primary Healthcare (PHC): What, Why, and How?

A road map (also referred to as systematic plan) is operationally defined as a strategy that is targeted to achieve a specific goal with inclusion of milestones, plans, or major steps required to reach the desired outcome. Sometimes a road map also serves as a tool for communication with documents that are mostly high level that help to express strategic thinking to achieve such goals using various tools and resources for beginner, intermediate, and advanced learners. For example, a road map is often built to align a company around its product vision, rationales ("Why" is there the need), or justifications with clear goals, themes, product metric as well as feedback mechanism to standardize, monitor, and analyze through collaborative powerhouse [5, 6].

This section elaborates on the authors' initiatives to develop a road map for PHC (with a special focus on health education and health promotion) integrating augmented reality (AR) and virtual reality (VR)-based technology in achieving sustainable development goal (SDG) no. 3 (Good health and well-being) and no. 4 (Quality education).

8.1.2.1 Methodologies Implemented

Based on the outlines set in Figure 8.1, systematic review (to be elaborated in the next section) with documentation of past records were conducted to explore what were done in the past, how health education and health promotion were being implemented in PHC settings, and what can be done in PHC integrating digital tools such as augmented reality (AR), virtual reality (VR), mixed reality (MR), wearable device, gamified apps, to name a few.

E-survey(s) were prepared and administered to elicit feedback from respondents in Malaysia and Indonesia. The instruments were validated using Rasch Model. Findings were analyzed using mixed-research methods and will be reported. Then after, the strategic plans are drafted with timelines and future plans charted to be elaborated in the final section.

8.1.2.2 Exploring the "What and How" of the Past and Present

Various tools used for the preparation of road map were explored. Figure 8.1 is an example of a tool that was used in response to the objectives set in this chapter.

What can be done in PHC especially on health education and health promotion integrating ICT?

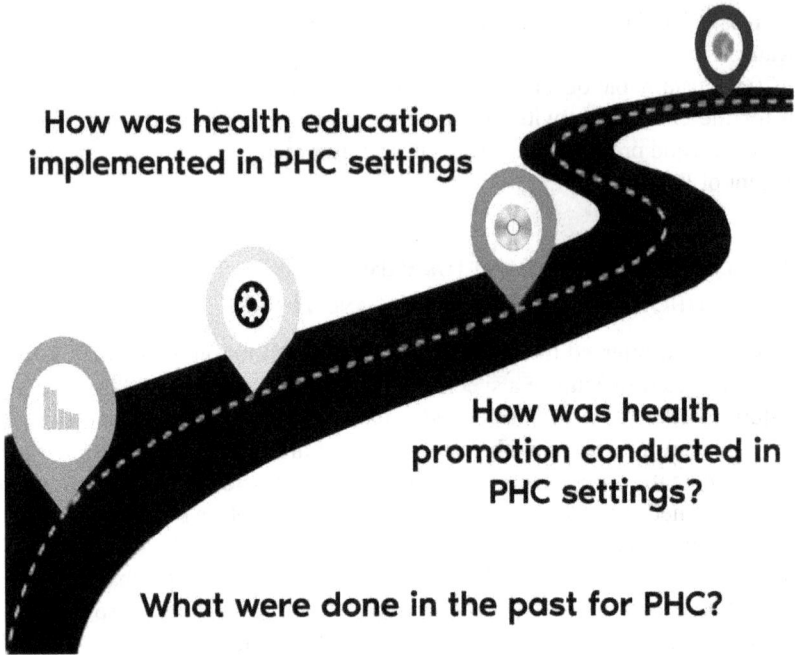

How was health education implemented in PHC settings

How was health promotion conducted in PHC settings?

What were done in the past for PHC?

FIGURE 8.1 Exemplary tool used for preparation of road map in response to the objectives set in this chapter

8.2   REVIEW OF RELATED LITERATURE

8.2.1   Systematic Review on Essential Elements of Primary Healthcare (PHC)

The systematic review on the eight essential elements of primary healthcare (PHC) and integration in augmented reality (AR)-based technology in safe water or sanitation as well as various socio-scientific issues (SSI) are explored through digital tools such as virtual learning AR-based technology in preventive healthcare.

8.2.1.1   Research on Integration of Technological/E-Tools in PHC

The heart of PHC is to improve the quality, affordability, and accessibility of the healthcare of communities (World Health Organization. A vision for primary healthcare in the 21st century. 2018). The future direction of PHC will be shaped by e-tools, technologies, and ICT integrated models to provide equitable and more comprehensive healthcare to communities as well as medical education training [Global Conference on Primary Health Care. Towards Health for All. Media centre. World Health Organization (www.who.int/mediacentre/events/2018/global-conference-phc/

en/, accessed 17 September 2018)]. There are vast opportunities in creation of technological tools and application of dynamic primary healthcare solutions which bring profound impact on primary healthcare [7–9]. In the realm of PHC, medical data and information can be collected and analyzed digitally to improve the effectiveness and efficiency of the healthcare systems. Accurate medical data and information can be obtained accurately and shared securely via electronic devices. Recently, the health development has been boosted with and supported by various digital technologies due to their utility, versatility, and ubiquity. Digital health cause a huge impact on primary healthcare, health services delivery, and running of health systems. Digital healthcare can provide better patient care management via secure usage and health information sharing. The technology and digital advancement improve the primary healthcare services such as the wearable devices to diagnose diseases in early stage and enable personalized treatments recommendation and telehealth technologies, which provide virtual communication between the patients and health professionals. Quality and cost-effective healthcare service can be provided to the communities with the developed secure and private electronic health devices and systems to enable the citizens to obtain their health information and records available electronically. Accurate and complete health information of the patients can be obtained to provide the best possible healthcare during a routine visit or medical emergency.

Practical applications of VR/AR/MR provide practical perspectives and different intelligent and immersive realities are being applied and utilized in real-world scenarios. The rapid development and integration of technologies and digital tools such as AR/VR/MR provide essential resources for PHC and essential public health functions with exponential growing potential as reported by [10] and [11]. Their common usages include search of medical knowledge resources and information, clinical support facilitation, monitoring of healthcare quality, tracking drugs or vaccines supplies and mapping or monitoring the infectious diseases spreading such as COVID-19, H1N1, SARS, to name a few.

With VR/AR/MR integration in healthcare system, accurate information in diagnosing health problems can be obtained to reduce medical errors. Digital healthcare provides comprehensive, equitable, and integrated health services that can manage the health of patients effectively and provide better disease diagnosing methods. The healthcare coordination ability and management are being improved and have revolutionary impacts to the patients, especially chronic cases. The patients can obtain safer healthcare at lower cost rates, clearer visualization, and understand more about their health condition and make proper decision. For example, the implementation of VR/AR/MR in healthcare provide alternative visualization path for magnetic resonance imaging (MRI) and involve in intervention procedures of the computerized tomography (CT) scanning. Patient safety can be ensured by using the advanced technologies to identify the risks and reduce the hazards in the setting of primary healthcare. Electronic sensors can be used to measure the vital signs and track the medical activity and monitor the patients at risk of falls and visualization can be monitored by using VR/AR/MR7 [12].

The revolutions of three-dimensional printing in manufacturing of orthotics, medical devices, and prosthetics empower the workforce and increase the quality of primary healthcare [13]. By integrating the VR/AR/MR with the 3D printing, the health information systems are improved. Timeliness and accuracy of public health data collection can be improved to report and facilitate disease monitoring and surveillance. Effective digital medical tools to support self-care and provide solutions to address health needs and enable the patients from the rural areas access to health services although the clinic or the health expertise is far away. The limitless possibilities of AR will transform the patient medical experiences in VR/AR/MR journeys.

8.2.1.2 Integration of Digital Tools With Reviews of Related Publications in the Areas of Total Health

The following Table 8.1 summarizes the integration of digital tools (e.g., AR, VR, wearable device, gamified apps etc.) with reviews of related publications by researchers in the areas of physical, psychological, and social health respectively.

The rapid rise of big data, Internet of Things (IoT), and artificial intelligence applications, in light of society's rising digitization, has enhanced the demand for experienced individuals in STEM fields. The craze surrounding these applications has presented STEM educators with a slew of new difficulties and opportunities [24]. The Internet of Things (IoT) is a global network that connects things and materials to the Internet to enable them to interact or communicate with their surroundings [23]. The Internet of Things (IoT) was introduced in education, allowing Internet-based communications to be used in between physical things, sensors, and controls. Massive changes were made to educational institutions by using embedding augmented reality, sensors in things, and incorporating cloud computing [25]. Arduino is an open-source platform used for building electronics projects. Arduino consists of both a physical programmable circuit board (often referred to as a microcontroller) and a piece of software, or IDE (Integrated Development Environment), that runs on your computer, used to write and upload computer code to the physical board. Introduced in 2005 the Arduino platform was designed to provide an inexpensive and easy way for hobbyists, students, and professionals to create devices that interact with their environment using sensors and actuators [26]. Arduino is an open source computing platform for building and programming electronic devices based on basic microcontroller boards. It can also operate as a little computer, taking inputs and regulating outputs for a range of electronic devices, exactly like other microcontrollers. Furthermore, the Arduino IDE makes programming easier by using a simplified form of C++.

8.2.1.3 Incorporating e-Platforms for Discussion of Socio-Scientific Issues (SSI) Related to Safe Water, Hygiene, and Sanitation

Over the turn of last few decades that promote Education for Sustainable Development (ESD), numerous international web-based learning programs [such as Science across the World (SAW) led by Association of Science Education (ASE), UK, as well as SEAMEO-UN Habitat Human Values-based Water, Sanitation and Hygiene Education (HVWSHE)] were initiated to raise awareness on the ways science and technology interact with society and environment through blended-mode learning program, as reported by [27] and [28] respectively. A lot of socio-scientific issues (SSI) are related to safe water, hygiene, and sanitation that will greatly impact human's health and sustainable living. Seeing the importance to tackle these issues

TABLE 8.1

Reviews of Research on Digital Tools Integration Related to Aspects and Effects on Primary Healthcare

	Research on Digital Tools With PHC Integration	Researches Related to Aspects and Effects on Physical Health	Researches Related to Aspects and Effects on Psychosocial Health
1	Augmented reality (AR) in health/science education	AR to illustrate the bad effect of influenza [14]	AR to improve students' motivation to learn [15]
2	Augmented reality (AR)/virtual reality (VR) in health/sport science education	Enhancing awareness on environmental and preventive healthcare for sports science supported by technology: a systematic review and suggested research [16]	The use of AR/VR/MR to improve performance in sports [17]
3	Wearable device–based and system	Detecting effectiveness and fatigue level of players [18]	With better physical health obtained from wearable devices, improvement was also seen in psychosocial health, e.g., reduced stress level and good mental health
4	Gamified app or gamification that enhanced attitude and motivation	Daily limit on prolonged play and learning through feedback [19]	Conditions for process with enhanced attitude [20]
5	Minecraft as digital tool for virtual reality/learning and mixed reality (MR)	Minecraft as digital tool that illustrates PHC settings in virtual world [21]	Mixed reality (MR) comes free with Minecraft and Windows, bringing all interesting features that motivate learning [22]
6	Internet of Things (IoT)	Exemplary projects on conservation of energy and/or other resources as well as waste reduction integrating IoT concept and technological tool(s) [16]	Internet of Things (IoT) is a global network that connects things and materials to the Internet to ease communication that improve psychosocial health [23]
7	Artificial intelligence (AI)	Trace of spreading area or infection rate of diseases such as COVID-19 AI for healthcare certificate; AI innovations are revolutionizing healthcare	The big data and the power of artificial intelligence are used by the researchers to support complex clinical decision-making and identify and report of adverse events

from early years in the digital era with expanded process of information sharing in classroom instruction with reference to a wide variety of complex challenges, the fifth co-author has initiated the development of a framework for an asynchronous discussion forum through an e-learning platform to facilitate students' discussions on SSI, such as "Climate Change and its impact on human's living" with input and video presentation as reported by [29].

8.2.1.4 Applications of AR and VR in the Health Industry and Medical Training

Interactive and immersive technologies such as AR/VR/MR involved in immersive, dynamic, adaptive, interactive world cause the pace of change in medical systems and medical training. Rote learning has been replaced with more clinically relevant, interactive, and practical digital learning tools. VR/AR/MR have gained momentum in experiential learning and knowledge delivery and become an integral part of healthcare and medical training. The development of VR/AR/MR enable the simulated clinical experiences to be shared virtually and to provide quality and effective interprofessional education at scale and transform the delivery of education to the medical students and clinicians. Implementation of AR/VR/MR in medical training such as virtual wards, virtual theater, robotic surgery, interaction and communication with patients, relatives, colleagues, and peers can be done similarly to real-time interactions. The medical students can learn in virtual world, move around and interact with the virtual environment and patient virtually in real life. The medical students or the learners can receive virtual debriefing by the educators' facilitating conversations via web-based videoconferencing platforms and view automatically-generated feedback on the performance. Blended learning can be carried out to examine learners' performance in detail. The peer learning can be facilitated, and feedback can be shared with the learners' classmates, trainers, mentors, and lecturers as a basis for discussion on specific learning topics.

Real-world usage, challenges, and limitless opportunities of AR/VR/MR interface, game, gamification software, or applications in the healthcare system medical education and training have been explored recently. The healthcare-relevant system (hospital-based system, clinical system, homecare-based system, institute and university, and industry) [30]. VR/AR/MR are emerging as new simulation delivery methods. Medical imaging VR support the safety of patients by reducing radiation dose exposure. AR involves in overlaying computer-generated images onto real world images. It is visible computer-generated imagery via the use of virtual visualization, where the images are overlaid onto real-life surfaces in the present environment. The standardization and scoring possibility of VR/AR/MR make it commonplace in continuing medical education and revalidation. It can be a benchmark to determine the patient safety and clinical competency across PHC systems. State-of-the-art innovation lab or surgery theater can explore emerging technologies to provide the best learning experience by using latest technologies of AR/VR/MR. More immersive and fully interactive healthcare training are provided using AR/VR technologies to improve patient care using cost-effective digital training programs with vast experience in enabling healthcare professionals [31].

8.2.1.5 Advantages of Implementation of AR/VR/MR in Health Industry

There is a positive educational impact of implementation of AR/VR/MR in primary healthcare area as revealed from literature [32], as summarized in Table 8.2.

Digital solutions are strengthened with VR, AR, and mixed reality (MR) technologies to enhance the data analysis and healthcare practices. With the effective technology integration in primary healthcare, it will bring a huge impact and provide most advanced cutting-edge solutions to support patient safety, direct patient care,

TABLE 8.2
Educational Impact of Implementation of AR/VR/MR in Primary Healthcare Area

Characteristics	Traditional Methods	Impact of AR/VR/MR
Realistic experience	There are difficulties in visualizing 3D features and related the relationship with 2D materials and components via paper-based learning. Visualization cannot be done clearly, and misunderstandings might occur and result in low learning rate.	Lifelike virtual object can be created to provide most realistic impression on the function and internal organs of the human body. Higher level of immersion can be provided to the patients, medical students and staff, doctors and surgeons, etc. so that interaction with virtual environment can be done in a realistic manner. The digital subjects can be manipulated easily with unlimited repetitions to identify spatial inter-relationships, and exploration can be done in three-dimensional space.
Low risk and high safety	The limitation of teaching and learning tools and resources.	Training with AR as compared with practicing on real patients can reduce medical errors, risky of patient and provides an opportunity to learn perfect skills. It can inspire higher confidence for the learners.
Cost-effective and affordable	The setting up cost of anatomy theatres is high. It costs a lot to provide specimens and cadavers for the medical students for medical training and practice.	AR apps cost is comparatively low, with the cost of setting up anatomy theaters. A relatively low-cost opportunity is provided by VR simulators for reproducible training under various environments and difficulty levels.
Accessible	They do not raise ethical issues compared with other animal and living tissue simulation models.	VR and AR-based medical education include teaching programs for individuals with reading disabilities (a barrier to traditional textbook-based learning).

(Continued)

**TABLE 8.2   *(Continued)*
Educational Impact of Implementation of AR/VR/MR in Primary Healthcare Area**

Characteristics	Traditional Methods	Impact of AR/VR/MR
Higher efficiency	Tablets, mobile phones, AR glasses, and other optimized devices can be employed as hardware for running AR applications. Thus, AR and VR provide standardized medical training on demand irrespective of geographical location, as opposed to the learners working in the laboratory where they have to rely on the schedule and the availability of disposable materials.	Augmented reality apps can easily connect trainees or remote workers with mentors or experts who can provide instructions or assistance in real-time. The use of VR/AR/MR applications increases in laparoscopic surgery training. Training in robotic surgery with VR simulators enables the medical professionals to attain better and transferable surgical skills and particularly benefited from training in robotic simulators. Open surgery simulator is developed for training and assessment. VR/AR simulators are commonly found in neurosurgery training.
Availability of expert assistance	Face-to-face learning cannot be done during COVID-19 pandemic and learning is shifted towards virtual mode due to restricted face-to-face access.	AR/VR are integrated in anatomy, with 3D visualization of hardly comprehensible structures, and physiology, with representation of mechanisms in 4D (in space and time dimensions). AR apps are used to connect the trainees or remote medical staffs with the mentors or medical experts to instruct or assist in real time.
Shortened training timelines	Face-to-face and physical explanation needs time.	Instead of long hour courses and training, AR/VR allow 3D animation and simulation. Learners will be able to learn anywhere and anytime, and hence the training timelines can be shortened

efficient communication, effective treatment, visualization data with possibility of live statistics, intense workflow handling, healthcare consultant, mobile medical services, logistics, management and maintenance of hospital and services, and reduction of waiting duration. The evolvement of VR, AR, and MR improves the effectiveness and efficiency of medical treatment and services critically and drastically. Implementation of AR, VR, and MR create a new vision such as healthcare mobile app to establish connections and maintain better communication with the patients during pandemic to provide remote medical consultant and personalized care. The medical training and the pre-surgery activities can be improved, and visualized explanation can be done to let the patients understand the flow of the surgery or treatment and the risk of the surgery and treatment can be measured. Organ transplants or dialysis treatment can be explained visually to the patients. When it comes to matters of life and death, the patients will feel more relaxed if they understand the treatment or surgery process. It will increase the confidence level of the patients.

Chronic patients feel uncomfortable during the treatment. Implementation of VR/AR/MR can reduce their uncomfortable experience and probably make it more exciting. AR helps the patients to keep track of the vital statistics so that the patients stay tuned with the therapy or treatment progress with higher confidence level and in an engaging manner. Awareness campaigns can be done to draw the public awareness regarding the prevention of diseases with application of AR/VR/MR at anytime and anywhere. The physical environments of the hospital, especially the operating rooms, theaters, and trauma rooms are full of virus, and sanitation is needed for the high-risk physical healthcare environments, and AR can help in identifying the sanitation process. Integration of AR/VR and MR has huge potential and implications in showing hospital layout design, equipment positioning, medical consultant, complex healthcare settings, explanation to the patients the surgery or process treatment and decluttering [33].

AR solutions can improve the patient experience significantly and reduce the problems by addition of pop-up information and navigation. The patients can get to the department using the shortest route, while the medical staff can manage the equipment and medicine in more proper ways. AR exploration in medicine can be done by scanning the QR code to remind the patients to consume the medicine. Numerous monitors are placed around the patients and control rooms so that the statistics can be shown directly and point out the problematic points of the patients and show medical data or statistics. The accurate and visually beautiful anatomy models can be shown by using VR and AR. 3D anatomy models for male and female contribute to drawing public health area of interest. VR/AR/MR are applied in the medical field like medical and training, surgical neurological psychotherapy, and telemedicine. However, the popularity of VR/AR/MR technologies are low level in worldwide healthcare facilities and clinics. The future and dissemination of VR and AR in healthcare and medicine are in progress and at early stages of adoption in healthcare with the ongoing research and development and investment. The disruptive potential of VR/AR/MR technologies drives the researcher, investors, and inventors to develop advanced digital healthcare solutions supported by VR/AR/MR technologies. The following Table 8.3 summarizes the involvement of stakeholder in healthcare integrating digital tools.

The following Table 8.4 summarizes the applications of VR/AR/MR in healthcare and medical field.

8.2.2 Exemplars on How AR Was Used in Health and STEM Education

Exemplars from Malaysia are illustrated on how AR was used in health and STEM education. Generally, teachers are known as the curriculum implementers in a school setting requiring teachers to adapt and be well-equipped with digital skills to integrate the use of technology in a classroom. According to [34], the integration of technology will provide a means to enhance students' learning and engagement in a classroom. Augmented reality (AR) is a new technology that has emerged with potential for application in education. According to [35], many research has been conducted on AR, mainly because AR provides an efficient way to represent a model

TABLE 8.3

Involvement of Stakeholder in Healthcare Integrating Digital Tools

Targets	Health Equity, Social Justice, Efficiency in Primary Healthcare With Digital Tools				
Communities	General knowledge on health.	Awareness campaign.	Immunization program.	Chronic diseases prevention.	Health campaigns/appointment and reminders can be sent via mobile telephones for medication visits.
Patients	Realize the medical treatments received is good for health.	Understand the health condition.	Core function of PHC and essential public health functions.	Obtain high quality treatment in shortest time.	Educated, aware, and engaged PHC.
Medical students	Communication devices, knowledge resources, management, and decision-support tools increase effectiveness and autonomy in studies.	Education and training can be monitored via digital tools.	Construct medical knowledge and skills via AR training modules and online courses to join the workforce in health.	Improve the ability to gather, analyze, manage knowledge, skill development, data, statistics, and information.	Improve knowledge sharing and networks to reinforces the knowledge and professional skills.
Healthcare team	Update immunization information. Provide healthcare to public by integrating digital clinical support tools and referral systems.	Digital technologies help to improve patients' journey to prevent duplication of care processes and enhance communication between providers as well as avoid unplanned hospitalizations and visits for urgent care.	Coordinate care and ensure its continuity across primary, secondary, acute, and aged care services.	Electronic health records capture information about an individual's health, medical conditions, medications, and key events, which can be shared for referrals and timely clinical decision-making.	Ensure the general public has access to timely, expert advice by telephone in health emergencies can save lives. Rapid, coordinated response in public health emergencies.
Doctors/surgeons/specialist	Communication with the patients can be conducted effectively.	Diagnose the diseases in the early stage.	Magnetic resonance imaging (MRI) and computerized tomography (CT) scanning	Better explanation provided to the patients regarding the surgery flow and treatment.	Provide better treatment and visualization to the patients and increase the confidence of the patients.
Ministry of Health and Family Welfare	Reform of medical education and provide high-quality primary care and essential public health functions. Central to strengthen public health action and support.		Focus on primary healthcare development.	Optimization of three pillars of primary healthcare.	Monitor policy impacts on population health/align stakeholders in digital health to develop digital health in the context of a country.

TABLE 8.3 *(Continued)*

Involvement of Stakeholder in Healthcare Integrating Digital Tools

Targets	Health Equity, Social Justice, Efficiency in Primary Healthcare With Digital Tools			
Policymakers	Investigate the best medical system.	Focus on PHC initiation. Integration of health services policy. Identify, assess, support, and oversee the implementation and integration of promising and proven AR or VR technologies.	Collect data for analysis. The users can feed back their healthcare experiences potential.	Design medical policy and propose to ministry of health and family healthcare.
AR/VR/MR developers	Healthcare information setup.	Invent and invest in 3D AR/VR/MR technologies.	Research and development to develop innovative digital technologies.	Test and data analysis.

TABLE 8.4

Applications of VR, AR, and Mixed Reality (MR) in Healthcare and Medical Fields

Applications	Functions
Medical training for medical students, doctors, therapists, surgeons, and medical staff	Perform better treatment to patients and carry out complex operations and reduce the risk of surgery mistakes
General diagnostics and medical training	Diagnostics and medical training can be effectively done with VR/AR/MR
Emergency treatment and emergency navigation	Medical centers, pharmacies, and healthcare facilities can be reached in shortest route with AR devices
Robotic surgery	High-precision operations of robotic devices can be controlled by a human surgeon with VR technology
Virtual doctor consultation	Virtual consultancy
Physical therapy performed with VR	Overcome high pain levels of the patients to ensure speedy recovery
Posttraumatic stress treatment	Traumatic situation and crisis situation can be overcome
Anxiety, phobia, and depression treatment	VR can be used for meditations and patients feel relaxed in safe VR environments
Body mapping	Examination process can be done without the doctors appearing physically
Personalized approach to patients	VR/AR/MR can help doctors better explain to their patients how their operations will be performed, or which steps a patient should take for more effective recovery
Medical immersion with AR	VR/AR/MR technologies improve customer experiences to engage effectively in healthcare activities
Self-diagnostics	Self-diagnostics can be improved with AR
Ophthalmology	Patients are provided with an AR for visual stimulation with specific conditions such as cataract or AMD
Virtual reality in medicine statistics	Data collection and analysis can be done systematically and visually
Floor plan	The entrance of the huge hospital can be accessed easily with AR signboards and layout plan

that needs visualization. Consequently, teachers must share knowledge on AR to provide greater support and collaboration in terms of research findings as well as workshops and training programs.

One such workshop is conducted in SEAMEO RECSAM for Penang secondary science schoolteachers in 7 April 2021 virtually (see Figure 8.2), also attended by RECSAM's staff on-site (Figure 8.3). It was conducted in blended mode due to the pandemic, that limited the number of on-site participation. Thirty-three teachers from the state of Penang, Malaysia, attended this one-day workshop on the use of AR using the metaverse application with interactive workshop activities that produced learning output (see Figure 8.4). The metaverse application enabled teachers to do quizzes in the form of 3D.

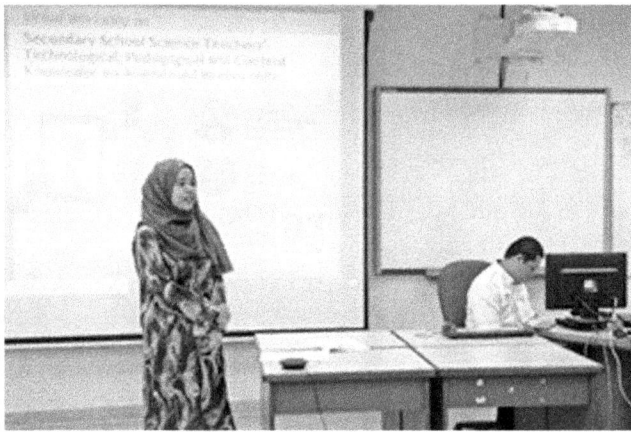

FIGURE 8.2   Penang secondary science teachers (mostly online) attended a workshop conducted by a facilitator (on-site)

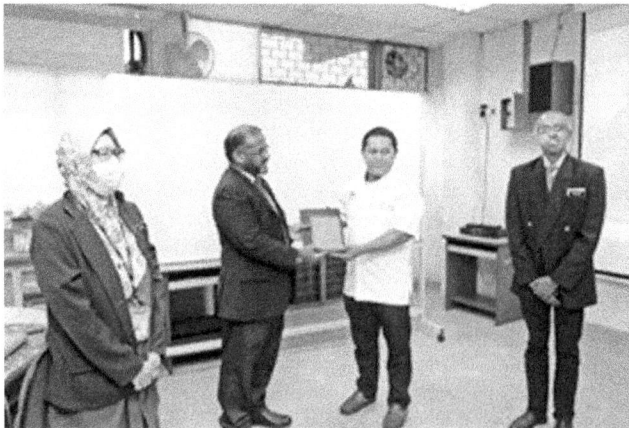

FIGURE 8.3   Staff attending AR workshop (onsite)

Apart from experiencing the metaverse application, the participants were also exposed to many AR instances embedded in the Malaysian secondary science textbook as presented in Table 8.5.

In the areas of healthcare, aspiring health professionals could learn the anatomy of humans using the AR health application (see Figure 8.5). The application allowed users to see the different systems found in the human body. Users could also zoom in on parts of the human structure for a better 3D view. The 3D view is equipped with labels for students' knowledge making learning anatomy a better experience than 2D anatomy textbooks.

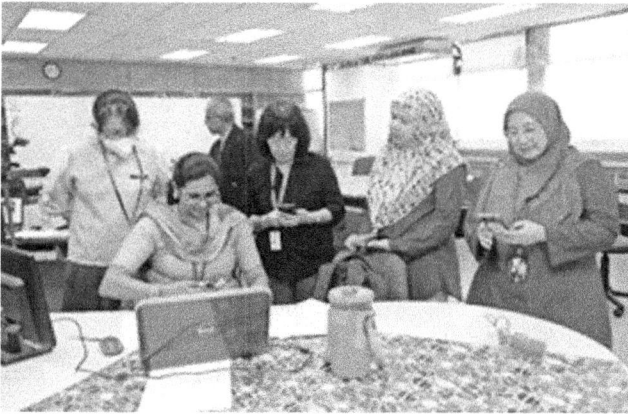

FIGURE 8.4 Exemplary workshop activity output integrating AR created by workshop participant

TABLE 8.5

Excerpt of Malaysian Lower Secondary Science Textbook With AR Instances

Title of Textbook	Page Number	Title of Diagram or Figure Incorporating Augmented Reality Feature
Science Form 1	51	Animal cell and plant cell
	108	Process of fertilization
	260	Earth's main layers
Science Form 2	62	Flow of food in the digestive tract
	275	Protecting the earth from asteroid impacts
	215	Model of a fire alarm
	252	Solar system
Science Form 3	4	Structure of human nervous system
	86	Structure and function of the human heart
	260	Prominences

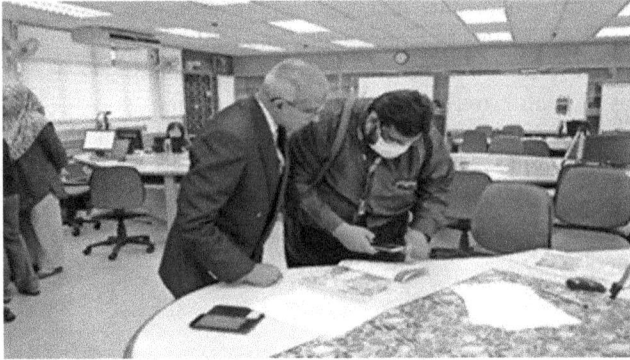

FIGURE 8.5   AR health application

8.3   LESSONS LEARNED AND THE WAY FORWARD

8.3.1   LESSONS LEARNED FROM INTEGRATION OF AR IN HEALTH AND STEM EDUCATION

In this section, lessons learned from the initiatives to integrate AR in health and STEM education are elaborated.

SEAMEO RECSAM was involved in the training of trainers (TOT) event and subsequent three months' online training programs organized by SEAMEO Secretariat to introduce "The real world of Immersive Augmented Reality (AR)" from October to December 2017. Numerous output were produced, as reported by [36] and [37]. However, due to the high level knowledge and skills required to master the tools, much time had to be spent in the training and affected the participation of the schools in the midst of hectic schooling time.

In the recent AR workshop organized by the co-author, it was also found that the input given on use of AR-related tools such as Unity and Blender was not able to be completed under much constraints of time and technical support such as the accessibility to Internet connection.

For educators, using AR is quite easy, but creating one can be a moderate to difficult task. The creator must first be equipped with basic knowledge of the application or software before building one. The creation of these AR features will also depend on the educators' interest and motivation. Some educators believe using AR imposes long class time hours and are reluctant to use them. Thus, the educators will have to be exposed to the benefits of using AR towards a more successful understanding via a 3D visualization. Thus, educators and aspiring health professionals may probably weigh on time and benefits before using the AR application.

Traditional curriculum needs evolvement to meet tomorrow's reality. VR/AR/MR technologies are powerful tools which can be applied to support and transform education so that the educators can create digital instructional tools or materials for active learning. Malaysia's new textbooks (physical and digital) have been upgraded with 3D AR animation in September 2022 and will be launched soon. The evolvement of classroom education at a faster pace and awareness are a draw among educators. Students need to develop new digital skills for future workforce. To meet the changes and evidence-based shifts in future classroom education, learning three-dimension (3D) Augmented Reality (AR)/3D Virtual reality (VR) and 3D features can develop computational thinking, problem-solving, coding, and science, technology, engineering, arts, and mathematics (STEAM) subjects to help to prepare students to address future challenges. This can expose the educators (pre-service and in-service teachers) and students in a wide range of digital tools or platforms related to 3D AR designs and prepare the teachers and students to integrate computational thinking (CT) skills as part of curriculum and promote active learning. It is aligned with SEAMEO Education Agenda Priority Area 7 "Adopting 21st Century Curriculum" as well as Priority Area 4 "Promoting technical and vocational education and training."

8.3.2 Suggestions for the Way Forward

Suggestions for the way forward are deliberated.

Much lessons were learned from the research and development (R&D) activities involved by the authors in this study. Among the suggestions for the way forward included the following aspects:

1. Bridging the gaps between educational, health, and industrial settings

   More R&D activities should be conducted to bridge the gap towards integration of AR-based technology in healthcare and industrial settings integrating transdisciplinary studies as reported by [38]. Providing proper training, considering matching proper knowledge and skills required for basic education in line with the governmental aspirations of local and global educational settings, plays an important role in this aspect.

2. Drafting of curriculum and training of trainers (ToT) for educators in AR applications

   Drafting curriculum outlines (as shown in Table 8.6) for educating young minds from basic to advanced level of learning with proper matching of knowledge and skills at appropriate levels with guidelines for "Project Completion and Creativity" in project-based program.

   Before using AR, trainer educators must first be equipped with relevant AR applications under their belt. These trainer educators will need to experience the strength and weaknesses of each application before conducting any lesson. Although the number of hours presented in Table 8.6 reflect the proposed duration of study, the hours depend on individual understanding and performing all tasks to ensure that the audience is well prepared.

The Figure 8.6 illustrates an exemplary road map prepared to summarize the suggestions for the way forward for AR/VR related research for PHC.

TABLE 8.6

Drafting of Curriculum Outlines Targeting "Beginner, Intermediate, Advanced" Levels of Learners

What Should Be Learned	Beginner	Intermediate	Advanced
Augmented Reality	Metaverse	Blender (Basic), Unity, Vuforia	Blender (Advanced) Unity, Vuforia
Justification	Considering the features of tools and minimum required training hours.		
Metaverse	Creating quizzes for educational purposes—3 to 4 hours; Dr. Loh to add more.		
Blender	Develop artistic skills and improve problem-solving skills by creating Blender video games; real-world application where the 3D creations using Blender can be translated into tangible objects through 3D printing. The main benefits of using Blender in school is zero cost. Blender is free, with nearly no-bar entry. Coolness: Blender is fun and students enjoy using it.		
Unity	Build an animation using Unity. Digital skills are developed and will be well versed in 3D as well as stay on top of digital and technology curve in future hobbies and professional careers. Learning transferrable skills and becoming very employable.		
Vuforia	Cognitive benefits are the students learn to create in 3D to improve spatial awareness. Synergies with subjects where students can create 3D visuals for science projects, practice principles of physics, biology, applied mathematics, etc.		

8.4 CONCLUSION

In conclusion, the study as reported in this chapter provided some insights with lessons learned from the initiatives to integrate AR in health and STEM education that were elaborated in the previous sections with suggestions made for the way forward. To conclude this chapter aiming at development of a road map for primary healthcare (PHC) integrating AR-based technology, a road map is charted to illustrate efforts towards achieving targeted output.

ACKNOWLEDGMENTS

The authors wish to express their profound gratitude to everyone in making this study possible with various support given to the past and recent events completed successfully. Special mention is given to the following who had contributed to the success of this study through the organization of AR workshop: (1) The facilitator Mr. Ahmad Afandi b. Yusri, postgraduate student from USM; and (2) academic and support staff of Training and Research Division (T&R) as well as Administration Division, especially ICT staff, with special mention to Dr. Mariam bt. Othman, Dr. Wan Noor Adzmin bt Mohd Sabri and Ms. Deva Nanthini a/p Sinniah from T&R division of RECSAM, Mr. Wahid Yunianto, ex-SEAQIM staff, as well as Mr. Baharulnizam Baharum and Mr. Mohd. Faizal Zainoldin (from Administration Division, SEAMEO RECSAM).

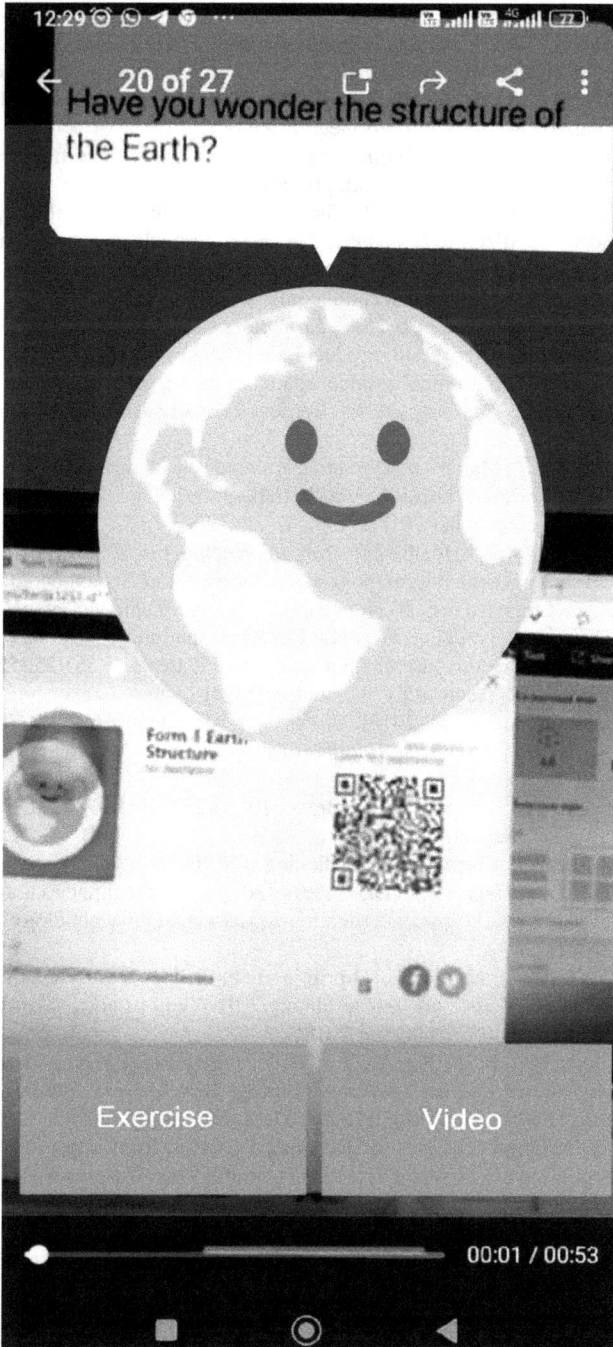

FIGURE 8.6 Exemplary road map prepared summarizing the suggestions for the way forward

REFERENCES

[1] Sheehan Health. (2021, January 28). *The Primary Health Care Approach.* Retrieved https://sheehanhealth.com.au/2021/01/28/the-primary-health-care-approach/.

[2] WHO. (2022). *Primary Health Care.* World Health Organization (WHO). Retrieved www.who.int/health-topics/primary-health-care.

[3] Pallipedia. (2022). *Primary Health Care (PHC).* Pallipedia: The free online Palliative Care Dictionary. https://pallipedia.org/primary-health-care-phc/.

[4] Du, S., Cao, Y., Zhou, T. et al. (2019). The knowledge, ability, and skills of primary health care providers in SEANERN countries: A multi-national cross-sectional study. *BMC Health Services Research*, 19, 602. https://doi.org/10.1186/s12913-019-4402-9. Retrieved https://bmchealthservres.biomedcentral.com/articles/10.1186/s12913-019-4402-9.

[5] McGuigan, B. (2020, November 25). *7 Examples of Excellent Product Roadmaps.* Product Management. San Francisco: Product Excellent Summit October 4, 2022. Retrieved www.productboard.com/blog/7-product-roadmap-examples/.

[6] ProductPlan. (2022). *Roadmap Basics.* Retrieved www.productplan.com/learn/roadmap-basics/.

[7] Hendricks, D. (2016, March 4). 3D printing is already changing health care. *Harvard Business Review.* Retrieved https://hbr.org/2016/03/3d-printing-is-already-changing-health-care (accessed 17 September 2018).

[8] Global Observatory for eHealth. *Directory of eHealth Policies.* World Health Organization. Retrieved www.who.int/goe/policies/en/ (accessed 17 September 2018).

[9] World Health Organization (WHO). (2016). *Global Diffusion of eHealth: Making Universal Health Coverage Achievable.* Report of the third global survey on eHealth. Geneva: WHO. Retrieved http://apps.who.int/iris/bitstream/10665/252529/1/978924151 1780-eng.pdf?ua=1 (accessed 17 September 2018).

[10] World Health Organization. (2016). *Global Observatory for eHealth. Global Diffusion of eHealth: Making Universal Health Coverage Achievable.* Geneva: World Health Organization.

[11] Retrieved http://apps.who.int/iris/bitstream/10665/252529/1/9789241511780-eng.pdf?ua=1 (accessed 17 September 2018).

[12] Oxehealth secures world-first accreditation for its vital signs technology. (2018, September 18). *eHealthNews.eu.* Retrieved www.ehealthnews.eu/industry/5630-oxehealth-secures-world-first-accreditation-for-its-vitalsigns-technology (accessed 17 September 2018).

[13] Hendricks, D. (2016, March 4). 3D printing is already changing health care. *Harvard Business Review.* Retrieved https://hbr.org/2016/03/3d-printing-is-already-changing-health-care (accessed 17 September 2018).

[14] Sari, N., Indarjani, R., & Ng, K. T. (2018). *Enhancing Effective Science Learning Through Augmented Reality: Challenges and the Way Forward.* Presentation compiled in the refereed Proceedings of ICRTSTMSD-18, August 4–5, 2018 at Kuta Central Park Hotel, Bali, Indonesia. Retrieved December 17, 2018, from https://drive.google.com/drive/folders/1DAUwL5K0OjaQEnMfP-rTLrimltPCDQ63?usp=sharing.

[15] Buzko, V. L., Bonk, A. V., & Tron, V. (2018, October 2) *Implementation of Gamification and Elements of Augmented Reality During the Binary Lessons in a Secondary School.* Paper presented at the Proceedings of the 1st International Workshop on Augmented Reality in Education Kryvyi Rih, Ukraine.

[16] Leong, W. Y. (Ed.). (2022). *Human Machine Collaboration and Interaction for Smart Manufacturing (Automation, Robotics, Sensing, Artificial Intelligence, 5G, IoTs and Blockchain).* Futures Place: The Institution of Engineering and Technology.

[17] *The Barça Innovation Hub Team.* (2019, September 2). The use of VR/AR/MR to improve performance in sports. Retrieved https://barcainnovationhub.com/the-use-of-vr-ar-mr-to-improved-performance-in-sports/.

[18] Westhuizen, E. J. V. D., & Haar, D. V. D. (2018, January). *A Wearable Device-Based Framework for Determining Player Effectiveness on the Football Pitch.* Retrieved www. researchgate.net/profile/Dustin_Van_der_Haar/publication/324814210_A_wearable_ device-based_framework_for_determining_player_effectiveness_on_the_football _ pitch/links/5ae94b4f0f7e9b837d3b18b3/A-wearable-device-based-framework-for-determining-player-effectiveness-on-the-football-pitch.pdf.

[19] Welbers, K., Konjin, E. A., Burgers, C., de Vaate, A. B., Eden, A., & Brugman, B. C. (2019). Gamification as a tool for engaging student learning: A field experiment with a gamified app. *E-learning and Digital Media*, 16(2), 92–109. Retrieved www.research-gate.net/publication/331384078_Gamification_as_a_tool_for_engaging_student_learning_A_field_experiment_with_a_gamified_app.

[20] Kiryakova, G., Angelova, N., & Yordanova, L. (2014). Gamification in education. *Proceedings of 9th International Balkan Education and Science Conference 2014*. pp. 1–5. Retrieved https://doi.org/10.4018/978-1-5225-5198-0.

[21] Pang, Y. J., Tay, C. C., Syed Ahmad, S. S., Ng, K. T., & Lim, S. H. (2021, December 16). Minecraft education edition: The perspectives of educators on game-based learning related to STREAM education. In Ng, K. T. & Lay, Y. F. (Eds.), *Learning Science and Mathematics Online Journal*. Penang, Malaysia: SEAMEO RECSAM. pp. 121–138. Retrieved http://www.recsam.edu.my/sub_lsmjournal/images/docs/2021/2021_8_PYJ_121138.pdf.

[22] Mojang. (2022). *Build, Explore and Battle Mobs*. Mojang Synergies AB. Retrieved www.minecraft.net/en-us/vr/.

[23] Abd-Ali, R. S., Radhi, S. A., & Rasool, Z. I. (2020). A survey: The role of the internet of things in the development of education. *Indonesian Journal of Electrical Engineering and Computer Science*, 19(1), 215. Retrieved https://doi.org/10.11591/ijeecs.v19.i1.pp215-221.

[24] Benita, F., Virupaksha, D., Wilhelm, E., & Tunçer, B. (2021). A smart learning ecosystem design for delivering Data-driven Thinking in STEM education. *Smart Learning Environments*, 8(1). Retrieved https://doi.org/10.1186/s40561-021-00153-y.

[25] Bagheri, M., & Movahed, S. H. (2016). The effect of the internet of things (IoT) on education business model. *2016 12th International Conference on Signal-Image Technology & Internet-Based Systems (SITIS)*. Retrieved https://doi.org/10.1109/sitis.2016.74.

[26] Louis, L. (2016). Working principle of Arduino and using it as a tool for study and research. *International Journal of Control, Automation, Communication and Systems*, 1(2), 21–29. https://doi.org/10.5121/ijcacs.2016.1203.

[27] Tan, K. A., Ng, K. T., Ch'ng, Y. S., & Teoh, B. T. (2007, November 13–16). *Redefining Mathematics Classroom Incorporating Project/Problem-Based Learning Programme*. Paper published in the International Conference on Science and Mathematics Education (CoSMEd) 2007 conference (indexed) proceedings, Penang, Malaysia, SEAMEO RECSAM. Retrieved https://scholar.google.com/citations?view_op=view_citation&hl=en&user= qewEkbgAAAAJ&citation_for_view=qewEkbgAAAAJ:IWHjjKOFINEC.

[28] Ng, K. T., Teoh, B. T., & Tan, K. A. (2007). Teaching mathematics incorporating values-based water education via constructivist approaches. In *Learning Science and Mathematics (LSM) Online Journal*. Penang, Malaysia: SEAMEO RECSAM.

[29] Durairaj, K., Assanarkutty, S. J., Ng, K. T., & Mohd Sabri, W. N. A. (2022). Development of a framework for an asynchronous discussion forum through an e-learning platform. *Dinamika Jurnal Ilmiah Pendidikan Dasar*, 15(2), 128–139. Universitas Mukammadiyah Purwokerto, Indonesia. http://dx.doi.org/10.30595/dinamika.v14i2.15274. Retrieved http://jurnalnasional.ump.ac.id/index.php/Dinamika/article/view/15274.

[30] Fu, Y., Hu, Y., Sundstedt, V., & Fagerström, C. (2021). A survey of possibilities and challenges with AR/VR/MR and gamification usage in healthcare, 733–740. http://dx.doi.org/10.5220/0010386207330740.

[31] Retrieved www.impelsys.com/.

[32] Retrieved www.impelsys.com/blog/the-role-of-ar-vr-technology-in-the-health-industry/.

[33] Bayramzadeh, S., & Aghaei, P. (2021, April). Technology integration in complex healthcare environments: A systematic literature review. Applied Ergonomics, 92, 103351. http://dx.doi.org/10.1016/j.apergo.2020.103351. Epub 2021 Jan 4. PMID: 33412484.

[34] Neumann, D. L., Neumann, M. M., & Hood, M. (2011). Evaluating computer-based simulations, multimedia and animations that help integrate blended learning with lectures in first year statistics. *Australasian Journal of Educational Technology*, 27(2), Article 2. https://doi.org/10.14742/ajet.970.

[35] Saidin, N. F., Dayana, N., Halim, A., & Yahaya, Y. (2015). A review of research on augmented reality in education: Advantages and applications. *International Education Studies*, 8(13). Retrieved June 8, 2023, from https://www.researchgate.net/publication/281336331_A_Review_of_Research_on_Augmented_Reality_in_Education_Advantages_and_Applications.

[36] Narulita, S., Perdana, A. T. W., Annisa Nur, F., Daru, M., Indarjani, D., & Ng, K. T. (2018, December 13). Motivating secondary science learning through 3D interactive technology: From theory to practice using Augmented Reality. *Learning Science and Mathematics (LSM) Online Journal*. Retrieved June 8, 2023, from http:// www.recsam.edu.my/sub_lsmjournal/images/docs/2018/(3)Sari%20Narulita%20p38-45_final.pdf.

[37] Ng, K. T., Baharum, B. N., Othman, M., Tahir, S. & Pang, Y. J. (2020). Managing technology-enhanced innovation programs: Framework, exemplars and future directions. *Solid State Technology,* 63(1s). Retrieved http://www.solidstatetechnology.us/index.php/JSST/article/view/741.

[38] Ng, K. T. (2017). Development of transdisciplinary models to manage knowledge, skills and innovation processes integrating technology with reflective practices. *International Journal of Computer Applications*, 975, 15–23. Retrieved https://pdfs.semanticscholar.org/9c1c/f423f6d2c5810c866ffbba64f65832179b5b.pdf.

9 Pressure Physiotherapy and Bio-signals

Kumar Avinash Chandra and Dr. Prabhat Kumar Upadhyay

9.1 INTRODUCTION

Almost everything we come across can be classified as a system, with some exaggeration. Lots of it comes down to such broad definition of the system, which is defined as "a series of operations or objects that interact towards a shared goal." Because we're interested in both signals and systems in this book, a system is described as a combination of actions or components which operate on or generate one or many signals. Many instances of well-defined systems dedicated to a shared goal may be found in the human body. The circulatory system transports oxygen-rich blood to the endothelial cells. The cardiopulmonary system is responsible for exchanging gases (mostly oxygen and carbon dioxide) between both air and blood. The renal system's job is to maintain water and ion equilibrium while also adjusting ion and molecule concentrations. The endocrine system aims for mass communication by distributing signaling molecules through the bloodstream, while the nervous system uses neurons and axons to analyze and transmit information encoded as electrical impulses in a closely controlled manner.

Organic systems, regardless of their type, must interact with other systems, and we bioengineers must have a mechanism to engage with these systems. Signals, or more precisely "Bio-signals," transport data and serve as a conduit for intrasystem communication. Signals, by definition, carry information that humans may use; noise, on the other hand, carries no valuable information. Professionals and medical scientists (who can be thought of as huge, complex systems) employ bio-signals evidence to determine or assess the state of a cardiovascular system. Changes in many organic-based variables produce bio-signals. Electrical impulses of the heart, musculature, and central nervous system; blood pressure; pulse rate; blood volatiles and concentration of certain other blood and its components; and sounds created by that of the heart and its chambers are all common signals examined in diagnostic medicine.

For reasons of experimentation or therapy, it is frequently useful to transmit signals into such organic system. Signals directed towards a certain physiological system are commonly referred to as "stimulus," whereas an output signal elicited by these inputs is referred to as a "response." In this context, the organic system behaves like input and output, as shown in Figure 9.1, which is a common paradigm in systems analysis.

Bio-signal "sources" are systems that provide an output without requiring an input stimulus, such as the heart's electrical activity. (Although stimuli such as exercise

DOI: 10.1201/9781003340133-9

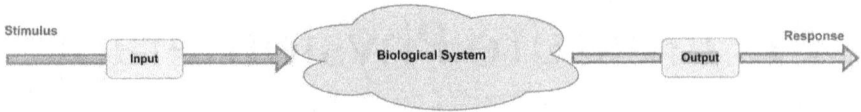

FIGURE 9.1 A physiologic mechanism system accepts an external electrical impulse or input signal and elicits a response or output in a classic systems view.

can modulate the heart's electrical activity, the basic signaling does not follow a particular stimulus.) Because the aim of a pulse is usually to generate some form of reaction, input-only systems, such as write-only memories, are not very practical. The placebo, on the other hand, is intended to elicit no physiological response. (However, it does occasionally generate significant results, most likely as a result of complicated, poorly understood neurological mechanisms.)

Because bio-signals are used throughout all of our encounters with physiological systems, the traits of these signals are extremely important. Signal processing technologies are also critical in bioengineering for extracting additional information from these signals. Indeed, most of the contemporary medical technology is focused on either collecting new physiological signals to the muscles or getting additional information from various bio-signals [1].

9.2 BIO-SIGNAL

Organic signals, also known as bio-signals, are recordings of an organic conjecture as in a heartbeat or a compressing muscle in space, time, or space-time. During these organic events, chemical, electrical, and physical activities often produce signals that may be monitored and evaluated. As a result, bio-signals include significant information which might be useful to decipher the underpinning mechanisms involved in a certain organic event or entity, as well as therapeutic diagnosis.

Bio-signals can be obtained in multifarious ways (as medical practitioner listening to a sufferer's heart sounds using a stethoscope or by any means of technically advanced biomedical equipment). Organic signals are evaluated after data collection so as to excerpt useful information. Many bio-signals can be analyzed using basic signal-analysis methods (as amplifying, winnowing, processing, digitalization, and storage). These methods are usually carried out using either facile electronic-circuit(s) or by means of digital-computers. Aside from the prevailing techniques, skeptical digital processing mechanizations are widely used and can greatly increase the aspect of the data reinstated. Signal smoothing, wavelet analysis, and ML techniques are among them.

9.2.1 CORPOREAL ORIGINS OF BIO-SIGNALS

9.2.1.1 Bioelectric Signals

Bioelectric signals are engendered by muscular along with nerves cells as a corollary of electrochemical alterations between and within the cells. An action potential is generated when a muscular along with nerves cell is activated by a stimulation sufficiently tenacious to achieve an imperative threshold. Employing intracellular or extracellular electrodes, the action potential, that reflects a short passage of ions astride cell membranes can be detected. An activated cell's action potentials can be passed through one cell to another through its axon. When a large number of cells become active, an external electric field that spreads throughout the organic tissue. Surface electrodes can be used to assess these variations in extracellular potential on the tissue or organism's surface. This phenomena can be seen in the electro-gastrogram (EGG), electro-cardiogram (ECG), electroencephalogram (EEG), and, electro-myogram (EMG) (Figure 9.1).

9.2.1.2 Biomagnetic Signals

All the human body organs produce or generate modest magnetic precincts or slow electromagnetic waves. The magnetic precincts (electromagnetic waves) generated from the human wave are sometimes very mild which are associated with the corresponding bioelectric signal (tocsin). "Biomagnetism," the study of magnetic-tocsins which are linked to peculiar corporeal activities and usually accompanied by electric precincts from a particular organ or tissue. It is able to precisely supervise magnetic activity out from peripheral nerves (magnetoneurography, MNG), brain (magneto-encephalography, MEG), heart (magnetocardiography, MCG), and gastrointestinal tract (magnetogastrography, MGG) using very concise magnetic sensors or magnetometers [2].

9.2.1.3 Biochemical Signals

Biochemical signals signal variations in the concentration of different chemical substances within the body. It is possible to measure and record the concentration of different ions in cells, like potassium, calcium, etc. To determine the normalcy of concentration for blood oxygen, variation in partial pressure of oxygen (pO_2) and carbon dioxide (pCO_2) inside the blood or wheezing system being frequently examined. These are all examples of organic signals. These signals can be utilized for a number of things, including detecting glucose, lactate, and metabolite levels, as well as providing info regarding working of many corporeal systems.

9.2.1.4 Biomechanical Signals

Motion, tension, displacement, flow, pressure, and force are all mechanical processes of organic systems that yield observable organic signals. For example, blood-pressure is the amount of force exerted by blood pushing counter the walls of the blood arteries. A waveform can be used to capture changes in blood pressure. The waveform's upstrokes reflect the contractions of a heart's ventricles as the blood being evacuated from the heart and the blood pressure rises to systole, or maximal blood pressure. As a blood pressure decreases to its lowest esteem, referred as the diastolic pressure, the waveform shows ventricular relaxation.

9.2.1.5 Bioacoustic Signals

Vibrations are involved in bioacoustic signals, which are subclass for biomechanical signals. Acoustic noise is produced by a variety of organic processes. The sound of blood flowing through to the heart valves, for example, is distinct. A heart valve's bioacoustic signal can be utilized to detect whether or not it is functioning properly. Bioacoustic signals are also produced by the respiratory, joints, and muscles, which are propagated through the organic medium and can be monitored at the epidermis facade with audile transducers like microphones, accelerometers, etc.

9.2.1.6 Bio-optical Signals

The optic, or light-coaxed, characteristics of organic-systems generate bio-optical signals. Bio-optical signals can arise naturally or be created artificially to assess an organic variable using an external light media. Measurement of the fluorescent qualities of the amniotic fluid, for example, can provide information on the health of a fetus. Dye-dilution technique, which embroil evaluating concentration for such a pigment since it recirculates into bloodstream, can be used to estimate cardiac output. Furthermore, red and infrared lights are utilized in a variety of applications, including detecting optical absorption from across epidermis or a specific tissue to provide exact measures of blood oxygen levels.

9.3 CHARACTERISTICS OF BIO-SIGNALS

Organic signals can be categorized based on a variety of criteria such as waveform shape, statistical schema, and temporal traits. Discrete and continuous signals are two types of signals that also are regularly encountered. Continuous signals are represented via continuous variable functions and span the continuum for time or space. Continuous-time-signal "x" which fluctuates as just function for the continuous-time "t" is represented by the notation x(t). Organic events provide signals that are almost invariably continuous signals. Voltage readings again from heart, arterial blood pressure readings, and brain electrical activity measurements are just a few examples.

Another signal type that is regularly found in today's healthcare situation is discrete signals. Whereas continuous signals are being construed over a continuous range of wide junctures in time or leeway, discrete-tocsin are construed at a subset of verily spaced junctures in time and/or leeway. Arrays or sequence of integers are used to represent discrete signals. A discrete consecution y which appears often at subset, the points in discrete-time n is denoted by the notation $x(n)$. Here, n being $\frac{1}{4}, 0, 1, 2, 3.....$ being an integer which illustrates nth of element within discrete-consecution. Despite the fact that since most organic signals really are not discrete in nature, these discrete signals play a vital part in today's digital technologies. The conversion of continuous signals of the human body into distinct digital sequences which could be evaluated and interpreted by a computer is typically done with sophisticated medical devices. CAT scans, for example, taking of digital samples from a patient's continuous x-ray images obtained from various viewpoint angles [3, 4]. These digitally enhanced, altered, and processed image segments are then used to create a comprehensive three-dimensional digital prototype of the patient's interior organs. These kinds of technologies are critical for clinical diagnosis.

Organic signals could also be divided into two categories: deterministic and random. Mathematical function or rules can be used to characterize deterministic signals. All deterministic signals are made up of periodic and transient signals.

Periodic-signals are often made up of summation of several sine waves or sinusoids and be penned as follows:

$$y(t) = y(t + aT) \qquad (9.1)$$

$y(t)$ denotes tocsin, represented by integer 'a', and the period denoted by 'T'. The period is the distance among successive replicas of a periodic signal along the time axis. Periodic signals have such a stereotyped waveform that repeats indefinitely and has a period of T units. Transient impulses are nonzero or change only for a short epoch of time before decaying towards a constant value as time passes. Because it repeats endlessly with a one-second repetition interval, the sine wave is just the simplest example of such a periodic signal.

Real organic signals nearly always contain some unpredictability in terms of noise or parameter changes and so are not completely deterministic. An illustration of a tocsin that looks to be practically continual and has dainty unexpected elemental is the ECG of a typical throbbing heart at rest. The T-wave, P-wave, and QRS complex create the basic waveform shape, which repeats. The exact patterns of the T-wave, P-wave, and QRS complex, on the other hand, vary from one pulse to the next. As a consequence of the *heart-rate whimsicality (HRV)*, the stretch of the time duration among QRS complexes, termed as R-R interval, varies over-time. HRV is a diagnostic technique that can be used to forecast the healthiness of the heart which has had a heart attack. Individuals with poor HRV typically have a worse long-term prognosis than those with high HRV.

The variables that describe random signals, often known as stochastic signals, are unclear. Mathematical functions could not be used to correctly explain random signals due to this ambiguity. Statistical techniques which involve the regimen of the arbitrary variables of the signals along probability density functions or elementary analytical measurements, as in the standard deviation and mean, are most commonly used to evaluate random signals. The electromyogram (EMG) is a random signal that is used to diagnose neuromuscular problems. It is an electrical record for electrical activity within skeletal muscle. Signals with stationary random statistics or frequency spectrum are those whose statistics or frequency spectrum do not change over time. Nonstationary random signals, on the other hand, have statistical traits or frequency spectrum which change over the time. The recognition of static parts of arbitrary signals seems critical for signal analysis, medical diagnosis, and pattern-recognition in many cases [5].

9.4   SIGNAL ACQUISITION

9.4.1   ANALYSIS OF BIO-SIGNAL DATA ACQUISITION

Organic signals are frequently quite tiny and often contain undesired noise or interference. As a result of this interference, valuable data that may be present within measured signal is obscured. Extraneous noise is noise that comes from external of the subject's body, including things like thermal noise from sensor(s) or notch-noise there in the electronic parts of data accession device induced by that lighting system. Noise can also come from neighboring tissues or organs inside the measuring location if the organic medium is intrinsically noisy. Bioelectric activity from nearby muscles, for example, can impact ECG results from the heart [6].

Sophisticated data gathering equipment and technology are routinely employed to extract relevant data from a tocsin which may be vital in comprehending a specific organic system or an event. To reduce the impacts of unwanted noise, high-precision low-noise technology is frequently required. Figure 9.2 shows a representation of the fundamental components of a bioinstrumentation system.

It is crucial that the original parent organic signal of interest's information and structure be faithfully preserved throughout the data collecting operation. The techniques of amplification, analogue winnow, and/or A-D conversions should not produce untraceable or misleading aberrations as these signals are frequently utilized to aid in the identification of clinical illnesses. Signal measurement distortions may result in an incorrect diagnosis.

9.4.2 SENSORS, AMPLIFIERS, AND ANALOG WINNOWS

Tocsins are at first recognized using a sensor in an organic medium, like a cell or on epidermis' surface. A sensor is such interface among organic systems and electrical recording equipment that turns a physical measurement into an electric output. The sensor will indeed be utilized depending on the bio-signal. Electrodes with a silver/silver chloride (Ag/AgCl) surface linked to the body detects the movement of ions, for example, are used to measure ECGs. A sensor which senses changes in pressure is used to gauge arterial blood pressure. It's critical that the sensor employed to capture the organic desired signal has no negative impact on the signal's traits and characteristics.

The bio-signal is typically amplified and winnowed after it has been detected using a suitable sensor. Operational-amplifiers comprise electronical circuits which are used to boost the size or amplitude of bio-signals. Bioelectric signals, for example, are frequently weak and need up to a thousand-fold amplification with such amplifiers. After that, an analogue winnow can be employed to reduce noise or adjust for sensor distortions. Amplification and filtration of the bio-signal might be required to suit the data acquisition system's hardware requirements. Before being digitized, including an ADC converter and stored in a digital computer, continuous signals might have to be restricted to a specific frequency band.

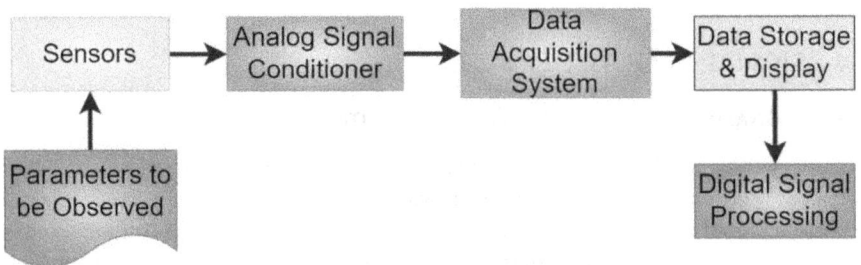

FIGURE 9.2 Signal measurement process

9.5 NEURONS

The human mind is thought to contain approximately 10 trillions of neurons divided into less than 1,000 various types in an orderly cadre with a fairly consistent appearance. It's worth noting that while there being two types of neuron: nerve cells and neuroglial cells, albeit this is not relevant to this chapter. Despite the fact that there can be 10 to 50 times the neuroglial cells as that nerve cells in human brain, the nerve cell is the center of attention here because the neuroglial cells are not engaged in signaling and largely serve as a support system for nerve cell. Because the primary objective is to perceive the signaling attributes of a neuron, the term neurons and nerve cell are often used interchangeably. Overall, the brain's complex capacities are best characterized by a neuron's linkages with those other neurons or either periphery, rather than by individual differences between neurons.

The cell body, axon, presynaptic terminal and dendrites, make up a typical neuron. A neuron's cell body, which is identical to that of other cells, houses the nucleus as well as other nutritive apparatus. The cell body of a neuron, unlike those of other cells, is linked to an aggregate of dendrites and a lengthy tube termed as axon, which links to cell body well to presynaptic terminals. The dendrites are the neuron's receptive shell, which receive impulses passive and without amplification from millions of other neurons. Receptor sites are found upon that dendrite and cell bodies and receive input from neighboring neurons' presynaptic terminals. Synapses are found in 10^4 to 10^5 neurons on average. A neurotransmitter that modifies membrane characteristics is used to communicate between neurons. An individual axon, which varies in lengths from 1 meter in the mammalian spinal cord down to few mm in brain is also attached to the cell body [7]. The axon's diameter ranges from less than 1 mm to 500mm. In general, the quicker the signal travels, the bigger the axon diameter. Axon signals travel at speeds ranging from 0.5 to 120 m/s xon acts as just a dissemination line for information to be sent through one neuron to the other at high rates. Hefty axons feature regular interstice called nodes of Ranvier, which enable the action potential to pass through one node to adjoining and also wrapped by such a fatty insulating mound called the myelin sheath. The action potential can be visualized as a continuous pulse which traverses the lengths of axon without diminishing in amplitude. The majority of the rest of this section is consecrated to elucidating this procedure. A system of up to 10,000 branching with presynaptic terminals can be found at the axon's end. All action potentials which travel through the axon are propagated to the presynaptic cell via each branch. These presynaptic terminals are the neuron's disseminating unit, which releases a neurotransmitter when activated, which travels across a $20nm$ gap to an adjacent cell, in which it meets with a postsynaptic membrane that also alters its potential.

9.5.1 Membrane Potential

The neuron, as any other cell in a human body, has an exterior membrane that separates charge. In a neuron, a cell membrane is positively polarized at the exterior side and negatively polarized at the inner side. The membrane potential is caused by charge separation caused by selective membrane permeability to ions. The potential differential all across the cell membrane of a neuron ranges from 60 *to* 90 millivolts, depending on the cell type. The outside potential is $14mV$ to $60mV$, while the restful potential is $40mV$ to $60mV$, according to convention. Because most signaling includes changes in this potential from across the membrane, this charge difference is of special relevance. Electrical disturbances of the membrane produce signals like action potentials. Hyperpolarization is defined as a decrease of membrane potential over restful potential (i.e., $60mV$ to $70mV$), whereas depolarization is defined as a rise of membrane potential over slumbering potential (i.e., $60mV$ to $70mV$).

9.5.2 ACTION POTENTIAL AND RELEGATED RESPONSE

By releasing its neurotransmitter, a neuron could also affect the membrane potential of that other neuron with which it's attached. The neurotransmitter travels over the synaptic gap or cleft, binds to receptor molecules with postsynaptic membrane of either the adjacent neuron's dendrite or cell body, and modifies the receptor neuron's membrane potential.

The conversion of neurotransmitter chemical energy into electric energy causes a shift of membrane potential just at postsynaptic membrane. The alteration in membrane potential is depolarizing or hyperpolarizing, depending as to how much neurotransmitter gets received. Because the volume of neurotransmitter received varies, this aspect in potential is known as a graded response. Another way to think about synapse activity is whether the neurotransmitter absorbed is consolidated or aggregated, resulting in a graded membrane potential response. A neuron's signal could either be inhibitory or excitatory; however certain synapses can be excitatory while others are inhibitory, allowing the nervous system to accomplish complicated tasks.

The action potential is the end outcome of nerve cell activation. The action potential seems to be a significant depolarizing signal that goes through the axon and lasts one to five milliseconds. A common action potential is seen in Figure 9.3. The action potential would be a one-of-a-kind signal which travels actively through the axon without diminishing in amplitude. Once the signal reaches the presynaptic terminal at the end of the axon, the shift in potential causes a package of neurotransmitter to be released. This is an extremely effective way to communicate over long distances. Following the introduction of various techniques for interpreting this phenomena, more specifics about just the action potential have been provided throughout the rest of this chapter.

9.6 BRAIN COMPUTER INTERFACE (BCMI)

The BCMI, a system which when measures and processes a user's brain activity patterns in order to transform those patterns into messages or directives for an application interface. Electroencephalography is commonly used to assess a BCMI user's brain activity (EEG) [8]. For example, by picturing left- or right-hand gestures, a BCMI can allow a subject to move a pointer to any direction around a computer screen. With the computer making control feasible even with no physical exercise, EEG-underpinned BCMIs affirms to revolutionize several more application aspects, prominently to facilitate gravely motor-impaired patients to operate technological

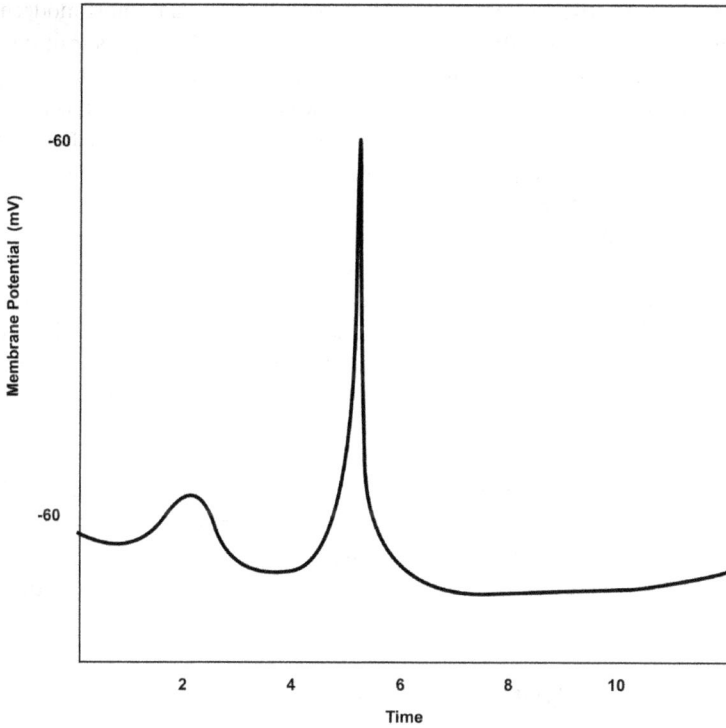

FIGURE 9.3 An action potential

devices, for example, textual input processes as well as assistive devices, as a reha-bilitation equipment for stroke survivors, and as for new gaming user input, to archi-tecture autonomous and intelligent interfaces which reacts with the user's state of mind, to name a few.

To use a BCMI, there are usually two phases: (1) offline training and testing wherein the device is overhauled or calibrated, also (2) an operational online-aspect, wherein the system could recognize hustle in the brain pattern and translate infor-mation into computer commands. The user creates a distinct EEG pattern, and these EEG signals are monitored in an online BCMI system, which is a closed loop [9–11]. The signals are then routinely preprocessed utilizing diverse multispectral and spa-tial winnow, and traits have been extracted from them in representing in a compact manner. Eventually, these EEG traits are classified prior to getting converted into an application command and before users are given feedback on whether a certain mental command was detected or not.

Although great work is being done to provide calibration-free operating modes, most BCMIs still require offline calibration in order to achieve a reliable system. The cataloguing system is calibrated at this point, and the best traits from various EEG channels are chosen. A training dataset from the user must be pre-recorded for this calibration. Because EEG signals are unique to each individual, most modern BCMI devices are gauged individually for individual subjects [12–14]. This training dataset consists of EEG tocsins captured as the subject repeated for every mental assignment of significance numerous epochs, as directed. The cataloguing algorithms (also known as classifiers) implemented to classify the liege's EEG waveforms based on EEG traits are one of the important aspects of the BCMI closed-loop. According to our 2007 analysis of classifier for EEG underpinned BCMIs, there was and still is a wide variety of classifier kinds that are utilized and have been researched to develop BCMIs [15]. Various new age algorithms have been devised and investigated so as to identify EEG data in BCMIs in the tens of years since this initial review was published. As a result, we believe the time has come to update our study of EEG classifiers. Consequently, in this chapter, various literature on BCMI and ML since 2007 were surveyed as in to identify the current EEG cataloguing algorithms for EEG cataloguing and which seems most significant [16–18]. Note that we include ML approaches for EEG extracting traits in this review, particularly for optimizing spatial winnows, which became a critical element of BCMI cataloguing systems. We combine these details in order to illustrate such methods, as well as how they were applied to BCMIs and what the results were. We also discuss advantages and disadvantages so as to provide advice on when and how to utilize each cataloguing approach, as well as some problems that must be overcome in order for EEG signal cataloguing to go further.

9.7 ELECTROENCEPHALOGRAPHY (EEG)

As of its non-invasiveness, greater temporal resolution, also lesser financial outlay, electroencephalography (EEG) is extensively utilized encompassing neural engineering, biomedical engineering, and neurosciences (e.g., BCMI), sleep exposition, and seizure detection. The categorization of such signals is a critical step toward making EEG more practicable in application and reducing the need on experienced specialists. Artifact removal, extraction of traits, and cataloguing are all part of a typical EEG cataloguing pipeline. An EEG dataset, at its most basic level is a 2D (time and channels) matrices of real measures that reflect brain-stemmed potentials measured on the scalp in response to certain task circumstances [19]. EEG data is excellent for ML because of its highly organized format. The EEG data has been lieged to a variety of classic ML and pattern-recognizing methods. For example, linear discriminant analysis (LDA) and decision trees are commonly used in neural cataloguing, and canonical correlation analysis (CCA) is often used in neural cataloguing (SSVEPs) [20].

As of practical challenges such that extended computation times and problems with vanishing/exploding gradients, NN(s) did not attract the same level of attention as they do now in neural cataloguing applications. Fortunately, the recent development of graphic processing units (GPUs) and the availability of big datasets provided NN(s) analysts with an affordable and powerful solution to their hardware limitation, allowing them to examine DL designs (NN-architectures consisting least of the two hidden layers). In the last decade, these advancements have resulted in a tenfold growth in interest in and uses of DL [21]. Indeed, it enhanced performance in a variety of previously difficult domains, including pictures, videos, voice, and text. Because NN(s) improve their parameters iteratively and automatically, they are expected to possess minimal prior technical expertise towards the dataset to operate adequately. This advantage prompted initial acclimation in the field of medical imaging that frequently consists of enormous datasets that are arduous to analyze even for professionals. DL frameworks have recently been used to the decoding as well as cataloguing of EEG signals that are typically characterized by meager signal-to-noise-ratios (SNRs) and computational complexity of the data due to the increasing accessibility of huge EEG datasets [22, 23].

9.8 EXTRACTION OF TRAITS AND SELECTION, AS WELL AS PERFORMANCE MEASURES

Several pattern recognition/ML systems, including BCMIs, include feature extraction/ selection approaches in addition to a classifier to represent EEG data in a compact and relevant manner. Before traits are recovered from the resultant signals, EEG signals are often winnowed in the spatial-domain (spatial-winnow) and temporal domain (band-pass winnow) for BCMI. Using feature selection techniques, the best subsets of characteristics are found, and these traits are then utilized to train the classifier [24]. Figure 9.4 shows how this method works. In this chapter, we'll go over which traits are commonly utilized in BCMI, how to choose the most important traits from among them, as well as how to assess the pattern recognition workflow that results.

9.8.1 FEATURE EXTRACTION

While EEG signals are sometimes represented in a variety of ways, frequencies band power characteristics and time point characteristics are the two most prevalent numerous criteria being used to represent EEG signals [25].

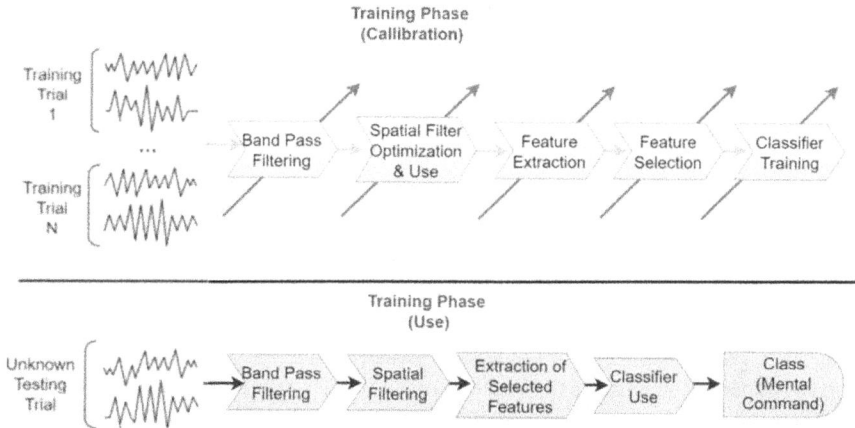

FIGURE 9.4 Typical cataloguing process in EEG underpinned BCMI systems

The average power (energy) of EEG tocsins for a specific frequency band across a specific channel over a given time window is represented by band power characteristics. Band power characteristics are widely employed in BCMIs that exploit oscillatory activity, such as variations in EEG rhythm amplitudes, and can be estimated in a variety of ways. As a result, for many passive BCMIs aimed upon deciphering mental states like psychological workload or emotional, or even for the Steady-State-Visually-Evoked-Potential (SSVEP) postulated BCMIs, band power attributes are the high standard traits.

EEG signals from all channels are concatenated to create time point characteristics. Pre-processing, such as band-pass or the low-pass filtration and down-sampling, is usually used to extract such information. They are the most common criteria used to categorize event related potentials (ERP), which become temporal fluctuations in the amplitudes of EEG signals that are time-locked to a specific event/stimulus. The majority of P300-based BCMIs have these qualities [26, 27].

Both types of attributes benefit from retrieval after spatial winnowing. Spatial winnowing is a technique of linearly integrating sensor data to create a signal with a higher SNR than distributed sources. Spatial winnowing can be based on the physical aspects about how EEGs signal data flow through to the epidermis and skull, for example, culminating in spatial winnows such as the Laplacian-Winnow or reverse solution-based spatial winnowing. PCA and independent component analysis (ICA) are two methods for obtaining spatial winnows that are data-driven and unsupervised. Finally, supervised learning, which would be arguably one of the most popular methodologies, can be used to obtain spatial winnows in a data-driven manner. Common spatial patterns (CSP), focused on band-power characteristics and oscillatory activity BCMI, as well as spatial winnows like xDAWN or Fisher spatial winnows for ERP categorization based on of time-point traits, are examples of supervised spatial winnows. Various variants for such methods have been created which will be greater in robust to noise or quasi signals, employing regularization techniques, rigorous data averaging, and/or new divergent metrics, due to the strong cataloguing results gained by so supervised spatial winnows in practice.

Extensions of these algorithms have also been proposed to jointly improve spatial and spectral winnows (e.g., the prominent Winnow-Bank CSP (FBCSP) technique [28] as well as others [29–31]). Finally, several approaches have coupled data-driven spatial winnows with physically driven spatial winnows built on inverse models.

9.8.2   Feature Selection

Following the feature extraction process, an attribute selection stage can be used to pick a subset of attributes with varied possible benefits. To begin with, some of the properties that can be extracted from EEG signals may be extraneous or unrelated here to mental states that the BCMI is designed to target. Second, the amount of traits is positively connected with the set of variables that the classifier must optimize. As a result of reducing the amount of characteristics, the classifier has fewer parameters to tune. It also decreases the risk of overtraining and, as a result, improves performance, particularly when the sample size is limited. Third, perhaps if a few traits are picked and/or graded, it is easy to see which traits are genuinely relevant to the intended mental states from an information retrieval standpoint. Fourth, because it should be way more efficient, a model featuring fewer traits and hence fewer parameters can generate faster estimates for a fresh sample. Fifth, the amount of data collected and stored will be decreased. The winnow, wrapper, and embedding techniques have been recognized as three feature selection techniques. For each strategy, a variety of alternate methods have been presented.

Winnow approaches, regardless of the classifier used, relies on measures of connection amongst each feature as well as the target class. As a feature ranking criterion, the coefficient of determination, and that is the square of the Pearson correlation coefficient estimation, might be utilized. In a two-class situation, its coefficient of determination can be used to designate classes as 1 or (+1). Correlation coefficient, on the other hand, can only find linear relationships between characteristics and classes. Applying nonlinear pre-processing, like calculating the log or square of the characteristics, is a straightforward way to exploit nonlinear correlations. Information-theory-based ranking criteria, such as the correlation between each characteristic and the set of possible [32, 33] can also be utilized. Many winnow feature selection methods necessitate data-based predictions of the probability density functions and combined densities of the feature and class label. Distinguishing the traits as well as class labels is one option. Another option is to use a non-parametric approach like Parzen windows to approximate their densities. When the densities are calculated using a normally distributed, the mutual information result will be similar to the correlation coefficient result. With regard to the number of traits, winnow techniques have a linear complexity. This, however, may lead to identification of redundant traits.

Wrapper and embedding techniques fix the problem, although they take longer to compute. A classifier is used in these methods to extract a feature subsets. Wrapper approaches choose a feature subsets, offer them as inputs to a classifiers for learning, monitor the results, and either end the search or suggest a new subgroup if the stopping criterion is not met. Embedded approaches combine the selection and assessment of characteristics in a single process, such as in decision tree and the multilayered perceptron having optimal cell damage.

The method is advantageous linear discriminant assessment (embedded process) for P300-BCMI as well as frequency spectra cataloguing for motor imagery utilizing maximum total similarity matrix (winnowing methods) are two examples of feature selection in BCMI. SVM for excerption, linear regressors for extracting knowledge, GAs for spectral selecting traits and P300-based feature extraction, and GA for selecting traits based on multiresolution assessment are also worth mentioning (all being wrapper methods). So as to escape the profanity of dimensionality, metaheuristic techniques (such as ant-colony, simulated annealing, swarms search, or tabu search) have been increasingly employed for selecting traits in BCMI [34].

Winnow approaches like maximal relevance minimal redundancy (mRMR) feature extraction or R2 extraction of traits are also commonly utilized in EEG underpinned BCMIs. Five feature selection approaches were tested on the BCMI competitions III datasets: gain ratio ranking, causal connection based extraction of features, Relief (an exemplar-based ascribe leaderboard strategy for of multiclass cataloguing), consistency premised feature engineering, and 1R-Ranking [35]. The best three feature selection procedures among ten classifiers are correlation premised feature extraction, gain ratio, and 1R ranking.

9.9 METHODS

9.9.1 METHODS FOR LOCATING STUDIES THROUGH SEARCHES

This evaluation of DL applications to EEG signal cataloguing uses PRISMA, a comprehensive review along meta-evaluation approach, to find studies and condense the collection. "Deep NN(s)*" or "DL" and "EEG" or Duplicate ion across the bi-databases were eliminated, as were research that did not satisfy the requirements for inclusion (described in the next section). The remaining papers' full texts were then examined.

Unqualified studies were excluded using the following criteria:

- Electroencephalography (EEG) only—Research involving multi-model datasets, such as EEG analysis paired with some other biomedical parameters (electrooculography, electromyography) or films, were omitted to limit variability in the studies.
- Task cataloguing—This study focuses entirely on the use of EEG data to classify tasks done by people. Other research were omitted, including power analyses, non-human investigations, and feature extraction with no end categorization.
- DL is described as NN(s)s including at minimum two hidden layers in this review.
- Time—Due to the rapid pace of research in this field, this evaluation only included articles published within the last five years.

2.2. Extraction and display of data
The following information was gathered:

a. *Task Information*
   - Task type
   - Quantity of test lieges
   - Total size for data analyzed
b. *Artifacts Removal Strategy*
   - Standard
   - Automated
   - Neither purification nor eradication
c. *Frequency Range has been used in the study*
d. *Formulation of input*
   - EEGs signal traits
   - Channel selection criteria
e. *The number of layers in the classifier, the output classes, and the fundamental characteristic of the DL strategy*
   - Number of layers in a Convolutional neural network (CNN) activation
   - Restricted Boltzmann machines (RBMs) and deep belief network (DBN)
   - Recurrent neural network (RNN), RNN layer number, RNN unit type

- Stacked auto encoders (SAE), hidden layer numbers, and activation
- MLPNN (multilayer perceptron neural network), hidden layers, activation
- Activation, hybrid architecture(s), varieties of algorithms, related main characteristics

f. *Accuracy rate or other model performance achieved*

9.10   EEG CATALOGUING METHODS

9.10.1   Adaptive Classifiers

9.10.1.1   Principle

When new EEG data becomes available, adaptive classifiers' parameters, such as the weights accredited to individual features in the linear-discriminant hyperplane, are sized and also changed over a time span. This then allows the classifiers to maintain track of potential changing feature distribution and hence remain successful even though dealing with non-stationary inputs as an EEG tocsins. Adaptive classifiers based on BCMI were first developed during the early 2000s and have now been shown to have limited utility in offline analysis. Since then, increasingly complex adaptation methods have been created and tested, including online tests.

Higher advanced adaptation methods, such as online experimentation, have been created and tested since then. As a result, unsupervised adaptation is relied on class-unspecific adaptation, such as updating the general across classes EEG signal mean or Covariance-Matrix in the classifier model, or on an assessment of its data labels to retraining/updating. Semi-supervised adaptation is a third type of adaptation that falls well within supervised and unsupervised approaches. Semi-supervised adaptation leverages contextually labelled data as well as unlabelled input to update the classifiers. In BCMI, semi-supervised adaptation is often achieved as (1) training of a supervised classification model on attainable annotated training data, (2) evaluating the labels of inbound datasets with a classification model, and (3) adapting the classifiers when using ultimately unlabelled datasets assigned to their ballparked labels conjunction with recognized accessible annotated training data. The technique is repeated as additional batch of unmarked inbound EEG dataset become available.

9.10.1.2   Pros and Cons

For several types of BCMI, adaptive classification techniques have been demonstrated to be superior than non-adaptive ones, most noticeably MoI BCMI, and for some ERP-based BCMI. It has access to genuine labels, supervised adaption is the most effective sort of adaptation. Unsupervised adaptation, on the other hand, has been demonstrated to outperform static classifiers in a number of experiments. It could also be utilized to reduce necessity calibration or perhaps eliminate it. Because the bulk of practical BCmI systems do not supply labels and so must rely on unsupervised approaches and the need for improved robust unsupervised adaption methods.

9.10.2 CLASSIFICATION OF EEG MATRIX AND TENSORS

9.10.2.1 Riemannian Geometry-based Cataloguing

9.10.2.1.1 Principles

Instead of just foretelling spatial winnows and/or tiny elite attributes, the Riemannian geometry classifier (RGC) concept would have been to map the data straight onto a geometric-shaped space fitted with such an apt metric; albeit without evaluating spatial winnows and/or choosing attributes, the RGC concept could be to map the document around a geometrical space accoutred with an apt metric. In this type of environment, dataset can be easily handled for a variety of purposes, including average, smoothing, linear interpolation, extrapolating, and categorizing. Mapping EEG data includes calculating many characteristics of data covariance. The hypothesis underlying this mapping is that for a given mental state, the amplitude and geographical dispersal of EEG sources are fixed and that this data may be stored using a covariance. The analysis of smooth curved spaces which can be estimated locally and also linearly is expressed as Riemannian geometry. The tangent space is the linear approximation of a manifold at every point. In a Riemannian manifold, tangent space has an integral (metric) which fluctuates gradually between point to point. As a result, a non-Euclidean notion of measure across two or more points (for example, each point could be a trial) and a concept of midline for any set of measurements emerges (Figure 9.5). As a result, rather than utilizing the extrinsic distance, that is, adjusted towards the geometry of all the manifold, the intrinsic distance is utilized, that is, adapted to the way information were mapped.

9.10.2.1.2 Pros and Cons

As described in Riemannian methodology, such RMDM have simpler processing procedures and mean fewer stages than more traditional approaches. Any BCMI paradigm (e.g., mental imagination BCMIs, SSVEP, and ERPs) can use Riemannian classifiers; only one variation is how sets of data are portrayed within SPD manifold. Furthermore, unlike most other cataloguing systems, the RMDM approach is parameter-free, meaning it does not require parameter tuning such as cross-validation.

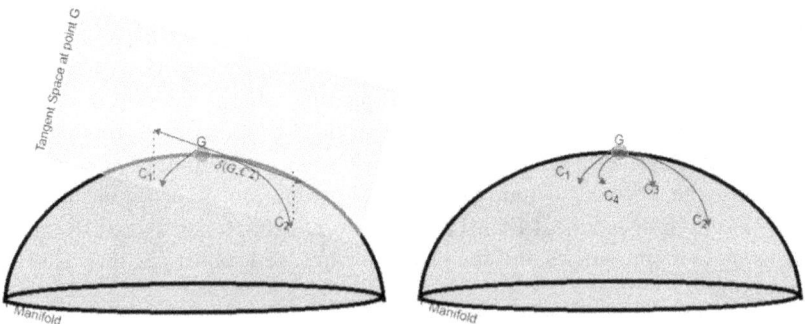

FIGURE 9.5 Schematic representation for Riemannian manifold

As a consequence, Riemannian geometry administers new tools for creating simple and accurate prediction models.

9.10.2.2 Feature Abstraction and Cataloguing by Applying Tensors

9.10.2.2.1 Principles

Higher cognitive tensor analyses and factorizations are emerging as possible (but unproven and understudied) approaches for EEG data processing, particularly for extracting features, categorizing, including cataloguing operations in BCMI. Tensorization seems to be the process of converting lower-order data formats into higher-order ordered tensors (multiway arrays), for a time-series EEG dataset collected vectors or matrices or vectors. Before retrieving and categorizing tensor (multiway) traits, this step is required.

The order of a tensor is determined by its quantity, often known as dimensions or ways (e.g., for that EEG-BCMI statistical dataset: spatial (channels), time, frequencies, people, conditions, trials, groups, dictionaries, wavelets). Several channels EEG signals are frequently represented as a third-order tensor with three main variants: spatial (channel), time, and frequency. To put it differently, S channels of EEG gathered over T time samples can be layered together to generate S matrix of FT dimensionality time-frequency spectrograms to build an FTS dimensionality third-order tensor. For many trials and multiple lieges, the datasets could've been simply described by higher-order tensors: for a 5th-order tensor, for example: trial liege space time frequency.

Elemental vector and lattice ML algorithms for extracting traits have indeed been expanded or adapted to convolution layers or could be extended or generalized towards tensors. The SVM has been naturally generalized into tensor supporting machine (TSMC), Kernel TSMC, and higher rank TSMC for cataloguing. Tensor Fisher discriminant analysis (TFDAN) and higher order discriminant analysis (HODAN) have been added to the traditional LDA method (HODA). Furthermore, because data structure information is often innate and is an innate constraint that allows for a decline in the amount of undisclosed features extracted in the categorization of a learning method, convolutional depictions of BCMI dataset are often quite useful in attempting to overcome the data sparsity conundrum in exclusionary subspace selection. In other words, anytime the number of EEG learning measurement approaches is circumscribed, tensor-based learning systems were always projected to outperform matrix or vector-based machine learning due to issues such as data leakage for structured dataset and overfitting for high-dimensional data.

9.10.2.2.2 Pros and Cons

There are advantages and disadvantages. In conclusion, recent improvements in BCMI technology have resulted in large volumes of brain data with high dimensionality, many modalities (physical modes including frequencies or time, numerous brain computed tomography or circumstances), and various coupling as brain functional data. Tensors offers powerful and intriguing tools enabling BCMI fusion and analysis of vast data, as well as an analytical backbone for the finding of abecedarian hidden complicated (time-space frequency) dataset structures due to their multiway nature.

Another benefit is that they can quickly compress large amounts of multidimensional dataset into low order factor-matrices and/or core-tensors that typically indicate decreased features, utilizing tensorization as well as low-rank tensor decomposition. Tensor approaches can also be used to differentiate prevalent from separate components in raw EEG data by analyzing linked (connected) blocks of events represented as matrix multiplication into tensors.

9.10.3 TRANSFER LEARNING (TsL)

9.10.3.1 Principles

For the most important hypothesis in ML would be of training dataset and test dataset correspond to a certain feature set and reflect having similar probability distribution. This concept is frequently broken in various areas, as in computer vision, bioengineering, and BCMIs. When data is collected from multi people and across different time sessions for BCMI, shift in data dissemination occurs.

TsL seeks to deal with that data which contradicts this notion by utilizing grasp gained while learning one task to solve a related but distinct one. To put it another way, transfer method is a combination of approaches for boosting the effectiveness of such a learned classifier training on one task (commonly known as domain) using knowledge gained as an act of learning a different task. Typically, the efficacy for TsL is highly influenced by the degree to which the two tasks are related. TsL across two P300 octavo activities taken up by two distinct individuals, for example, is more important than TsL across one P300 octavo challenge along MoI activities done by the dupe liege.

TsL is important for cases whenever there is enough annotated data for one job, referred to as a source domain, but data for said second task, referred to as a target domain, is rare or expensive to get. Transferring information from the given dataset to the objective domain functions as a regularizer or a bias for completing the objective task in such instances. Based on Pan et al.'s surveys, we propose a much more detailed explanation of TsL.

9.10.3.2 Pros and Cons

According to the findings mentioned previously, TsL is vital throughout every session and beholden decoding functioning. This will be required in the future in order to develop a successful calibration-free BCMI way of action that will supplement BCMI adoption. In actuality, it's widely accepted in the profession that the calibration huddle can be excessively exhausting for analytical individuals with limited cognoscible abilities, as well as annoying among healthy users in general. According to Sanelli et al., peer assessment from the start of a BCMI interaction is highly exhilarating and appealing for beginner users.

Then, before utilizing co-adaptive approaches, users can use TsL to achieve a good BCMI. In this vein, for a naive user, TsL might be applied for establishing a BCMI utilizing dataset obtained via differ liege(s), and for known users, dataset(s) from various periods. In any case, as when an initiation is inefficient, hence such an accession necessitates the classifier being adjusted while in the huddle.

To accomplish the desired purpose for the calibration-freed method of act, TsL with adaptivity must work together.

TsL seems robust by definition, even if it is suboptimal in general. For example, if liege-to-liege TsL is of poor quality, it can give better outcomes than liege-specific calibration. This is especially beneficial in analytic situations, where getting a better calibration can be difficult.

9.10.4 Deep Learning

DL is a part of ML technique as in where the classification technique as well as traits both being taught from the data itself. The model's design, which itself is centered on cascading of the nonlinearities and trainable traits extraction modules, gave rise to the phrase "DL." Learned traits being frequently linked with rising levels of concepts as a result of this cascade. The two most prominent DL algorithms for BCMI are CNN with limited Boltzmann machines, shown in Figure 9.6.

9.10.4.1 Benefits and Malefits

DNNs retains the ability to train simultaneously relevant attributes and classifiers out of raw EEG dataset at the same time. DNNs appear propitious leading to classifiers and stronger traits, therefore adding more of robustness in EEG categorization, based on their efficacy in other disciplines. However, the great review of available investigations while DNN(s) for EEG-adapted BCMIs has proved flimsy in establishing their substantive relevancy along advantage in practice over newfangled BCMI approaches. Indeed, various studies either did not equate the investigated DNN to newfangled BCMI methodologies or did so in a biased way, using either inadequate parameters for the

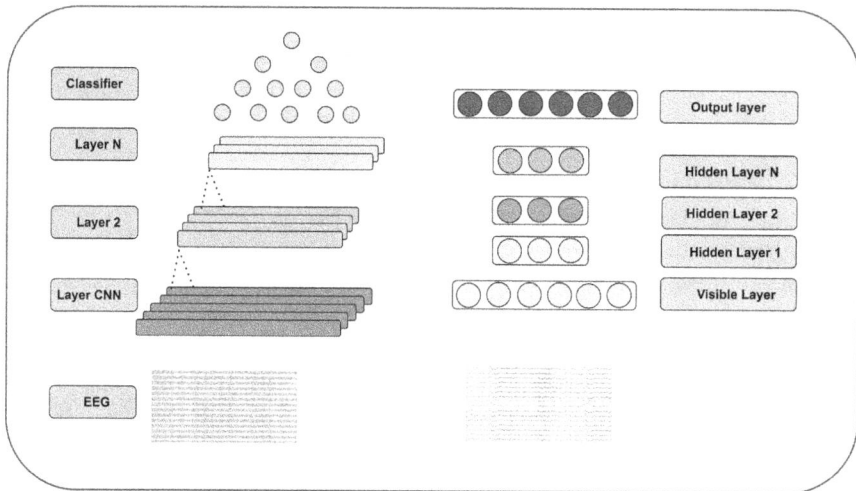

FIGURE 9.6 Architectures for two types of deep learning frameworks. In left: CNN. In right: stacked restricted Boltzmann machine.

newfangled competitors or gratuitous parameter volition regarding the DNN, preventing users from ruling out conventional tuning for these variables with the proficiency of the test set. As a result, it is necessary to ensure that such difficulties are addressed in future DNN for BCMI publications. A notable exception being worked on demonstrated that a superficial CNN may outperform FBCSP in a rigorous and compelling manner. This shows that one of DNN's primary drawbacks for EEG underpinned BCMI being such a network that has a huge number of parameters, necessitating a number of training instances to overhaul them. Ineptly, conventional BCMI set(s) of data and experimentations have a limited number for training examples because BCMI users cannot be requested to complete millions of cognitive instructions beforehand utilizing the device. In fact, DNNs have been shown to be suboptimal and among the lamest classifiers with limited training sets outside of the BCMI sector. Unfortunately, when it comes to designing BCMIs, only modest training sets are usually available. This could explain why shallow networks, with many fewer parameters, have proven to be the most effective for BCMI. In the future, either limited parameter NNs, alternatively, BCMI applications with large training datasets, such as multi-liege metadata, will be required.

9.10.5 Multilabel Classifiers

9.10.5.1 Principles

To generate a multiclass cataloguing function, two major approaches can be employed to classify more than two mental activities. The first method involves employing multiclass approaches like decision trees, k-NN, multilayered perceptrons, or naive Bayes classifiers to estimate the class directly. The second method entails breaking the problem down into a series of binary collocation tasks. This disintegration might also be achieved in a variety of fashion, including employing (a) pairwise classifiers that are one-against-one, (b) one-contra-the-rest (one-vs-bar none) classification techniques, (c) hierarchic classification techniques comparable with binary decision tree, and lastly (d) multi-label-classifier. Each class is associated with a subset of L labels (or attributes) in the latter scenario. The smallest proximity among the cataloguing results, and every subset of labels specifying a class is used to determine the predicted class.

9.10.5.2 Pros and Cons

As a result, multiclass and multi-label techniques try to recognize several commands. In both circumstances, the increased number of recognized classes may provide the user with additional commands to interact with the system more quickly, potentially eliminating anything like a drop-down menu, for example. Because it only needs learning a limited handful of labels, the multiclass cataloguing approach makes learning easier and less tiresome. Because there are so many different combinations of these labels, there are a lot of classes and thus a lot of commands. The multi-label technique also allows for variability in the markers, which portrays a class, which aids in class bifurcation. Typically, the number of labels is necessarily less than the total count of classes. Eventually, multiclass and multi tag systems offer reduced computational complexity than typical methods because they can exchange parameters, such as multilayer perceptron or class descriptor.

9.11 CONCLUSION

9.11.1 SUMMARY

We extracted the following for picking proper cataloguing based on the many studies covered in this chapter:

- Adaptive cataloguing techniques, among both classifiers as well as spatial winnows, should be chosen over static ones when it comes to cataloguing performance. Albeit only unsupervised adaptability is possible for the specified application, this should be the case.
- DL networks do not consider to be impactful for EEG signal categorization in BCMI at this time, given the circumscribed training dataset accessible. Shallow convolutional NN(s) appear to be more promising.
- For minimal training data, shrinkage linear discriminant analysis (sLDA) should be applied rather than of regular LDA because it's more effectual and resilient.
- If there is not much training data, use transfer learning, random-forest, sLDA, or Riemannian minimal distance to the mean (RMDM) classification techniques.
- Domain acclimation can be utilized to increase classifier rendition provided lieges' tasks are comparable. However, when something comes to the effectiveness of TsL, caution is warranted because it can sometimes hinder from performance.
- Riemannian geometry classifiers (RGCs) seem extremely propitious and are now state-of-the-art for a variety of BCMI tasks, including motor imaging, P300, and SSVEP cataloguing. To improve their effectiveness, they should be implemented and researched further.
- Tensor techniques are new and may be promising, but additional study is needed to make them practical in practice, online, and to compare their performance to certain newfangled methods.

Numerous EEG cataloguing application submitted that have evolved since early 2007 are discussed in this chapter. Adaptive classifiers, tensor classifiers and matrix, DL and TsL methods, and being the primary kinds of methodologies that investigated.

According to our findings, dynamic classifiers, both unsupervised and supervised, handily beat static classifiers in accustomed fashion. Matrix and/or tensor-classifiers have also shown promise in enhancing BCMI reliability; nonetheless, Riemannian geometry classifiers remain the present avant-garde for many BCMI designs. TsL tends to be beneficial as well, particularly when training data is insufficient, but its efficacy is highly variable. More research is needed to discover if this can be incorporated into standard BCMI designs. Random Forest and Shrinkage LDA are two other BCMI algorithms that work well with little training datasets. Finally, notwithstanding their effectiveness in other sectors, DL models have yet to show a consistent and unambiguous enhancement of avant-garde BCMI techniques.

REFERENCES

[1] Lotte F, Bougrain L and Clerc M 2015 Electroencephalography (EEG)-based brain–computer interfaces *Wiley Encyclopedia on Electrical and Electronices Engineering* (New York: Wiley).

[2] Lotte F and Congedo M 2016 *EEG Feature Extraction* (New York: Wiley) pp 127–43.

[3] Lotte F and Jeunet C 2017 Online cataloguing accuracy is a poor metric to study mental imagery-based BCMI user learning: An experimental demonstration and new metrics *International Winter Conference on Brain-Computer Interface*.

[4] Lotte F, Jeunet C, Mladenovic J, N'Kaoua B and Pillette L 2018 *Signal Processing and ML for Brain-Machine Interfaces* (Stevenage: Institution of Engineering and Technology (IET)).

[5] Toshihisa T and Arvaneh M, ed *Brain-Machine Interfaces* (Stevenage: Institution of Engineering and Technology (IET)).

[6] Lotte F, Larrue F and Mühl C 2013 Flaws in current human training protocols for spontaneous brain–computer interfaces: Lessons learned from instructional design *Front. Human Neurosci.* **7**.

[7] Mayaud L et al. 2016 Brain-computer interface for the communication of acute patients: A feasibility study and a randomized controlled trial comparing performance with healthy participants and a traditional assistive device *Brain-Comput. Interfaces.* **3** 197–215.

[8] McFarland D J, McCane L M, David S V and Wolpaw J R 1997 Spatial winnow selection for EEG underpinned communication *Electroencephalogr. Clin. Neurophysiol.* **103** 386–94.

[9] McFarland D, Sarnacki W and Wolpaw J 2011 Should the parameters of a BCMI translation algorithm be continually adapted? *J. Neurosci. Methods.* **199** 103–7.

[10] Meng J, Yao L, Sheng X, Zhang D and Zhu X 2015 Simultaneously optimizing spatial spectral traits based on mutual information for EEG cataloguing *IEEE Trans. Biomed. Eng.* **62** 227–40.

[11] Meng J, Zhang S, Bekyo A, Olsoe J, Baxter B and He B 2016 Noninvasive electroencephalogram based control of a robotic arm for reach and grasp tasks *Sci. Rep.* **6** 38565.

[12] Millán J, Renkens F, Mouriño J and Gerstner W 2004 Noninvasive brain-actuated control of a mobile robot by human EEG *IEEE Trans. Biomed. Eng.* **51** 1026–33.

[13] Mladenovic J, Mattout J and Lotte F 2017 A generic framework for adaptive EEG underpinned BCMI training, operation *Handbook of Brain–Computer Interfaces* ed C Nam et al (London: Taylor & Francis).

[14] Morioka H, Kanemura A, Hirayama J I, Shikauchi M, Ogawa T, Ikeda S, Kawanabe M and Ishii S 2015 Learning a common dictionary for liege-transfer decoding with resting calibration *NeuroImage.* **111** 167–78.

[15] Mühl C, Jeunet C and Lotte F 2014 EEG underpinned workload estimation across affective contexts *Front. Neurosci.* **8** 114.

[16] Washizawa Y, Higashi H, Rutkowski T, Tanaka T and Cichocki A 2010 Tensor based simultaneous feature extraction and sample weighting for EEG cataloguing *International Conference on Neural Information Processing, ICONIP 2010: Neural Information Processing. Models and Applications* (Berlin: Springer) pp 26–33.

[17] Waytowich N, Lawhern V, Bohannon A, Ball K and Lance B 2016 Spectral TsL using information geometry for a user-independent brain–computer interface *Front. Neurosci.* **10** 430.

[18] Wei Q, Wang Y, Gao X and Gao S 2007 Amplitude and phase coupling measures for feature extraction in an EEG underpinned brain–computer interface *J. Neural Eng.* **4** 120.

[19] Yi W, Qiu S, Qi H, Zhang L, Wan B and Ming D 2013 EEG feature comparison and cataloguing of simple and compound limb motor imagery *J. Neuroeng. Rehabil.* **10** 106.

[20] Woehrle H, Krell M M, Straube S, Kim S K, Kirchner E A and Kirchner F 2015 An adaptive spatial winnow for user-independent single trial detection of event-related potentials *IEEE Trans. Biomed. Eng.* **62** 1696–705.

[21] Wolpaw J, Birbaumer N, McFarland D, Pfurtscheller G and Vaughan T 2002 Brain-computer interfaces for communication and control *Clin. Neurophysiol.* **113** 767–91.

[22] Wolpaw J and Wolpaw E 2012 *Brain–Computer Interfaces: Principles and Practice* (Oxford: Oxford University Press).

[23] Wolpaw J R, McFarland D J, Neat G W and Forneris C A 1991 An EEG underpinned brain–computer interface for cursor control *Electroencephalogr. Clin. Neurophysiol.* **78** 252–9.

[24] Yger F 2013 A review of kernels on covariance matrices for BCMI applications *IEEE International Workshop on ML for Signal Processing* pp 1–6.

[25] Yger F, Berar M and Lotte F 2017 Riemannian approaches in brain–computer interfaces: A review *IEEE Trans. Neural Syst. Rehabil. Eng.* **25** 1753–62.

[26] Antoniades A, Spyrou L, Took C C and Sanei S 2016 DL for epileptic intracranial EEG data *2016 IEEE 26th International Workshop ML Signal Processing* pp 1–6.

[27] Zhang J and Wu Y 2018 Complex-valued unsupervised convolutional NN(s)s for sleep stage cataloguing *Comput. Methods Programs Biomed.* **164** 181–91.

[28] Liu M, Wu W, Gu Z, Yu Z, Qi F and Li Y 2018 DL based on batch normalization for P300 signal detection *Neurocomputing.* **275** 288–97.

[29] Sakhavi S, Yan S and Guan C 2018 Learning temporal information for brain–computer interface using convolutional NN(s)s *IEEE Trans. Neural Netw. Learn. Syst.* **29** 5619–29.

[30] Moon S-E, Jang S and Lee J-S 2018 Convolutional NN(s) approach for EEG under-pinned emotion recognition using brain connectivity and its spatial information *2018 IEEE International Conference on Acoustics, Speech and Signal Processing (ICASSP).*

[31] Waytowich N R et al 2018 Compact convolutional NN(s)s for cataloguing of asynchro-nous steady-state visual evoked potentials *J. Neural Eng.* **15** 066031.

[32] Supratak A, Dong H, Wu C and Guo Y 2017 DeepSleepNet: A model for automatic sleep stage scoring based on raw single-channel EEG *IEEE Trans. Neural Syst. Rehabil. Eng.* **25** 1998–2008.

[33] Bashivan P, Rish I, Yeasin M and Codella N 2015 Learning representations from EEG with deep recurrent-convolutional NN(s)s (arXiv:1511.06448).

[34] Dong H, Supratak A, Pan W, Wu C, Matthews P M and Guo Y 2018 Mixed NN(s) approach for temporal sleep stage cataloguing *IEEE Trans. Neural Syst. Rehabil. Eng.* **26** 324–33.

[35] Teo J, Hou C L and Mountstephens J 2017 DL for EEG underpinned preference cata-loguing *AIP Conf. Proc.* **1891** 020141.

10 Smart Mobile Healthcare
Unlocking the Potential of Blockchain and IoMT

Sandhya Avasthi, Ayushi Prakash, Tanushree Sanwal, Shweta Roy, and Shelly Gupta

10.1 INTRODUCTION

The present world is facing challenges in the form of a pandemic, and many others' healthcare needs with its growing life expectancy. As the growth is exponential in the field of information technology, healthcare applications, security, and confidentiality are any user's primary concerns. Enhanced diagnostic technologies allow for more innovative patient care, and smart healthcare devices improve healthcare quality in real-time. The objective of intelligent healthcare is to inform individuals about their health conditions and treatment options. Individuals are better prepared for potential medical emergencies thanks to intelligent healthcare. A remote checkup service is given, which reduces treatment costs and provides medical practitioners with additional options to serve patients in different regions. To ensure patients' access to necessary medical care as smart cities proliferate, a robust smart healthcare infrastructure is required. As Internet of Things (IoT) is evolving and other new technologies are giving rise to smart ecosystems everywhere that enable interconnection between living entities. The interconnection facilitates capturing, storage of data, communication, and fast sharing of information.

As per the report of "The India Brand Equity Foundation (IBEF)" India is growing to become the largest "healthcare industry" in terms of revenue and job opportunities. IoT will change healthcare and make medical devices cheaper. 5G networks will be a big part of making IoT deployments more widespread. One of the most important uses of 5G networks is smart healthcare [1–4]. The building of the 5G-based smart healthcare network and its most important elements are shown in Figure 10.1. The Internet of Things (IoT) can help with telemedicine, assisted living, smarter medication, monitoring behavioral change, remote monitoring, and asset management for hospitals. Shortly, these applications will be essential to the medical sector. The IoT business in healthcare is anticipated to reach approximately US\$ 117 billion by 2020. Numerous integration applications for mobile, eHealth, and/or web services have been presented. In [5], for instance, a portable health application that electronically stores health data is suggested. The key objectives of [6] are health examinations and dietary tracking. In [7], the author suggests a novel approach for mobile health applications. With mobility assistance, wearable solutions for the living environment

DOI: 10.1201/9781003340133-10

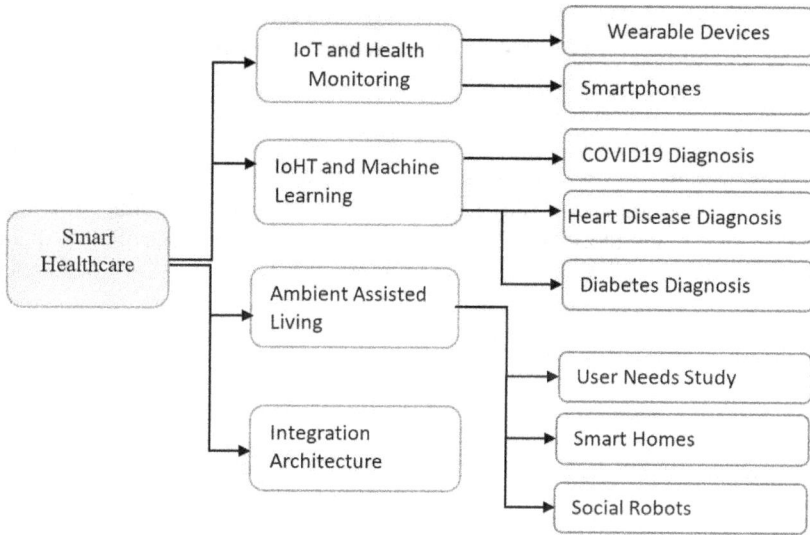

FIGURE 10.1 Smart healthcare and various types of systems

are offered [8]. In [8], an IoT application for intelligent assistance in the mobile health setting is presented.

The healthcare market in India will surpass US$ 372 billion by the year 2022, and the healthcare industry will see tremendous growth and is estimated to reach US$ 133.44 billion in the year 2023. The rising income of people is directly impacting how they spend money on the use of the latest gadgets and smart devices. This is also driving the healthcare market. In addition, this is bringing changes in the technological boom in the form of applications and policies by the government. In the current scenario led by technological advancement that is moving toward Industry 4.0, smart mobile healthcare is a promising solution to many healthcare needs. The penetration of smart mobile healthcare in the remotest areas is only possible if social and technological barriers are dealt with utmost care. Some social barriers are reluctant to adopt changes, irrational mindset, absence of basic infrastructure, and uneducated population. Many studies on smart healthcare have been conducted, each focusing on a different facet of the topic. The main objectives of the research are to provide an overview of the Internet of Things, blockchain technologies, virtual reality, and augmented reality and their uses in smart healthcare solutions.

- A classification system for intelligent medical care that includes communication systems, networks, services, applications, needs, and features.
- A comprehensive overview of the smart healthcare industry is explaining how diverse technologies can be integrated to advance smart healthcare.
- Studying the need for blockchain and augmented reality in monitoring healthcare quality.

- To discuss the current applications of IoT and blockchain.
- To identify and discuss current challenges and vulnerabilities in smart healthcare.

The overall chapter is divided into six sections. Section 10.1 gives an introduction to the healthcare area and recent technologies being used in improving healthcare solutions. In Section 2, we discuss smart mobile healthcare and remote monitoring. The Internet of Things, IoMT, and blockchain technology, background, and types of blockchain are explained in Section 10.3. In Section 10.4, blockchain applications, their features, and their need in the mHealth domain are provided. In the section 10.5, we examine some of the issues and unanswered problems. Concluding remarks are presented in Section 10.6.

10.2 SMART MOBILE HEALTHCARE AND REMOTE MONITORING

The healthcare sector is growing due to the use of mobile devices and IoT-based gadgets. It is now possible to create intelligent healthcare applications thanks to the convergence of computer science, electronics, and other related sciences. Thanks to the Internet of Things (IoT), artificial intelligence (AI), machine learning (ML), cloud computing, robotics, and big data analytics (BDA), the smart healthcare system is improving. Sharing of data and records is common in this Internet-dependent world, and this is giving rise to malicious attacks and all kinds of risks. In emerging Industry 4.0, sharing and storing data has become easier, and the risk associated with it is increasing. However, this increases the risk of attacks and the chance that private information could get out when shared. Smart gadgets that make health information easy to access have caused patients to see more doctors [9, 10]. This makes sharing and keeping this information private a concern. Figure 10.1 illustrates broad areas of use of IoT in the healthcare sector.

10.2.1 MOBILE HEALTH (MHEALTH) AND INCLUSION OF AUGMENTED REALITY

Primary components in mobile healthcare systems are low-power body-area wireless networks, small sensors, and ubiquitous cell phones. mHealth is plagued by many of the same issues as large, centralized server systems for healthcare. Sharing data and managing consent, regulating access, establishing one's identity, and gaining the trust of users are unique issues [11]. However, healthcare information that is improperly managed or compromised might "harm" the patient and the future of mobile healthcare applications. These dangers stem from the fact that healthcare institutions employing this technology may lack the expertise necessary to safeguard patient information [12]. Some other dangers include malware attacks whenever a device is connected to an unencrypted network. The main use of augmented reality in both training and medicine is the visualization of internal organs in patients as well as other objects that are usually invisible to the human eye.

10.2.2 REMOTE HEALTH MONITORING

The world's aging population and the rise of chronic diseases demand cost-effective and high-quality healthcare solutions. As a platform for remote health monitoring systems, the Internet of Things (IoT) has drawn a lot of research attention. Hospitals and healthcare providers may be relieved of some of their burdens, and healthcare costs may be lowered, especially for elderly and chronically ill patients [13]. IoT tiered architecture (IoTTA) was proposed as a technique for converting sensor data into clinical feedback as a result of this research [14]. Everything from sensing to transmission to processing to storage to data mining is included in this approach. It is hoped that this approach will make it easier to design IoT healthcare application systems that are both practical and efficient. The fastest-growing areas of healthcare IoT applications were found to be data mining and machine learning.

10.2.3 Prime Entities in Smart Mobile Healthcare

Any smart healthcare system work with blockchain technology deployment at the core. The sensitive health data is stored and maintained on cloud platforms coming through various sensors from mobile devices in a distributed manner. The main entities that are part of such a smart system are IoT-based wearable devices, EHRs data, standards of encryption/decryption, blockchain mechanisms, and end users. *Wearable devices* send the information of a patient and are monitored by doctors. Examples of wearable devices are wristbands, watches, or sensors attached to the patient being monitored. The sensors in the IoT network record patient vitals and other movements such as blood pressure, temperature, heartbeat, pulse rate, ECG, speech, dilation in the eye, etc.

The sensors' data have many formats, come in multimodal versions, and so to have proper analysis with good results, standard formats for all kinds are a must. The *encryption/decryption* unit encrypts all the data using a blockchain mechanism. Smart contract development helped in accumulating digitally signed copies from all involved stakeholders of the healthcare system in a secure manner. In addition, this smart contract is temper proof with providing security, transparency, privacy, and consistency. The data from transactions are stored in immutable storage blocks, and access to the data is given to only legitimate users. The data exchange systems make it possible to have a secure exchange without compromising the privacy of the users. The smart contracts eliminate the overheads in data reconciliation when participating users access real-time patient data. Patients, doctors, clinicians, pharmacists, insurance companies, and analysts are *end users*.

10.2.4 Inclusion of Augmented Reality and Virtual Reality in Healthcare

AR displays pertinent information in the form of text, images, or animations on a device, like a smartphone or a headset, by using sensors and cameras to detect the user's environment and position. Both augmented and virtual reality has emerged as powerful technologies changing the way shopping, healthcare, and entertainment applications works. In augmented reality (AR), also called mixed reality, virtual objects are mapped to real-world objects, and elements are augmented with inputs from sensors. Past research evaluated the use of computer-assisted surgeries based on AR; computer-assisted drawing helps in making accurate data models [15, 16]. Applications for augmented reality in medicine help with patient education, health condition assessment, treatment planning, and even training future surgeons.

AR is proving to be helpful in the healthcare system where remote monitoring or long-distance treatment needs to be supervised. The system provides support in managing the pain of the patient and helping with other health-related issues during COVID-19 pandemic times. Telemedicine is one prevalent application supported by AR technologies [17–19]. Virtual reality use in physical rehabilitation started way back in the year 2000 and continuously experimenting to provide an effective cure for Parkinson's disease. The study shows VR potential in mimicry and further uses the result to reveal neurological autism spectrum disorder. Online collaboration between experienced physicians and those just starting in the field allows for immediate feedback and guidance. According to the findings of one case study, the latency of the effective communication of augmented reality technology between participants is only 237 milliseconds.

10.2.5 Existing Challenges in Smart Healthcare System

Even though smart healthcare systems offer state-of-the-art services to stakeholders around the world, they still can't handle their risks. Since there are so many sensitive medical records on connected medical devices, cyber criminals want to break into them the most. In situations like these, it is easy to put the privacy of sensitive information about patients at risk. Worst case, hackers could take full control of wearable IoT devices and use them for bad things. In one such case, Johnson & Johnson had already told patients that one of its insulin pumps was weak and could be used by hackers to cause patients to overdose [15–16]. These devices that have been hacked can also be used as a passport to get into a network that would be safe otherwise. "European Union Agency for Network and Information Security (ENISA)" recent report states that to steal information from smart healthcare systems in general, malware is being used.

10.3 CONVERGENCE OF THE INTERNET OF THINGS (IOT) AND BLOCKCHAIN

The main characteristic of a blockchain network is that it modifies records only after a common consensus, similar to a ledger network in a distributed manner. The technique behind is a cryptographic hash that connects newly added information block records with each data block. The data is maintained on the network instead of a database.

10.3.1 Internet of Things (IoT)

As more consumers are willing to participate in health decision-making, IoT technology is becoming increasingly commonplace in the healthcare industry [17]. Additionally, patients are increasingly eager to take more initiative to personalize their healthcare. Personalizing healthcare and treatment can be aided by the use of smart devices and sensors that record and send critical health data to a physician for the remote monitoring and analysis of chronic ailments [18]. Smartwatches, contact lenses, fitness bands, microchips beneath the skin, and wireless sensors are a few examples of IoT applications in healthcare that enable people to make better decisions regarding their health [19].

Two types of assaults can be made against wireless IoT systems: *active* and *passive*. When data packets are routed through a system and an attacker can modify where the packets are moving or mess with the routing protocols, this is an example of a passive attack [19]. Additionally, a hacker can intercept the packets as they pass through a network or wireless area and "sniff" them to discover the data they contain. Active assaults are when an attacker actively locates, steals, modifies, or obtains information about the user of the device or network via a vulnerability in the device or network.

10.3.1.1 Internet of Medical Things (IoMT)

The term "Internet of Medical Things" refers to the collection of medical devices, wearables, and applications that connect them to a healthcare system. This collection includes both traditional and nontraditional medical technologies (IoMT). The vast majority of these applications necessitate the use of cloud storage as well as an analytics platform to analyze the data generated by the IoMT devices. The main applications include remotely monitoring patients with chronic or long-term conditions, tracking medication purchases, patient locations, and wearable mHealth devices. The information gathered through active devices is sent to healthcare providers. Hospital beds that have sensors to track patients' vital signs and infusion pumps that are connected to analytics dashboards are just two examples of medical items that can be upgraded to or used with IoMT technology. TechTarget has defined the Internet of Medical Things (IoMT) as follows:

> The Internet of Medical Things (IoMT) is the collection of medical devices and applications that connect to Health Care IT systems through online computer networks. Medical devices equipped with Wi-Fi allow the machine-to-machine communication that is the basis of IoMT. IoMT devices link to Cloud platforms such as Amazon Web Services, on which captured data can be stored and analysed. IoMT is also known as Health Care IoT.

The consumer's mobile devices are equipped with near-field communication (NFC) radio frequency identification (RFID) tags, enabling them to share information. A smartphone and a medical gadget, for example, that are both NFC-enabled can share data. Near-field communication (NFC) technology is a short-range wireless communication system. In the Internet of Medical Things (IoMT), NFC technology is employed in a variety of ways to increase the effectiveness and efficiency of healthcare delivery. The medical equipment with RFID tags is capable to record the supply levels always. The IoMT devices monitor the patient remotely when they are at home through telemedicine. When a patient receives this type of care, they are spared from visiting a hospital or doctor's office every time they have a medical inquiry or a change in their condition. Healthcare providers are becoming increasingly concerned about the security of sensitive data, such as protected health information, which is governed by the Health Insurance Portability and Accountability Act and moves through the IoMT. To continually monitor health vitals utilizing wearable technology and smartphone solutions, smart sensors are first coupled in an IoMT environment. Machine learning approaches analyze and deliver predictive analytics, such as forecasting sicknesses, once the data has been gathered using smart sensors. Additional algorithms are employed to track persistent disorders like diabetes and heart disease, as well as to find irregularities in the patient's health.

10.3.1.2 Internet of Health Things (IoHT)

Internet of Healthcare Things refers to the recognizable, Internet-connected equipment that can be employed in the medical industry. By offering medical assistance and error detection, these technologies raise the bar for safety. They conduct remote medical consultations and automatically evaluate the data gathered by the gadgets. The world has already been altered by the Internet of Things. It has had an impact on people's lives and jobs. Other industries have connected the IoT and gadgets more swiftly, which will increase the automation and efficiency of their job in the future. Some devices making an impact in IoHT are summarized in Table 10.1.

TABLE 10.1
Medical Devices Included in IoHT

Devices name	Usage
Glucose monitoring and insulin pens	A CGM (glucose monitor) continually examines diabetics while periodically checking blood glucose levels. Users of smart CGMs like Freestyle Libre can check their health status and have blood glucose levels sent to their Apple Watch or Android device. The time and the kind of insulin administered are automatically recorded by insulin pens like Esysta. These gadgets are linked to smartphones and keep persistent data.
Inhalers	Healthcare practitioners can access the reports produced by connected inhalers. Patients can receive temperature alerts via connected inhalers to help prevent asthma. It accurately assesses the existing situation and averts impending assaults.
Smartwatch monitors depression	Apple watches enable more dialogues about treatment and provide patients and healthcare providers with information about their condition. Additionally, it tracks the patient's depression level and uploads information to the cloud.
Connected contact lenses	In addition to detecting changes in eyeball size, linked contact lenses also offer presbyopia correction.
Hearing aid	Users of hearing aids can listen to several conversations at once. Additionally, it facilitates hearing in a noisy setting. For listening to doorbell rings and other uses, a hearing aid can be connected to the Internet.
Implanted devices and wearable devices	Medical implants support and replace biological structures that are damaged or absent. It includes things like glucose monitors and medicine delivery systems.
Treatment devices	These gadgets assist doctors to monitor patient medication adherence and enhance the quality of life for chronic patients. The Philips drug dispensing service, which was developed for senior citizens, is the best illustration of an automated treatment device.

10.3.2   BLOCKCHAIN BACKGROUND

The blockchain concept, which was originally intended to be used for maintaining a financial ledger, can be expanded to provide a broader framework for constructing decentralized computational resources [20]. Consider each computing resource to be a singleton state machine capable of changing states via secure cryptographic transactions. When nodes create a new state machine, they encapsulate the logic that specifies acceptable state transitions and uploads it to the blockchain. Following that, the blocks record a series of legitimate transactions that, when carried out incrementally with the state from the previous block, transform the state machine into its current state. The proof of work consensus process and its associated safeguards protect the state machines and transitional logic from manipulation. The blockchain is illustrated in Figure 10.2.

Due to its ability to generate and transmit irreversible, permanent transaction records in a safe manner, blockchain is gaining appeal. The new Bitcoin mania may reignite public interest in blockchain, the technology that makes Bitcoin possible. Blockchain, often known as digital ledger technology, is not itself a cryptocurrency. It generates blocks (transaction sequences) and stores them in a sequence of actions that network participants can share. Because the blocks are secured with cutting-edge cryptographic technology, blockchain supporters claim that the records are nearly impossible to alter. Every transaction taking place between nodes or devices is logged and verified to make sure that all nodes agree on a specific time and date. The result is a single shared source of facts accessible to all.

Healthcare industry faces problems of inefficiency that can be improved by blockchain technology with its decentralized structure to provide security and privacy to sensitive medical data [21]. In addition, it can streamline claims adjudication, speed up medical insurance enrolment, and by augmenting the B2B process in the healthcare system value chain. In combination with IoHT, the blockchain can further reduce risks through proper control of a chain of possession of medical devices. Not only tracking of products is possible by healthcare organizations, but alert messages can also be sent in case of harmful events like extreme environmental conditions,

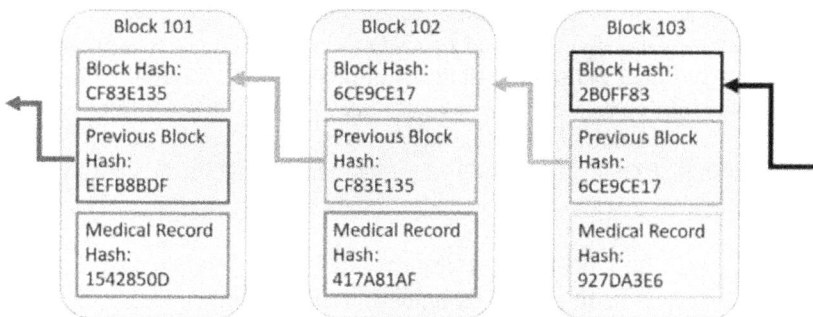

FIGURE. 10.2   A blockchain is depicted diagrammatically. Each block here is a medical record. This block combines data of patient vitals and biometrics through IoT devices.

careless handling, and tampering. For handling quality issues related to a delivered product, the system provides a valuable forensic trail.

10.3.2.1 Types of Blockchain

Public, private, hybrid, or consortium are types of blockchain, and each type has some unique qualities that influence its optimal applications [21, 22]. Blockchain and its various types and generations cater to the needs of the developer's building applications.

- **Public Blockchain:** This technique removes the limitations of centralization, for example, security risks, and transparency. DLT sends data in a distributed manner throughout the P2P network rather than storing it in a single location. Due to decentralization, DLT needs an authentication method for data. In this type of blockchain, permissions are not required, and everyone has access to the application.
- **Private Blockchain:** This blockchain operates under a centralized authority, and permission is required to use it. It performs similarly to a public blockchain network in terms of P2P connectivity and decentralization, but it is much smaller. In a private blockchain, the network's creator is always aware of who the users are and what type of transactions are allowed. A public web does not allow for the development of permission-based solutions, and users are completely anonymous.
- **Hybrid Blockchain:** To govern who has access to certain data kept on the blockchain and what data is made public, it enables organizations to construct both a private, permission-based system and a public, permissionless system. This operates under the leadership of a group, and participants are preapproved. Banking applications are mostly based on this type.

10.3.2.2 A Comparison Between Blockchain and Traditional Database

The blockchain utilizes the cryptography technique to provide data reliability, which is possible via distributed trust network. This network does not depend on a master copy. Blockchain technology is designed in the form of an append-only structure. The main operations associated with blockchains are *read* and *write* [23, 24]. Traditional databases are mainly based on client-server architecture. Any user which has access to this data can modify data stored in a central location. In a blockchain, the database is decentralized, where each node is part of the administration. The verification of new additions is done by the node which can insert new data into the system. To make changes in the system, the nodes must reach a consensus. The mechanism of consensus in blockchain also guarantees security.

10.3.2.2.1 Why It Is Becoming Imperative in Healthcare

Examples include expediting claims adjudication, accelerating medical insurance enrolment, and boosting B2B activity throughout the healthcare value chain [25].

- When combined with IoHT, secure, immutable blockchains can reduce risks by monitoring the possession chain of medical devices and medications.

- Companies can easily track progress throughout their supply chains to check authenticity or discover potentially damaging in-transit events, such as signs of manipulation, severe environmental conditions, or careless handling. This information provides a vital forensic trail if quality issues arise after delivery.
- Blockchain can aid vendors in expediting recalls if a manufacturer uncovers a problem with a gadget or medication by rapidly tracking inventory throughout the supply chain and removing it from circulation.
- Other blockchain-based opportunities include faster and more efficient employee credentialing, made possible by the ability to confirm caregivers' immutable records, and the use of smart contracts to automatically carry out contractual agreements, such as pre-authorizations between payers and providers.

10.4   BLOCKCHAIN AND IOT IN HEALTHCARE

The two of them employ many kinds of electronic information security maintenance approaches. Furthermore, research shows how both technologies can work together. The combination procedure was observed to achieve this goal. These services vary from combining blockchain technology into data exchanges among IoT devices to simply storing metadata on it. Smart cities are the most frequently discussed IoT application, with blockchain being used to improve data exchange in real-time systems, power merchandise, and so on.

The combination of the two technologies allows blockchain technology to be used in an IoT environment. The function of blockchain in the entire system, the degree to which blockchain technology is connected to data exchanges between IoT, as well as the severity to which processes illustrate blockchain for service provision, differs between integration approaches. Security is one of the gains that blockchain technology can bring to healthcare and the Internet of Everything. One such benefit addresses a wide range of issues, which include data, system, and network security. There are many reasons why all data management procedures in IoT and healthcare settings need to be improved. In healthcare, for example, impediments include the lack of a unique patient identity, messaging standards that allow for syntax and semantic connectivity between systems, in addition to data-encoding standards.

10.4.1   Need for Blockchain in Healthcare

A blockchain network is beneficial for storing, sending, and receiving patient data in medical domain applications. In the medical system, a blockchain is used to contain and transfer patient information among healthcare institutions, health professions, pharmacist firms, and doctors. The blockchain does not keep data in a single position. Instead, a network of computers is used to attempt to duplicate and disseminate the blockchain. To symbolize the addition of a new block to the blockchain, every Internet-connected machine must update its blockchain technology. The basic workflow of blockchain in IoMT is illustrated in Figure 10.3.

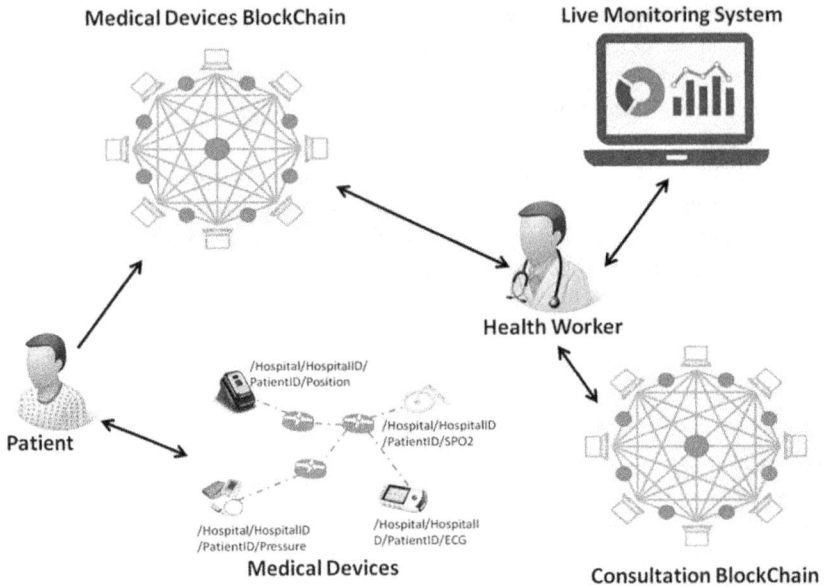

FIGURE 10.3   Illustration of workflow in IoMT blockchain

Blockchain technology is essential in transforming the medical sector. Also, the landscape of the healthcare system is shifting in favor of a patient-oriented strategy that emphasizes two essential elements: consistently available services and enough healthcare resources. Blockchain encourages healthcare businesses' capacity to simply deliver adequate patient safety and superior healthcare facilities. With the help of this technology, another time-consuming and redundant process that raises healthcare costs can be promptly finished. Using blockchain technology, citizens can participate in health research programs. Furthermore, improved public well-being research and data sharing will improve treatment for a wide range of communities to handle the entire healthcare system and organizations, a knowledge resource is used in healthcare organizations and systems [26–30].

A blockchain application in the medical field can detect serious, even dangerous, errors. Blockchain applications in the medical field can identify precisely harsh and even acute errors. Because of this, it can upgrade medical data-sharing performance, security, and transparency in the medical management and care system. Blockchain supports hospitals and clinics in gaining awareness and improving medical record analysis. To improve healthcare outcomes, blockchain technology is critical in dealing with deception in clinical trials. Blockchain is critical in dealing with deception in clinical trials and has the potential to improve data efficiency in healthcare. It provides flexibility in data access, interconnection, accountability, and authentication.

10.4.2   BLOCKCHAIN CAPABILITIES TO SUPPORT HEALTHCARE

By regulating the drug supply chain, facilitating the safe transfer of patient medical records, and facilitating the safe transfer of patient medical records, ledger technology aids healthcare experts in deciphering genetic codes. The diverse range of traits and key blockchain concept enablers in a variety of healthcare and related disciplines are shown in Figure 10.4. Some of the outstanding and technically derived factors used to develop and apply blockchain technology include medical records security, diverse genome management, electronic data management, interoperability, digitalized tracking, problem outbreak, and others [4, 31]. The healthcare sector's adoption of blockchain technology is largely attributable to its applications and completely digital components.

The full course of the medication, from manufacturing to drugstore shelves, is transparently monitored using blockchain technology. Using IoT and blockchain, it is possible to monitor traffic, freight direction, and speed. It enables proper planning of purchases to reduce delays and deficiencies in pharmacies, clinics, and other medical services that employ a specific prescription. Digital structures built on the blockchain should be used to stop unauthorized changes to logistical data. It fosters confidence and discourages individuals interested in purchasing narcotics from illegally manipulating papers, finances, and prescriptions. The technique can effectively improve patients' conditions while keeping competitive pricing. There are no hurdles or restrictions that prevent multilevel authentication [28–29]. Figure 10.4 describes various key application areas of blockchain technology.

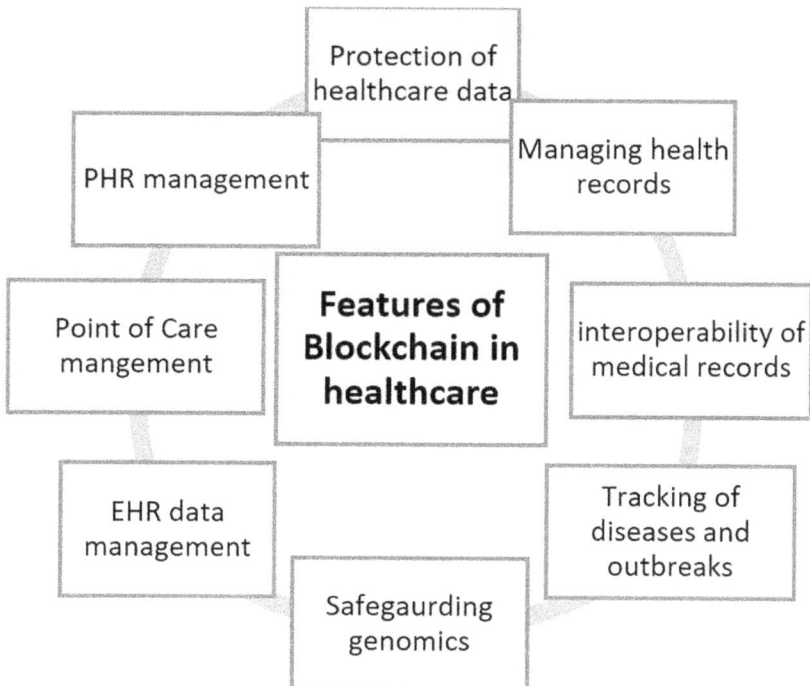

FIGURE 10.4   Blockchain technology and its various key application areas

10.5 CURRENT ISSUES AND CHALLENGES IN BLOCKCHAIN, IOT

The blockchain, which is a paradigm shift, is changing all of the major IoT application sectors right now. It does this by providing a decentralized environment where transactions are anonymous and reliable. When IoT systems are combined with blockchain technology, their operational costs go down, their resources are managed in a more decentralized way, they are more resistant to threats and attacks, and they have other benefits. Blockchain and IoT are working together to solve these huge problems and make the IoT platform a reality in the future. Due to the complexity of blockchain, which includes high calculating costs and interruptions, it is hard to combine blockchain with IoT devices, which have limited power and storing space [15]. Figure 10.5 shows some of the problems with managing IoT data on the blockchain. Here, we'll talk briefly about those problems.

Choices between how much power is used, how well it works, and how safe it is: Blockchain algorithms need a lot of computing power to work, which has slowed

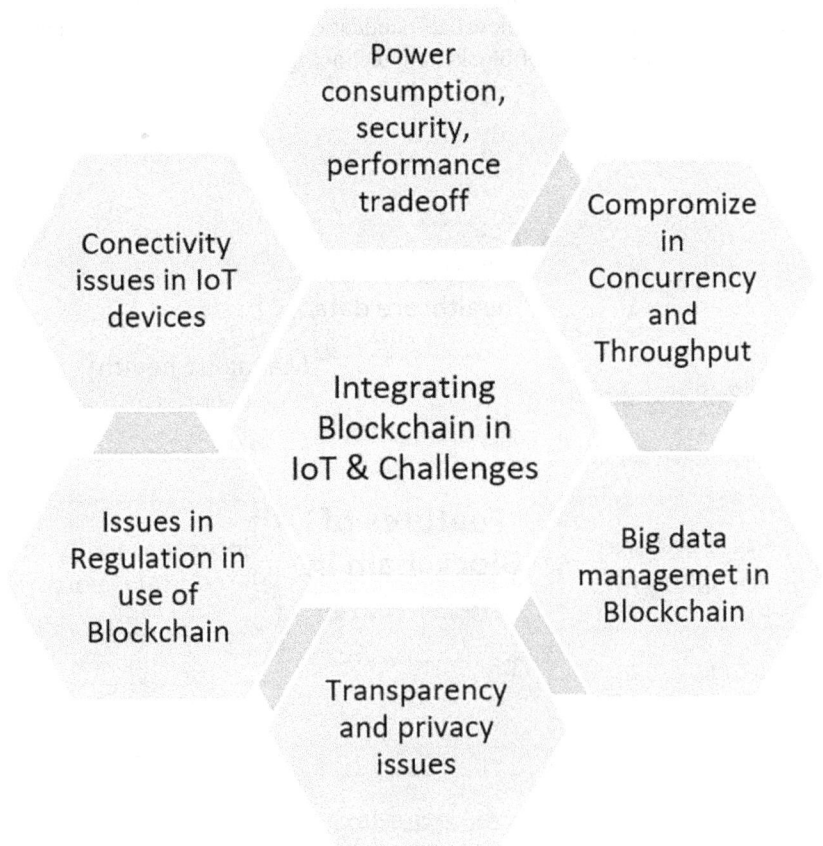

FIGURE 10.5 The challenges in the Internet of Things while integrating blockchain technology

down the development of apps that use this technology on devices with few resources. IoT devices can't do things that Bitcoin can do, which Irish homes can do using less energy [16]. Zhou et al. [11] say that the whole Bitcoin network uses a lot more energy than in some countries, like Colombia and Austria. Researchers have also questioned how well blockchain processes IoT data and proposed improving its fundamental algorithms to boost the rate at which confirmed blocks are created [9]. For example, if the PoW consensus mechanism is taken out of the blockchain, it can use less power and work better [17]. On the other hand, proof of work makes it hard to change the blocks and stops malicious Sybil attacks. So the goal is to improve how blockchain works in a way that strikes a good balance between speed and safety [10].

IoT systems have a lot of people using them at the same time because IoT devices constantly send out data [18]. This is bad for concurrency and performance [9]. The blockchain's throughput is limited by how hard it is to reach a consensus and how it uses cryptography for security. In a chain-structured ledger, faster organization of new blocks across all blockchain nodes requires extra bandwidth, which can increase throughput [11, 19]. It is challenging to raise the throughput of blockchain in order to handle the demand for frequent transactions in IoT devices.

IoT connectivity issues [32] include the fact that IoT devices should be linked to storage, high computing, and networking capabilities so that IoT data can be shared with probable stakeholders. The Internet of Things' (IoT) limited ability to interact with blockchain technology stops new business opportunities from making new services and apps in a wide range of industries. Because each participant keeps a copy of the whole distributed ledger, the blockchain can handle a lot of information. When the transaction is confirmed, a new block is sent out to the whole P2P network, and each node adds the confirmed block to its ledger. This autonomous storage system boosts productivity, eliminates bottlenecks, and does away with the need to rely on a third party. However, participants have to pay a fee to store IoT data on the blockchain [33]. According to the research in Ref. [34], a blockchain node would require about 730 GB of storage space per year if 1,000 users used a blockchain app to exchange just one 2 MB image per day. So it's hard to keep up with the growing need for data storage when using blockchain to handle IoT data.

Privacy and transparency are also problems. Blockchain can make transactions transparent, which is important in many fields, including finance. But when IoT data from certain IoT systems, such as eHealth, is stored and retrieved from the blockchain [23], user privacy may be at risk [35–37]. To find a good balance between privacy and openness, access control for the Internet of Things (IoT) must be built with the help of blockchain technology.

Decentralization, immutability, anonymity, and automation are just some of the technological features of blockchain that could help make IoT applications more secure. However, when these features are combined, they also create several new regulatory challenges [24]. On the distributed transaction ledger (DTL-immutability), data is supposed to be posted for good and can't be changed or deleted. Also, since there is no government, papers can't be checked for privacy before they are put on the blockchain because there is no one in charge. When a smart contract is run on a DTL, it could lead to actions that break the law. Because the DTL is anonymous, it is hard to find the people involved in transactions for illegal services. Even though the fact that the blockchain is automated is helpful in many ways, it's not always clear who is in charge of things like coding errors and making code hard to read. Existing IoT laws and rules must be changed so that the DTL can be used, especially since new disruptive technologies like blockchain have come out [25].

Researchers have recently written about how blockchain technology can be used in IoT for smart cities and homes, agriculture, eHealth, supply chains, and industries. Miglani et al. [25] looked at recent state-of-the-art studies on the technology to give readers a complete picture of how blockchain could be used and applied in the Internet of Energy (IoE) industry. They talked about several energy management blockchain smart contract applications, such as automatic data exchange, energy transfers, energy demand, and trading on the protected blockchain P2P network [38, 39]. [26] put together a list of different ways that blockchain technology can be used in unmanned aerial vehicle (UAV) systems. They also looked closely at how blockchain features can help solve problems with the UAV system. UAVs are a group of robots that can carry payloads and bring out attack missions by remote control or on their own. UAVs have caused a lot of new problems, such as cyber-physical attacks on UAVs, more air traffic, controlling UAV swarms, route optimization, flight planning, emergency management, and other things. According to research, using disruptive technologies like blockchain could help solve these problems.

10.6   CONCLUSION

The healthcare business could also profit from the implementation of blockchain technology. The distributed and block-related infrastructure made it possible to provide security, integrity, decentralization, availability, and authentication in healthcare application that is grounded on blockchain technology. The healthcare industry struggles to adapt to an expanding digital infrastructure that includes Internet-enabled devices, the Internet of Things (IoT), smart gadgets, and sensors. To sum up, the healthcare industry can benefit from the use of blockchain technology in a variety of ways. Security, integrity, decentralization, accessibility, and authentication are the most promising uses of blockchain technology in the healthcare industry. The privacy and security of IoMT could benefit from blockchain. The confluence of blockchain technology and the Internet of Medical Things can control an ever-growing number of IoMT devices through its decentralized mechanism. The blockchain-based IoMT architecture addresses the vast majority of security and privacy threats.

A blockchain's immutable data permits the establishment of a digital data ledger based on a verifiable consensus. Thus, blockchain protects the real-time integrity of a patient's clinical history and grants every node in the IoMT network access to tamper-resistant open data. The healthcare sector will have a difficult time adjusting to an IoT-based, smart device, and sensor-based technical infrastructure. Bad actors may take advantage of flaws in these technologies (as well as processes and users) to access and duplicate data, making it more challenging for healthcare providers to exchange patient records in an increasingly networked world. If a patient's medical documents contain out-of-date information that could result in health issues or inaccurate diagnoses, their identity may be compromised.

REFERENCES

[1] Hölbl, M., Kompara, M., Kamišalić, A., & Nemec Zlatolas, L. (2018). A systematic review of the use of blockchain in healthcare. *Symmetry*, 10(10), 470.

[2] Pazaitis, A., De Filippi, P., & Kostakis, V. (2017). Blockchain and value systems in the sharing economy: The illustrative case of Backfeed. *Technological Forecasting and Social Change*, 125, 105–115.

[3] Tan, T. M., & Salo, J. (2021). Ethical marketing in the blockchain-based sharing economy: Theoretical integration and guiding insights. *Journal of Business Ethics*, 1–28.

[4] Tripathi, G., Ahad, M. A., & Paiva, S. (2020, March). S2HS-A blockchain based approach for smart healthcare system. *Healthc (Amst)*, 8(1), 100391. doi: 10.1016/j.hjdsi.2019.100391.

[5] Rodrigues, J. J., Pedro, L. M., Vardasca, T., de la Torre-Díez, I., & Martins, H. M. (2013). Mobile health platform for pressure ulcer monitoring with electronic health record integration. *Health Informatics Journal*, 19, 300–311.

[6] Rodrigues, J. J., Lopes, I. M., Silva, B. M., & Torre, I. D. (2013). A new mobile ubiquitous computing application to control obesity: SapoFit. *Informatics for Health & Social Care*, 38, 37–53.

[7] Yang, G., Urke, A. R., & Øvsthus, K. (2018, March 22–23). Mobility support of IoT solution in home care wireless sensor network. In *Proceedings of the 2018 Ubiquitous Positioning, Indoor Navigation and Location-Based Services (UPINLBS), Wuhan, China* (pp. 475–480).

[8] Santos, J., Rodrigues, J. J., Silva, B. M., Casal, J., Saleem, K., & Denisov, V. (2016). An IoT-based mobile gateway for intelligent personal assistants on mobile health environments. *Journal of Network and Computer Applications*, 71, 194–204.

[9] Avasthi, S., Chauhan, R., & Acharjya, D. P. (2021). Processing large text corpus using N-gram language modeling and smoothing. In *Proceedings of the Second International Conference on Information Management and Machine Intelligence* (pp. 21–32). Springer, Singapore.

[10] Avasthi, S., Chauhan, R., & Acharjya, D. P. (2022). Information Extraction and Sentiment Analysis to gain insight into the COVID-19 crisis. In *International Conference on Innovative Computing and Communications* (pp. 343–353). Springer, Singapore.

[11] Kotz, D., et al. (2016). Privacy and security in mobile health: A research agenda. *Computer*, 49(6), 22–30.

[12] Sahi, M. A., Abbas, H., Saleem, K., Yang, X., Derhab, A., Orgun, M. A., . . . Yaseen, A. (2017). Privacy preservation in e-healthcare environments: State of the art and future directions. *IEEE Access*, 6, 464–478.

[13] Alshamrani, M. (2021). IoT and artificial intelligence implementations for remote healthcare monitoring systems: A survey. *Journal of King Saud University-Computer and Information Sciences*, 34(8), 4687–4701.

[14] Abdullah, W. A. N. W., Yaakob, N., Elobaid, M. E., Warip, M. N. M., & Yah, S. A. (2016, March). Energy-efficient remote healthcare monitoring using IoT: A review of trends and challenges. In *Proceedings of the International Conference on Internet of Things and Cloud Computing* (pp. 1–8).

[15] Parekh, P., Patel, S., Patel, N., & Shah, M. (2020). Systematic review and meta-analysis of augmented reality in medicine, retail, and games. *Visual Computing for Industry, Biomedicine, and Art*, 3, 1–20.

[16] White, J., Schmidt, D. C., & Golparvar-Fard, M. (2014). Applications of augmented reality. *Proceedings of the IEEE*, 102(2), 120–123.

[17] Ara, J., Karim, F. B., Alsubaie, M. S. A., Bhuiyan, Y. A., Bhuiyan, M. I., Bhyan, S. B., & Bhuiyan, H. (2021). Comprehensive analysis of augmented reality technology in modern healthcare system. *International Journal of Advanced Computer Science and Applications*, 12(6), 840–849.

[18] Patel, G. S., Tripathi, S. L., & Awasthi, S. (2018, November). Performance enhanced unsymmetrical FinFET and its applications. In *2018 IEEE Electron Devices Kolkata Conference (EDKCON)* (pp. 222–227). IEEE.

[19] Mendiratta, N., & Tripathi, S. L. (2022). 18nm n-channel and p-channel Dopingless asymmetrical Junctionless DG-MOSFET: Low power CMOS based digital and memory applications. *Silicon*, 14(11), 6435–6446.

[20] Wood, G. (2014). Ethereum: A secure decentralised generalised transaction ledger. *Ethereum Project Yellow Paper*.

[21] Haleem, A., Javaid, M., Singh, R. P., Suman, R., & Rab, S. (2021). Blockchain technology applications in healthcare: An overview. *International Journal of Intelligent Networks*, 2, 130–139.

[22] Avasthi, S., Chauhan, R., & Acharjya, D. P. (2022). Topic modeling techniques for text mining over a large-scale scientific and biomedical text corpus. *International Journal of Ambient Computing and Intelligence (IJACI)*, 13(1), 1–18.

[23] Kuo, T-T., Kim, H-E., & Ohno-Machado, L. (2017). Blockchain distributed ledger technologies for biomedical and health care applications. *Journal of the American Medical Informatics Association*, 24, 1211–1220. https://doi.org/10.1093/jamia/ocx068.

[24] McBee, M. P., & Wilcox, C. (2020). Blockchain technology: Principles and applications in medical imaging. *Journal of Digital Imaging*, 33, 726–734. https://doi.org/10.1007/s10278-019-00310-3.

[25] Rao, A. R., & Clarke, D. (2020). Perspectives on emerging directions in using IoT devices in blockchain applications. *Internet of Things*, 10, 100079.

[26] Avasthi, S., Chauhan, R., & Acharjya, D. P. (2022). Significance of preprocessing techniques on text classification over Hindi and English short texts. In Unhelker, B., Pandey, H. M., & Raj, G. (eds) *Applications of Artificial Intelligence and Machine Learning. Lecture Notes in Electrical Engineering* (Vol. 925). Springer, Singapore.

[27] Avasthi, S., Chauhan, R., & Acharjya, D. P. (2021). Techniques, applications, and issues in mining large-scale text databases. In *Advances in Information Communication Technology and Computing* (pp. 385–396). Springer, Singapore.

[28] Aravinth, S. S., Arepalli, G., Sakthivel, P., Kumar, V. D., & Kumar, S. J. (2022). AI technology in lifestyle monitoring: Futuristic view–AI technology and IoT. In Arti Jain, John Wang, Sailesh Suryanarayan Iyer. (eds) *Handbook of Research on Lifestyle Sustainability and Management Solutions Using AI, Big Data Analytics, and Visualization* (pp. 338–351). IGI Global, Hershey, PA.

[29] Chauhan, R., Avasthi, S., Alankar, B., & Kaur, H. (2021). Smart IoT systems: Data analytics, secure smart home, and challenges. In Bhavya Alankar, Harleen Kaur, Ritu Chauhan. (eds) *Transforming the Internet of Things for Next-Generation Smart Systems* (pp. 100–119). IGI Global, Hershey, PA.

[30] Avasthi, S., Sanwal, T., Sareen, P., & Tripathi, S. L. (2022). Augmenting mental healthcare with artificial intelligence, machine learning, and challenges in telemedicine. In Sailesh Suryanarayan Iyer, Arti Jain, John Wang. (eds) *Handbook of Research on Lifestyle Sustainability and Management Solutions Using AI, Big Data Analytics, and Visualization* (pp. 75–90). IGI Global, Hershey, PA.

[31] Agbo, C. C., Mahmoud, Q. H., & Eklund, J. M. (2019, April). Blockchain technology in healthcare: A systematic review. *Healthcare*, 7(2), 56.

[32] Nasr, M., Islam, M. M., Shehata, S., Karray, F., & Quintana, Y. (2021). Smart healthcare in the age of AI: Recent advances, challenges, and future prospects. *IEEE Access*, 9, 145248–145270.

[33] Yin, H., Akmandor, A. O., Mosenia, A., & Jha, N. K. (2018). Smart healthcare. *Foundations and Trends® in Electronic Design Automation*, 12(4), 401–466.

[34] Zhang, Y., Chen, M., & Leung, V. C. (2017). Topical collection on "smart and interactive healthcare systems". *Journal of Medical Systems*, 41(8), 121.

[35] Torre, I., et al. (2016). A framework for personal data protection in the IoT. In *Internet Technology and Secured Transactions (ICITST), 2016 11th International Conference for IEEE*. IEEE. doi: 10.1109/ICITST.2016.7856735.

[36] Al Ameen, M., Liu, J., & Kwak, K. (2012). Security and privacy issues in wireless sensor networks for healthcare applications. *Journal of Medical Systems*, 36(1), 93–101.

[37] Srivastava, G., Parizi, R. M., & Dehghantanha, A. (2020). The future of blockchain technology in healthcare internet of things security. In *Blockchain Cybersecurity, Trust and Privacy* (pp. 161–184). Springer International Publishing, Cham. doi: 10.1007/978-3-030-38181-3_9.

[38] Gupta, R., Tanwar, S., Tyagi, S., Kumar, N., Obaidat, M. S., & Sadoun, B. (2019, August). HaBiTs: Blockchain-based telesurgery framework for healthcare 4.0. In *2019 International Conference on Computer, Information and Telecommunication Systems (CITS)* (pp. 1–5). IEEE. doi: 10.1109/CITS.2019.8862127.

[39] Avasthi, S. (2019, December). Topic modeling on twitter data and identifying health-related issues. In *International Conference on Information Management & Machine Intelligence* (pp. 57–64). Springer, Singapore.

11 Blockchain in Healthcare
Some Use Cases

Girish Kumar Sharma, Anant Bhardwaj,
Shwetank Arya, and Manoj Singhal

11.1 INTRODUCTION

Retrospectively, the Hippocratic Oath is one of the oldest texts available for a medical practitioner, which is the core ethical framework for healthcare workers worldwide. But now, the scenario has changed significantly. Especially in the COVID time, the Internet and smartphones have changed the entire scenario. The world is becoming an online-centric world [1, 2]. In line with the Internet of Things (IoT), cloud computing, etc., have come up for many people around the world with a new invention, the Internet of Trust (blockchain). Irrespective of all the issues, this has the potential to change lives and everything people encounter. This is especially true for the healthcare sector, where the properties and characteristics of the blockchain are highly desired not only for health issues but also for maintaining the privacy and security of their profiles lying with the different stakeholders like hospitals, insurers, etc., which are critical for the life of patients. In the subsequent sections of this chapter, we will focus on the basics of blockchain technology and see how blockchain technology could impact our current healthcare systems [3].

11.1.1 BLOCKCHAIN TECHNOLOGY

This is required to understand how blockchain technology works since there is still a myth that blockchain technology is tightly connected to Bitcoin and whenever we talk of blockchain, people start thinking about Bitcoin only. Although there is nothing wrong with this connection, most people do not know that blockchain technology is much more than "just" Bitcoin. The technology was first introduced in October 2008 with the publication of the Bitcoin white paper [4]. Launched in early 2009, it was the first implementation utilizing blockchain technology.

Although the idea of making a secure time-stamped hash chain of transactions started many years before the Bitcoin white paper was published by scientists Stuart Haber and W. Scott Stornetta in 1991[5], they tried to introduce a computationally practical solution for time-stamping digital documents so they could not be back-dated or tampered cryptographically. At its core, it is a decentralized distributed

DOI: 10.1201/9781003340133-11

ledger where data of any form (e.g., transactions) is stored in blocks chained together and cryptographically secured using asymmetric cryptographic algorithms like SHA 256 [6] etc.

One of the major advantages of blockchain technology is that there is no centralized control, rather than the ledger is residing, maintained, and authenticated by every participant (nodes) of the network resulting in no single point of failure as in centralized systems, where a failure of one single node could lead to a complete loss of data. Also, blockchain technology enables direct access without intermediary or third-party intervention since every participant has a cryptographically secured hash address with an anonymous identity.

This leads to defining two types of networks: public permissionless and private permission in the case of public, where nobody can prevent others from participating. While on the contrary, in the case of a private blockchain, the participant has to have permission before becoming part of the network, and sometimes control occurs.

Now, it can be concluded that every blockchain-based network is not permissionless. Along with public open blockchain networks like Bitcoin or Ethereum, there are private (corporate) permissioned blockchain networks, which can provide significant throughputs, especially in comparison to the permissionless private blockchain networks since they can give a significantly increased speed (e.g., processing transactions), network capacity, and scalability. Along with this, the security can be comfortably implemented by only allowing selected participants to access and use the network. This is important if we consider susceptible data like genetic records and other sensitive data of the patient and people. Immutability is another critical characteristic that is often talked about in blockchain technology [7]. It is used to describe the property of being resistant to change.

Sometimes there is a confusion that the blockchain architecture is a distributed network. The answer is no, because in distributed although the replica of a database lies at every node, it also has a local administrator who has the full authority to make a change in the database, while on the contrary, in blockchain, nobody can change or alter the data because the change in one block will l lead to a change in another block. It is one of the key advantages over earlier databases, where anybody can make alterations if we think about a spreadsheet. In blockchain-based networks, the entries in the ledger or database residing at every node cannot be changed by anybody except the node's owner. A consensus mechanism leads this process of validating the transactions.

Another beautiful concept of securing data or transactions in a blockchain is lying on Merkle Tree, which was first introduced in 1992. Merkle Trees [8] were incorporated into the design, which makes blockchain more efficient by allowing several documents to be collected into one block. The hash function calculation using $H(x) = X$ mod n illustrates the concept. This is a one-way function, where given an X(Message) and a considerable value n, one can find $H(x)$, but given $H(x)$, it is almost impossible to find X. There is no deterministic algorithm existing to date for this. Typically a block in a blockchain contains some transactions, the hash of the previous block and the hash of the current block along with the mere root. The previous block's hash is used to create the hash of the next block in a cascaded manner. These are used to create a "secured chain of blocks." It stored a series of data records connected to the one before. The newest record in this chain contains the history of the entire chain. However, this technology went unused, and the patent lapsed in 2004.

The architecture of blockchain technology is mechanized in such a cascaded way that editing entries in a single block would need a change in the subsequent blocks because for making the hash of the new block, the hash of the old block is also used along with other parameters which are residing in block header of every block to be added on top of the block afterward. The mechanism involves the process of mining, where some of the nodes in the network act as miners. To find and make consensus in the network, prospective miners will solve a nonce (Mathematical Puzzle). The miners who will first solve the puzzle will be given the privilege to add this block to the blockchain, and all other participants in the blockchain are to make a consensus [6]. Depending on the underlying consensus mechanism, which refers to the algorithm used to find consensus between the network participants in validating new blocks, excessive amounts of energy or resources would be needed to change blocks. Although not completely impossible, the chances of someone challenging the immutability of well-adopted and thought-out blockchain networks are often diminishingly low. Blockchain networks are also called trustless due to the ability to direct interactions with network participants (e.g., sending transactions, exchanging information, or data) without the need for any central authority or third party involved [9].

Due to the cited attributes, many enterprises and companies are increasingly interested in utilizing blockchain technology. Here it is pertinent to mention that it is not the case that blockchain technology can be applied anywhere. Some projects have faced complete failure in the implementation of this. Besides, the financial industry, especially healthcare, focuses on utilizing blockchain technology in various ways [10].

11.1.1.1 Smart Contracts

Now another important thing includes the execution and implementation of this technology. Things can be better understood if we take the case of a manual supply chain system where multiple participants like seller, buyer, insurer, bank, and transporter are part of the ecosystem, and every participant has its mechanism, which leads to the crunch of the data available to another participant. Every participant has their way of doing business and transactions. The standardization includes a need for a piece of code containing terms and conditions, which are to be mutually agreed upon by all the participants. This piece of code is called smart contract. In the blockchain for enterprises, this smart contract plays a key role in participating in the network. Many languages like solidity and Golang and Java are used to write smart contracts and can be further deployed into the blockchain. A smart contract allows a completely new level of autonomy. The was first introduced by Nick Szabo in the early '90s [11]. The actions executed by smart contracts are predefined through a specific rule set. Smart contracts found widespread adoption and usage after the launch of the Ethereum protocol in 2015. It was the first protocol to enable native support of smart contracts, enabling completely new functionality and automatization. One of the prime use cases of smart contracts, demonstrating how smart contracts can be used, was the distribution of tokens on the Ethereum protocol during a so-called

"Initial Coin Offering (ICO)." Today, smart contracts found widespread adoption and are present everywhere if we think about the blockchain industry.

This section includes the possible usage of blockchain technology in healthcare systems, where smart contracts will enable completely new ways of digitalization. This will become especially evident if we consider sharing patient data with institutions [12]. The other new technologies like AI, ML, and IoT, combined with blockchain technology smart contracts, will enable new ways of using data.

11.1.2 Medical Healthcare System

It is evident that the healthcare system in every country is assumed to be the backbone of every society and economy; therefore, a considerable amount of budget is allotted and spent to sustain a properly working healthcare system. Also, studies estimate that in the last few years, several countries in the world spent more than 10% of their gross domestic product (GDP) on healthcare [13]. It becomes more of a matter of concern in the current scenario, where the average age of society is constantly rising, and hence governments are therefore looking for new ways to reduce general healthcare expenses. In our age of automation, new inventions like blockchain technology, AI, or big data could dramatically reduce the amount of money spent in the healthcare sector.

The main constituents of most healthcare systems are mainly three. The first part of the healthcare system comprises patients, or recipients of medical services, including the general public [14]. The last parts of most healthcare systems are medical health insurances or research institutions. So it is evident that looking at the interaction of different stockholders, the healthcare system is the best-suited process for implementing blockchain where there are higher possibilities for improvement by technological progress. It will also be cost-effective since the studies estimate that a considerable amount of money could have been saved concerning general health expenses by automating the healthcare system in Germany [13].

Due to this fact, many companies around the world are starting to explore blockchain-based solutions in the healthcare sector. The area of business and interest includes maintaining electronic health records, telemedicine, or pharmaceutical supply chain management. This leads not only to the huge possible economic benefits but also the integration of blockchain technology could bring significant benefits for the patient and the general public.

The properties like data availability, the trustless and immutable architecture, the increased usage of blockchain technology can directly improve the lives of many people around the world due to better research, traceability, and healthcare in general [15].

11.1.3 Objective and Methodology

As stated earlier, new technologies like blockchain are often claimed to be the solution to every existing problem. Although blockchain technology has the potential to change different sectors significantly, it would not be the solution to every problem or challenge we currently face. To understand where the implementation of blockchain technology in the healthcare sector makes sense and where possible limitations are, we will focus on the following objective throughout the following pages:

Why does it make sense to implement blockchain technology in the healthcare system?

An extensive literature survey is conducted for the same, and it is being found that healthcare and other sectors like finance will give us the best use cases for implementing this technology.

11.2 IMPLEMENTATION OF BLOCKCHAIN TECHNOLOGY IN THE HEALTHCARE SYSTEM

Since the publication of the Bitcoin white paper, followed by the launch of the network in early 2009, blockchain technology has come a long way. But even today, blockchain technology is tightly connected to Bitcoin and cryptocurrencies for the broad public. It is not surprising that the vast majority of people do not know what blockchain technology is, rather than which benefits an implementation could have on a broad range of sectors and companies. New technologies always take time to reach adoption and are heavily influenced by the opinion of mainstream media in the early years. Various types of research suggest that blockchain technology is still at a very early stage of adoption.

But that is why it is appreciable to see companies and startups increasingly interested in the technology rather than focusing on Bitcoin and cryptocurrencies alone. Market analysis and research suggest that around 49% of companies in the healthcare sector are already working on blockchain projects or have increased interest in implementation [13]. Although early companies only focused on the implementation in the financial sector, the healthcare sector is surely one of the key sectors to get profit from the integration of blockchain technology.

We need to focus on the general advantages of blockchain technology and how it compares to traditional solutions. Although blockchain technology is often propagated to be the solution to every modern-day problem, especially by the general media, there are still many use cases where traditional solutions, like databases, are more efficient. In the past, blockchain technology was commonly used to attract investors or create the impression of being a modern technological company. Most proposed projects and startups focusing on blockchain failed, mostly due to a lack of knowledge. It is, therefore, really hard to define for the majority of people where implementation of blockchain technology makes sense. This is significantly harder for projects targeting the healthcare sector as medicine and healthcare are often quite complex and existing structures are hard to define [16].

We need to focus on the core values of blockchain technology and the comparison to traditional databases. In traditional databases, which are often client-server based, one central entity controls the database. The user can access the database stored on a central server and only execute certain actions that the administrator predefined. Depending on the user rights, the end-user and the administrator can change, delete, or create existing entries. In blockchain-technology-based networks, there is no central authority to control the network and no central form of record-keeping fully. A full copy of the database is stored by the participating nodes of the network [17].

Most participating nodes will need to reach a consensus to confirm actions or add new entries to the database. In addition, one of the main differences to existing databases is that only entries can be added. Old entries will remain intact. This feature originates in the key architecture of blockchain technology, where new transactions are added in blocks, cryptographically chained together with existing entries to create a chain.

Therefore, blockchain technology is often considered immutable, which is one of the key differences from traditional databases. Therefore, blockchain technology is the technology of the choice for use cases in the healthcare sector, where immutability plays a crucial role in enabling more trust and transparency. Suppose we focus on supply chain management in the pharmaceutical industry very briefly, which is the first use case presented in the following section. Blockchain technology can lead to significantly more transparency and especially security for pharmaceutical drugs and medical products of all kinds. Without only one central authority in control of the database, saving the records or entries throughout the supply chain, every step becomes tamper-proof and accessible for every participant in the process [18]. Everybody can rely on blockchain-based entries, which will build trust and enable transparency.

Immutability provided by blockchain technology is one of the key advantages for medical use cases. Blockchain technology might be a suitable implementation if you think about the need for tamper-proof record-keeping, preventing any participant from cheating or abusing the system. This is, for example, especially important if we think about distributing organs for transplantation purposes. In the past, many participants abused the system, which heavily relied on trust. By using blockchain technology, entries cannot be changed without breaking the chain completely, which might restore some of the much-needed trust in the system over time.

Transparency is one of the additional core attributes of blockchain technology. Stepping away from the healthcare sector for a moment, transparency is one of the key advantages of Bitcoin and cryptocurrencies. In public permissionless networks like Bitcoin, for example, no one can stop you from accessing the network. From a network perspective, everyone is the same, having the same rights to participate. As a result, anyone can access the ledger and every recorded transaction at any time. This is one of the main advantages over traditional ways of transferring value. If we think about the financial sector and banks, most people cannot access information other than their bank accounts. Even the amount shown in the bank account is not verifiable as there is no way to prove that the bank owns the money. In addition, the whole process of transacting money is completely nontransparent. Coming back to the healthcare system and possible use cases of blockchain technology, the availability of transparency has been one of the most important challenges in our existing system. If we focus on the "hot topic" of blockchain-technology-based applications, digital patient record-keeping, features like transparency and immutability can completely change our understanding of modern-day medicine. Although it is apparent that a well-adopted blockchain-technology-based digital patient record-keeping solution is still several years away in the majority of countries, it definitely will be one of the prime use cases of blockchain technology in the future. In our current healthcare system, there are countless participants like hospitals, physicians, specialists, health insurances, the government, pharmaceutical companies, and research institutions. As this list is far from exhaustive, it only shows how distributed the current healthcare landscape in most countries is. Especially in most Western countries like Germany, the general healthcare system is very conservative and slow to adopt new technologies or any form of change [14].

Due to the distributed nature of the healthcare system, patient-related data is currently not stored in any central form and, therefore, not readily accessible in most cases. In addition, the current system is mainly paper-based, which makes it even harder to access all available data. As a result, the current healthcare system is very inefficient, leading to an incredible waste of resources and countless disadvantages for every participant in the system, especially the patient. Patients are often under- or over-diagnosed due to the lack of available patient data. Whereas the problem of over-diagnosis might not severely impact the patient's health if we think about the additional physical examination or blood samples, it can lead to serious consequences in terms of additional X-rays or computer tomography. The availability of a digital patient record, where all patient data is stored securely, would therefore be a huge improvement for every participant in our current traditional healthcare system [19].

Moreover, this will lead to serious changes in our understanding of ownership of data and the role of patients in our healthcare system. The patient will be the sole owner of the data, able to decide with whom the data should be shared. This will change the role of our current understanding of the patient completely, as in the current system, the patient is more like a spectator to their health. Transparency will be established as the patient can see who accessed the data and which entries are being made. But blockchain technology will not only enable immutability and transparency, which are prerequisites for digital patient records to be successful, but it will also offer integrity. The term *integrity* is used to describe the ability of users to be sure that the data is genuine.

This is especially important in the medical field as everyone needs to be sure that the data they receive is original and has not been tampered with. Only if integrity is ensured can the necessary level of trust be established and rely on the available data to make important decisions. In addition to being decentralized, attributed to integrity, immutability, or transparency, it will facilitate the adoption of blockchain technology in the healthcare sector and provide significant improvements over existing solutions. Due to a higher level of automatization (e.g., smart contracts), administrative costs can be cut extensively in addition to the more efficient availability of data. Another major advantage of blockchain technology for patients and participants in the current healthcare system is the ability to reduce the need for third parties or intermediaries. In our current health system, several intermediaries are interacting with patient data. One of the possible use cases that reduce the need for intermediaries and greatly benefit the patients will be presented as a use case in the next section. With the help of digital patient records, patients can directly share their medical data for research purposes without relying on third parties to share and use the data precisely as agreed. Without the need for intermediaries and a central institution in sole control of all data, blockchain technology provides an entirely new way for patients to control their data and revolutionize the healthcare sector in a way never been possible before [20].

In addition to the benefits presented previously, blockchain technology will provide additional advantages if combined with other emerging technologies like AI, IoT, or big data. Blockchain technology provides the necessary framework to enable large amounts of (real-time) data to become available and be used. As such, blockchain technology might be the necessary next step in digitalizing medicine and the healthcare sector. Especially where attributes native to blockchain architecture, like immutability or transparency, can lead to significant improvements over existing systems, integration should be considered. Although some implementations of blockchain technology in the healthcare system, like digital health records, might still be years away, some use cases could still be realized shortly. Some of the most promising blockchain technology-based use cases are presented in the below sections.

11.2.1 Selected Use Cases of Blockchain Technology in the Healthcare System

There are some selected use cases of blockchain technology in the healthcare sector [13, 15, 17, 18]:

- Secure storage and transfer of medical data
- Monitoring diseases and reporting outbreaks in real-time
- Securing genetic data and improving research
- Democratization and acceleration of clinical trials
- Medical supply chain management and drug traceability/safety
- Blockchain-based vaccination certification (COVID-19)
- Medical record management
- Smart contracts for insurance and supply chain settlements
- Increasing IoT security in healthcare
- Medical staff credential verification
- Rabies vaccine tracking with blockchain in Mali and Ivory Coast
- Patient-centric healthcare and personalized medicine

It is worth noting that the provided list is far from being exhaustive, as the current interest in blockchain-based use cases in the healthcare sector is high. As already mentioned, the need for innovation in the healthcare sector is accelerating due to the high costs for governments and health insurance. It, therefore, is not surprising that many reputed organizations and companies are working on new ways to digitalize the healthcare system and implement blockchain technology. Some of the most popular and promising initiatives and companies working on blockchain technology for the healthcare system and medicine are shown here:

- IBM
- SAP
- ConsenSys Health
- Centers for disease control and prevention (CDC)
- HIT Foundation (to be renamed into Health Foundation) Patientory
- Nebula Genomics
- Doc.Ai

- Chronicled
- Factom
- Akiri

Especially in light of the ongoing pandemic, the relevance of blockchain technology and the interest in implementation in the healthcare sector are constantly on the rise. Due to the limited quantity of vaccination available worldwide and inefficient and nontransparent distribution, blockchain could offer significant benefits over existing solutions. To reduce the possibility of fraud in the distribution process and minimizing the possibility of counterfeit vaccinations, the first selected use case focuses on implementing blockchain technology in drug supply chain management.

11.3 USE CASE: BLOCKCHAIN TECHNOLOGY FOR PHARMACEUTICAL DRUG SUPPLY CHAIN MANAGEMENT

11.3.1 BACKGROUND AND SIGNIFICANCE

The healthcare system's first blockchain-technology-based use case targets the global problem of counterfeit pharmaceutical drugs and medical products. Counterfeit drugs have a significant impact on healthcare systems and especially on patients all around the world due to the potentially lethal consequences. Studies suggest that around 15% of all pharmaceutical drugs in circulation could be counterfeit [18]. As the amount of non-genuine drugs greatly varies between countries and societies, the percentage is even higher in developing countries. As such, studies estimate that in some countries, even up to one-third of the circulating drugs could be counterfeit. With some pharmaceutical drugs costing more than several thousand USD (e.g., chemotherapeutics, antibodies, genetic treatments), the market for counterfeit drugs is incredibly huge. Besides any economic impact, the consequences for patients all around the world are potentially lethal in every "treatment." Not only do counterfeit drugs prevent the patient from receiving adequate medication, which leads to life-threatening conditions in the case of chemotherapeutics, antibiotics, or several other classes of drugs, but the products sold also are often of minor quality and even contain harmful substances themselves [21]. This is especially important if we think about situations where only minutes or hours will significantly impact the patient's life (e.g., snake bites). In addition, most counterfeit drugs are non-sterile, which can lead to severe infections if administered through injection. Still, despite the significant consequences on millions worldwide, the economic impact shouldn't be neglected. The development process for new pharmaceutical drugs typically takes several years and requires more than the equivalent of one billion USD in funding. If the economic impact on pharmaceutical companies is too high, they could focus on easier methods of producing pharmaceutical drugs, neglecting the costly and complex process of conducting excessive research needed to identify entirely new classes of pharmaceutical drugs. Although this might not seem too important at first glance, the consequences can be fatal for millions of people around the world. With the growing antibiotic resistance of bacteria, new ways of treatment are needed more than ever. Overall, the impact of counterfeit drugs worldwide is significant, and current security measures are far from being protective in the vast majority of cases. End-users currently cannot prove the authenticity of their medication, for example, which is highly important even in Western countries due to the rise of online pharmacies and drug distributors. In addition, many companies and people are involved in distributing pharmaceutical drugs or products from the manufacturer to the patient [22]. All these steps could be highly improved through the implementation of blockchain technology. One possible solution for the implementation is presented next.

11.3.2 BLOCKCHAIN TECHNOLOGY SOLUTION

Since the inception of blockchain technology in early 2009, supply chain management has been one of the prime use cases for revolutionary technology. The integration of blockchain technology in the supply chain management of pharmaceutical drugs has the potential to significantly decrease the number of counterfeit drugs in circulation as it introduces the possibility for companies, governments, and patients to check whether their medical product is genuine. Although especially Western countries have identified the problem of counterfeit drugs and their potentially fatal consequences on the population, the solutions in place often lack the possibility of end-user/patient validation. In addition, as most introduced solutions are costly and only introduced in Western countries, developing countries, where the number of counterfeit drugs is even higher, often lack additional security measures.

By implementing blockchain technology, the pharmaceutical drug manufacturer would use a newly developed interface (e.g., smartphone/scanner app or web client) to interact with the underlying blockchain and create unique QR codes (unique identification numbers). With the creation of the QR code, which is directly printed on the package containing the pharmaceutical drug or medical drug for better safety, the underlying blockchain is updated, creating an immutable time-stamp and tamper-proof record entry. On a side note, to increase security even further, every package should be sealed to provide the possibility of checking whether the package has been opened or not.

As in the vast majority of cases, the packages will be packed together and aggregated; a new QR code for every bigger package should be created too. This will allow any step of the shipment the process to be tracked, providing proof on the blockchain. At every step in the supply chain, from the manufacturer to the patient, the QR codes would be scanned, and the blockchain would be updated. As soon as the product reaches a pharmacy, authenticity can be checked before handing the pharmaceutical drug to the patient. But even if the product is purchased over the Internet or distributed through intermediaries, the patient or end-user can prove its authenticity on their own. Every step of the supply chain could be retraced, enabling new levels of trust. A visualization of the process is shown in Figure 11.1. To reduce the number of counterfeit drugs in circulation, each manufacturer labels the newly produced.

Besides the significant impact on the security of pharmaceutical drugs worldwide, providing entirely new ways of traceability and trust, the integration of blockchain technology into the supply chain of pharmaceutical drugs and medical products will enable even more possibilities in combination with other new emerging technologies like IoT, big data or AI.

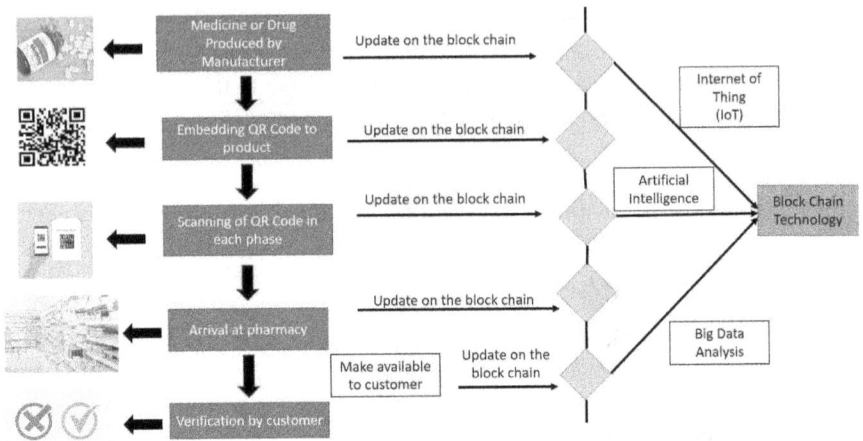

FIGURE 11.1 Schematic overview of the implementation of blockchain technology for the supply chain management of pharmaceutical drugs and medical products

In combination with AI and big data, for example, by providing reliable real-time data, blockchain technology could be used to predict possible disease outbreaks in a certain region of the world by tracking the sales process of a certain pharmaceutical drug. This might enable significant advantages over existing solutions if we keep the possibility of new pandemics in mind. In addition, the tracking process could identify possible shortages early, providing necessary information to suppliers or manufacturers. Thinking about IoT, the integration of blockchain technology would enable a higher level of automatization, as logistics companies participating in the distribution of pharmaceutical drugs could be paid automatically after fulfilling the shipment. The process will largely benefit from other features, such as smart contracts, providing significant benefits over existing solutions.

11.3.3 TECHNICAL SPECIFICATIONS

At the core of the implementation described previously is the blockchain. A hybrid blockchain is proposed, where interoperability between a public permissionless and a private permissioned blockchain is assured. The blockchain would be run and governed by a consortium made of every participating member in the use case solution (e.g., pharmaceutical companies, logistic companies, pharmacies), in addition to the government (e.g., EU) and pro-patient-related organizations (e.g., the WHO, ICMR, CDRI). The different distributed validators committed to the network will allow important features, such as scalability, governance, and the protection of user rights. To be more precise, it will be better to propose that the blockchain utilizes proof-of-stake as an underlying consensus mechanism, where the stakeholders are the respective participants/validators of the use case. Using a hybrid blockchain solution has the advantage that the private network will allow better scalability, faster finalization, block time, and higher throughput. At the same time, the public blockchain would allow third-party developments and increase security and trust. Generally, the stakeholders/validators of the network would run full nodes to allow light client functionality on the end-user side without downloading the whole blockchain. This is crucial to facilitate adoption, as downloading the whole blockchain significantly reduces usability.

In general, the application or web client has to be as user-friendly as possible to allow easy and intuitive usage and facilitate adoption. In addition, extensive user education needs to happen to provide further trust and adoption. One of the main advantages of the proposed use case is that the necessary technological framework for a successful implementation is already existing. The participating companies could use their existing server infrastructure to run the blockchain.

Although the hardware or server requirements should be sufficient in most countries, the lack of knowledge of blockchain solutions could slow the implementation. As such, either internal training or external contracting should be conducted. Besides the points mentioned previously, sufficient Internet coverage is needed to implement and run the use case as proposed. This might not be a significant problem in most Western countries, but it could reduce the solution's benefits in some developing countries. This applies to smartphones or electronic devices connected to the Internet, enabling the possibility to use the provided app or web client.

In summary, the technical requirements to implement the solution are comparably low if we consider the possible huge benefits for every participant, especially patients worldwide.

11.3.4 LIMITATIONS

Although implementing blockchain technology in the described use case could provide significant benefits over currently existing solutions, there are still limitations. One of the key points of successful integration and usage is that the QR Code is scanned at every possible step during the distribution process. While many steps could be automatized in the future, the integration currently relies on the people working in the logistics companies. Although the implementation would still increase security and trust, even if the package was never scanned during the whole distribution process and the recipient could only see that a certain manufacturer produced the drug, further proof of authenticity and trust is still lacking. Extensive public education is needed to prevent criminal organizations from selling their counterfeit drugs and products by creating their app and mimicking the whole distribution process. Participating companies, countries, health insurance, and governments should coordinate their efforts by creating a consortium to increase the overall level of trust and adoption in society. This consortium would not only be able to govern and run the blockchain, but it would also make it even harder for counterfeit drugs to be sold due to the uniform framework (e.g., app and web client) established [23].

This becomes even more evident if we focus on the level of adoption of blockchain technology in our current society. Although many companies have increasingly started to look into implementing blockchain technology, we are still early in overall adoption [24].

The healthcare system can greatly benefit from blockchain technology as it will provide more transparency, security, and trust for all participants. But even with all the advantages of blockchain technology named throughout this chapter, we should always keep in mind that it still has some vulnerabilities due to the rather new age of the technology. Like with every software application, even if audited by several independent entities, there can still be bugs, hacks, or exploits. As a result, the chosen blockchain for the presented use cases in this chapter should be tested extensively. Although blockchain technology has the potential to change our healthcare system permanently, there are still possible limitations. Besides the relative immaturity of the technology in case of adoption and security, blockchain technology will not answer every existing problem.

This becomes even clearer if we think about the huge amount of medical data produced every day and their need for extensive storage capacity in the case of computer tomography (CT) or magnet resonance therapy (MRT). Although blockchain protocols are already available, where huge amount of data can be stored (e.g., Filecoin, Sia), it would neither be efficient nor lead to any cost reduction. As such, hybrid solutions must be developed to combine blockchain technology with the storage capacity of traditional databases. Blockchain technology could, for example, assure the integrity of the data stored in databases. This is only one limitation of current use cases of blockchain technology in the healthcare sector, and this is the reason it is assumed that holistic and widely adopted blockchain-based digital health record solutions will still need years to reach the market.

Another major limitation of blockchain-technology-based use cases in the healthcare system is that most solutions are developed for people that are not very tech-savvy. In contrast to younger generations that grew up with the Internet, many people in our society lack technological knowledge. Although most of the currently proposed use cases, like the digital patient record solution, could benefit the younger generation, the people of older generations are statistically the ones to have more impact on current healthcare systems. This is a significant problem to consider as most people could be overwhelmed by implementing new technologies. As a result, even the best-developed technological improvement, possible to provide significant benefits for patients, could still find no major adoption. Especially in healthcare, where existing structures are complex, the lack of adoption from the patient side often results in a step back to previous lesser digitized solutions.

Overall, the implementation of blockchain technology in the healthcare system has the potential to change existing structures permanently, leading to huge benefits for every participant and especially the patients.

11.4 CONCLUSION AND DISCUSSION

Current solutions in the healthcare sector feature a low level of interoperability, which is inefficient and time-consuming. Blockchain technology can offer significant advantages over existing solutions in the healthcare sector due to its more decentralized, transparent, and immutable architecture. Blockchain technology can provide the framework for emerging technologies like big data or IoT in the healthcare system. Increased digitalization and the implementation of emerging technologies such as blockchain or AI can completely change our understanding of modern-day medicine. Blockchain technology minimizes the need for third parties or intermediaries to interact with sensitive patient data.

REFERENCES

[1] Vogel, S. L. "Digitizing healthcare—risks and opportunities of blockchain in the healthcare system". Published in Global Block Chain Initiative in September 2021.

[2] Khan, D., Low, T. J., & Hashmani, M. A. "Systematic literature review of challenges in blockchain scalability". *Applied Science*, 2021, 11, 9372. https://doi.org/10.3390/app11209372.

[3] Agbo, C. C., Mahmoud, Q. H., Eklund, J. M. "Blockchain technology in healthcare: A systematic review. In healthcare". *Multidisciplinary Digital Publishing Institute*, June 2019, 7(2), 56.

[4] "Digital transformation of healthcare: A blockchain study". *IJISET—International Journal of Innovative Science, Engineering & Technology*, May 2021, 8(5), ISSN (Online) 2348–7968.

[5] Dagher, G. G., Mohler, J., Milojkovic, M., Marella, P. B., & Marella, B. "Ancile: Privacy-preserving framework for access control and interoperability of electronic health records using blockchain technology". *Sustainable Cities and Society*, 2018, 39, 283–297.

[6] Glaser, F. "Pervasive decentralisation of digital infrastructures: A framework for blockchain-enabled system and use case analysis". In *Proceedings of the 50th Hawaii International Conference on System Sciences | 2017*.

[7] Brodersen, C., Kalis, B., Leong, C., Mitchell, E., Pupo, E., Truscott, A., & Accenture, LLP. *Blockchain: Securing a New Health Interoperability Experience*. 2016. http://www.investdata.com/eWebEditor/uploadfile/201801141109264457 9769.pdf.

[8] Benchoufi, M., Porcher, R., & Ravaud, P. "Blockchain protocols in clinical trials: Transparency and traceability of consent". *F1000 Research*, 2018. https://doi.org/10.12688/f1000research.10531.5.

[9] Crawford, M. "The insurance implications of blockchain". *Risk Management*, 2017, 64(2), 24.

[10] Roman-Belmonte, J. M., De la Corte-Rodriguez, H., Rodriguez-Merchan, E. C. C., la Corte-Rodriguez, H., & Carlos Rodriguez-Merchan, E. "How blockchain technology can change medicine". *Postgraduate Medical*, 2018, 130, 420–427.

[11] Georges, N. "Blockchain or distributed ledger technology what is in it for the healthcare industry". In *Proceedings of the 11th International Joint Conference on Knowledge Discovery, Knowledge Engineering and Knowledge Management* (IC3K), 2019, pp. 277–284. ISBN: 978-989-758-382-7, 10.5220/0008348902770284.

[12] Ahram, T., Sargolzaei, A., Sargolzaei, S., Daniels, J., & Amaba, B. "Blockchain technology innovations". In *Proceedings of the 2017 IEEE Technology & Engineering Management Conference* (TEMSCON), Santa Clara, CA, June 8–10, 2017, pp. 137–141.

[13] Zhou, L., Wang, L., Sun, Y. M. I. "A blockchain-based medical insurance storage system". *Journal Medicine System*, 2018, 42(8), 149.

[14] Clark, S. A. "The impact of the Hippocratic Oath: The conflict of the ideal of the physician, the knowledgeable humanitarian, versus the corporate medical allegiance to financial models contributes to burnout." *Cureus*, 2018, 10(7), e3076.

[15] Nakamoto, S. "Bitcoin: A peer-to-peer electronic cash system". *Decentralized Business Review*, 2008, 21260. https://bitcoin.org/bitcoin.pdf.

[16] Iansiti, M., & Lakhani, K. R. "The truth about blockchain". *Harvard Business Review*, 2017, 95(1), 118–127.

[17] Kormiltsyn A., Udokwu, C., Karu, K., Thangalimodzi, K., & Norta, A. *Improving Healthcare Processes with Smart Contracts.* Springer, 2019, pp. 500–513. 10.1007/978-3-030-20485-3_39.

[18] Szabo, N. *Smart Contracts: Building Blocks for Digital Markets.* 1996. http://www.truevaluemetrics.org/DBpdfs/BlockChain/Nick-Szabo-Smart-Contracts-Building-Blocks-for-Digital-Markets-1996-14591.pdf.

[19] Kuo, T. T., Kim, H. E., & Ohno-Machado, L. "Blockchain distributed ledger technologies for biomedical and health care applications". *JAMIA*, 2017, 24(6), 1211–1220.

[20] Linn, L. A., & Koo, M. B. "Blockchain for health data and its potential use in health it and health care-related research". In *ONC/NIST Use of Blockchain for Healthcare and Research Workshop.* Gaithersburg, MD: ONC/NIST, 2017.

[21] Moreira, C. et al. "A prescription for blockchain and healthcare: Reinvent or be reinvented". 2018. https://www.pwc.com.au/digitalpulse/report-blockchain-healthcare-disruption.html.

[22] Ben Fekih, R., & Lahami, M. "Application of blockchain technology in healthcare: A comprehensive study". *The Impact of Digital Technologies on Public Health in Developed and Developing Countries: 18th International Conference, ICOST 2020, Hammamet, Tunisia Proceedings, 12157*, June 24–26, 2020, pp. 268–276.

[23] Bhavnani, S. P., Narula, J., & Sengupta, P. P. "Mobile technology and the digitization of healthcare". *European Heart Journal*, 2016, 37(18), 1428–1438.

[24] Leible, S., et al. "A review on blockchain technology and blockchain projects". *Fostering Open Science. Frontiers in Blockchain, Sec. Blockchain for Science,* 2019, 2(16), https://doi.org/10.3389/fbloc.2019.00016.

Index

For Product Safety Concerns and Information please contact our EU
representative GPSR@taylorandfrancis.com
Taylor & Francis Verlag GmbH, Kaufingerstraße 24, 80331 München, Germany